GENETIC CONNECTIONS™

A GUIDE TO DOCUMENTING YOUR INDIVIDUAL AND FAMILY HEALTH HISTORY

DANETTE L. NELSON-ANDERSON, R.N., B.S.N.
CYNTHIA V. WATERS

SONTERS PUBLISHING

WASHINGTON, MISSOURI

"**W**hile leafing through your family photo album can bring back fond memories, taking the time to trace your family health tree can offer a lifesaving picture of your future. If people would take a proactive role with their health, many could live 15 years longer. One of the best ways to do that is to be aware of your family's medical past.

"I could perform numerous and expensive tests, and it wouldn't give me nearly the information that a person's medical history can. I suggest that people organize their medical records in the same form as their taxes and canceled checks. It's that important."

Joseph Thompson, D.O.
Family Practice
DePaul Health Center
St. Louis, MO

"**A**lmost every day we learn more about the 'genetic connections' to our health. Yet too few of us have the time to document our family's health history or to learn about the diseases we might some day inherit. By knowing our genetic predisposition for disease and by understanding risk factors, however, we can better control our health destiny.

"This book can make the task much easier. Everyone who reads this book will learn more about how the human body should function and what can cause it to dysfunction. Included are instructions for creating a family health history and determining individual health risk.

"In 1992, medical genetics was officially recognized as a bona fide specialty in clinical medicine. Maybe it's now time for each of us to examine our own genetic health history."

Denton A. Cooley, M.D.
Surgeon-in-Chief
Texas Heart Institute
Houston, TX

GENETIC CONNECTIONS™

A GUIDE TO DOCUMENTING YOUR INDIVIDUAL AND FAMILY HEALTH HISTORY

BY
DANETTE L. NELSON-ANDERSON, R.N., B.S.N.
CYNTHIA V. WATERS

FIRST EDITION JULY 1995

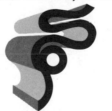

SONTERS PUBLISHING

WASHINGTON, MISSOURI

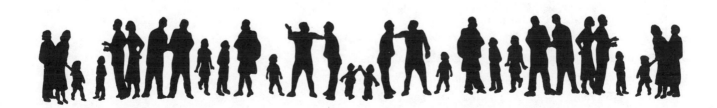

DISCLAIMER: This book is designed to help readers compile health information useful in managing family health by explaining how to prepare a family health history. This guide is not intended to be used in self-diagnosis or to replace the services of a health-care provider. All readers are urged to consult with their personal physician regarding any medical condition about which they have concerns, rather than use this book as a source of diagnosis. Author and publisher disclaim responsibility for any adverse results due to misuse of information obtained in this book. To more fully understand the family health pedigree created by using this book, seek the advice of a physician or geneticist.

Publisher:	Sonters Publishing, Inc., dba Sonters Publishing Ink P. O. Box 109 Washington, MO 63090-0109
Author:	Danette L. Nelson-Anderson, R.N., B.S.N.
Concept Originator:	Cynthia V. Waters
Contributions by:	Carol Isaacson Barash, Ph.D.
	Beverly J. Connor, R.N.
	Penny S. Smith, B.S.N., J.D.
	Roberta J. Weseman, R.N., M.S.N.
Content Editor:	Maureen A. Connolly, B.S.
Manuscript Editor:	Chris Roerden, M.A.
Assistant Editor:	Pat Meller, B.S.
Typesetting & Layout:	Chuck Ramsay and Chris Roerden
Illustrations:	Janice Saliba
Cover Design:	Alex Paradowski Graphic Design

Publisher's Cataloging in Publication

Nelson-Anderson, Danette L.
    Genetic connections : a guide to documenting your individual and family health
history / author, Danette L. Nelson-Anderson, R.N.; concept originator, Cynthia V. Waters.
    p. cm.
    Includes bibliographical references and index.
    Preassigned LCCN: 94-67892
    ISBN 0-9639154-1-X (Wire-O-Binding, hardcover)
    ISBN 0-9639154-2-8 (casebound)
    ISBN 0-9639154-3-6 (softcover)

    1. Health. 2. Medical genetics. 3. Self-care, Health. I.
Title.

RA776.N45 1995   613
                                  QBI94-21218

CONTENTS

UNIT I – YOUR UNIQUENESS / YOUR HEALTH

CHAPTER 1 – GENETIC INHERITANCE

CHAPTER 2 – THE PRENATAL HISTORY

CHAPTER 3 – BIRTH HISTORY

CHAPTER 4 – PHYSICAL ATTRIBUTES

CHAPTER 5 – GENERAL HEALTH INFORMATION

UNIT II – YOUR BODY SYSTEMS

CHAPTER 6 – THE EYES AND EARS

CHAPTER 7 – THE NERVOUS SYSTEM

CHAPTER 8 – MENTAL ILLNESS

CHAPTER 9 – THE CARDIOVASCULAR SYSTEM

CHAPTER 17 – THE MUSCULOSKELETAL SYSTEM

CHAPTER 18 – THE INTEGUMENTARY SYSTEM

UNIT III – YOUR HEALTH PEDIGREE

CONTRIBUTORS

CAROL ISAACSON BARASH, Ph.D.
Foreword: Keeping Genetic Information Confidential and Avoiding Discrimination
Genetics, Ethics & Policy Consultant, Boston, Massachusetts

Consultant:	American Association for the Advancement of Science for the United Nations Commission on Human Rights
	Colorado Osteopathic Association, Education
	Facing History and Ourselves National Foundation
Past Director:	Studies in Genetic Discrimination, The E.K. Shriver Center for Mental Retardation
Committees:	Boston Women's Health Collective
	Council for Responsible Genetics
	Human Genome Project, New England Regional Genetics Group
	The Genetic Screening Study Group

BEVERLY J. CONNOR, R.N.
Gastrointestinal Disorders Research

Administrator:	Tri-County Outpatient Surgery Center, Washington, Missouri
Staff:	Reservation Coordinator, St. Louis University Hospital, St. Louis, Missouri
	Post-Anesthesia Care Unit, St. Joseph's Hospital, Kirkwood, Missouri
Member:	American Society of Post-Anesthesia Nursing

PENNY S. SMITH, B.S.N., J.D.
Accessing Your Medical Records; Respiratory Disorders Research
Nurse Attorney in Private Practice, Atlanta, Georgia

Member:	Georgia Association of Women Lawyers
	American Association of Nurse Attorneys, Georgia Chapter

ROBERTA J. WESEMAN, R.N., M.S.N.
Chapter 8: Mental Illness

Nurse Educator:	Associate Degree Nursing Program, East Central College, Union, Missouri
Staff:	Psychiatric Care, St. John's Mercy Hospital, Washington, Missouri
Member:	American Nurses Association
	Missouri Nurses Association
	Missouri State Allied Health Occupations Educators
	Missouri Vocation Association
	Sigma Theta Tau International

REVIEWERS

JEAN A. AMOS, Ph.D.

Molecular Genetics, *reviewed complete text*

Director: DNA Diagnostic Laboratory, Center of Human Genetics, Boston University School of Medicine, Boston, Massachusetts

Assistant Professor: Department of Pathology and Laboratory Medicine, Boston University School of Medicine, Boston, Massachusetts

Diplomate: Clinical Molecular Genetics, American Board of Medical Genetics

Certification: American Board of Medical Genetics

THOMAS R. ANDERSON, M.D.

Psychiatry, *reviewed complete text*

Private Practice: Psychiatric Services, Inc., Columbia, Missouri

Consultant: Audrain Medical Center, Mexico, Missouri

Past President: Boone County Medical Society

Central Missouri District Branch of the American Psychiatric Association

Missouri Psychiatric Association

Diplomate: American Board of Psychiatry and Neurology

Fellow: American Psychiatric Association

Certification: American Board of Neurology and Psychiatry

SUNIL M. APTE, M.D.

Urology, *reviewed urinary system, male reproductive system*

Private Practice: Washington, Missouri

Certification: American Board of Urology

HEIDI A. BEAVER, A.B., M.P.H.

Genetic Counseling, *reviewed complete text*

Director: Genetic Counseling Services, Genetics Division, Department of Obstetrics and Gynecology, Washington University School of Medicine, St. Louis, Missouri

Diplomate: American Board of Medical Genetics

Certification: American Board of Medical Genetics

American Board of Genetic Counseling

JONATHAN D. BORTZ, M.D.

Endocrinology, *reviewed endocrine system*

Private Practice: St. Louis, Missouri

Assistant Clinical Professor of Medicine: St. Louis University School of Medicine, St. Louis, Missouri

Director: Diabetes Services, St. Mary's Health Center, St. Louis, Missouri

Diabetic Foot Center, St. Mary's Health Center, St. Louis, Missouri

Certification: American Board of Internal Medicine

Board Certification, Endocrinology and Metabolism

British Medical Council

New South Wales Medical Board, Australia

South African Medical and Dental Council

BARRY D. BROWN, M.D.

Gastroenterology, *reviewed gastrointestinal system*

Chief: Department of Gastroenterology, Deaconess Health Center, St. Louis, Missouri

Assistant Clinical Professor: St. Louis University School of Medicine, St. Louis, Missouri

Certification: American Board of Internal Medicine

Board Certification, Gastroenterology

DENTON A. COOLEY, M.D.

Cardiology, Cardiovascular Surgery, *reviewed cardiovascular system*

Surgeon-in-Chief: Texas Heart Institute, Houston, Texas

Founder: Texas Heart Institute

Cooley Surgical Society

Distinguished Alumnus:

University of Texas

Johns Hopkins University

Honorary Fellow: The Royal Colleges of Surgery in Scotland, Australia, Ireland, and England

Certification: American Board of Surgery

American Board of Thoracic Surgery

Recipient: The Medal of Freedom

Theodore Roosevelt Award

Rene Leriche Prize

8 honorary degrees

45 honors and awards

ROBERT A. GOOD, Ph.D., M.D., D.Sc., F.A.C.P.

Immunology, *reviewed blood and immune systems*

Physician- in-Chief: All Children's Hospital, St. Petersburg, Florida

Head: Allergy and Clinical Immunology, Department of Pediatrics, All Children's Hospital, St. Petersburg, Florida

Distinguished Research Professor: University of South Florida, Tampa–St. Petersburg, Florida

Past President: American Association of Immunologists

American Society of Clinical Investigation

Association of American Pathologists

Central Society of Clinical Research

Reticuloendothelial Society

Society of Experimental Biology and Medicine

Certification: Board Eligible, American Board of Pediatrics

Recipient: 12 honorary doctorate degrees

80 major awards

DAVID R. KRAUSS, M.D.

Neonatology, *reviewed neonatology content*

Director: Division of Neonatology, Scott & White Memorial Hospital, Temple, Texas

Staff: Senior Staff, Department of Pediatrics, Scott & White Memorial Hospital, Temple, Texas

Professor: Department of Pediatrics, Texas A & M University College of Medicine, Temple Campus

Certification: National Board of Medical Examiners

American Board of Pediatrics

Sub-Board of Neonatal–Perinatal Medicine of the American Board of Pediatrics

ABOUT THE CREATORS OF
GENETIC CONNECTIONS™

Concept Originator **Cynthia V. Waters** attended Southeast Missouri University of Cape Girardeau, Missouri. As an ancillary health care professional she has held administrative, supervisory, and purchasing positions in both hospital and ambulatory care settings.

Two family medical emergencies led Waters to the conclusion that keeping personal and family health records is essential.

"I realized how little I knew about my parents' health histories or that of other family members. Working in the health-care profession, I knew that health disorders occurring in blood relatives had a direct impact on my risk factors for developing these same disorders. I told myself I should collect a family health history to share with my health-care provider and one day pass on to my children. The problem was I didn't know how or where to start."

That is when Waters approached an associate, Nelson-Anderson, about writing **GENETIC CONNECTIONS™**. Experience in both nursing and education made Nelson-Anderson immediately recognize how valuable Waters' concept was, and she agreed to author **GENETIC CONNECTIONS™**.

Author **Danette Nelson-Anderson**, R.N., B.S.N., received her Bachelor of Science in Nursing from the University of Mary Hardin-Baylor, Belton, Texas. As a past nurse educator with East Central College, Union, Missouri, Nelson-Anderson has worked as a registered nurse in both hospital and ambulatory care settings.

She has practiced in a variety of areas, including newborn and neonatal intensive care nurseries, perinatal outreach education, adult cardiac catheterization, angiography, ambulatory surgery, and nursing education.

"Together we have created a book we feel no individual or family should be without."

ACKNOWLEDGMENTS

This book would not have been possible without the support of many colleagues, friends, family members, and the helpful members and volunteers of numerous professional health and support organizations.

We thank our **contributors:**

Carol Isaacson Barash, Ph.D., for her foreword on genetic ethics and discrimination;

Beverly J. Connor, R.N., for hours contributed to gastrointestinal system research;

Penny S. Smith, B.S.N., J.D., for information on legal rights in accessing medical records, and hours contributed to respiratory system research; and

Roberta J. Weseman, R.N., M.S.N., for Chapter 8, Mental Illness.

We thank our many **reviewers** (listed on the preceding pages) for their expert input and comments, professional dedication, and invaluable critique of the text.

We thank the following **professionals** and **professional organizations** for granting us permission to reprint valuable information in this book:

Alliance of Genetic Support Groups and Mary Ann Wilson: compiling and allowing the partial reprint of their directory of health organizations and support groups;

Aubrey Milunsky, MB.B.Ch., D.Sc., F.R.C.P., D.C.H., and the Johns Hopkins University Press: material from *Heredity and Your Family's Health*, by Aubrey Milunsky, M.D.;

J. B. Lippincott Company: formula for approximating daily calorie requirements and determining healthy body weight, from *Nutrition Handbook for Nursing Practice*, 2nd edition, by Susan G. Dudek, R.D., B.S.;

Mosby-Year Book, Inc.: modification of congenital heart defect illustrations from *Waley & Wong's Essentials of Pediatric Nursing*, 4th edition, Donna L. Wong, R.N., Ph.D., P.N.P., C.P.N., F.A.A.N.;

National Society of Genetic Counselors and Robin Bennett: standardized human pedigree symbols as recommended and published by the Society's Pedigree Standardization Task Force;

American Journal of Human Genetics, Dr. Peter Byers, Editor: modification of symbols from *Recommendations for Standardized Human Pedigree Nomenclature*, R. L. Bennett, et al.

National Retinitis Pigmentosa Foundation, Inc.: information from *The Inheritance of RP and Allied Retinal Degenerative Diseases*, Jill C. Hennessey, M.S.;

The Trustees of Columbia University in the City of New York and The College of Physicians and Surgeons of Columbia University, and G. S. Sharpe Communications: glossary reprint from *The Columbia University College of Physicians & Surgeons Complete Home Medical Guide;*

National Center for Learning Disabilities: information on specific learning disabilities as published in *General Information Packet On Learning Disabilities;*

U.S. Department of Agriculture, Public Information Office, Food & Nutrition Service: use of the Food Pyramid;

U.S. Departments of Agriculture and Health and Human Services: use of excerpts from *Nutrition and Your Health: Dietary Guidelines for Americans.*

We thank Chris Roerden, editor, for her professional expertise and eye for detail.

We thank Maureen A. Connolly, content editor, Janice Saliba, illustrator, and Chuck Ramsay, typesetter, for agreeing to take on such a tremendous task, for never-ending support, and for jobs well done.

Special thanks to Brenda Garrison for many hours of data entry and moral support.

With special affection and gratitude we thank our families for their love, patience, and support while we pursued this calling. Thank you Mark, Chris, Brett, and Ashley Anderson; Dr. Thomas R. and Mary Elizabeth Anderson; William H. and Kathryn L. Nelson; John E. Waters III; John Waters II; Jeannine and John Moroney; Howard Moore; Dan and Guinevere Yoest; Lester L. Moore; and Dale and Priscilla Strohbehn.

Thank you to special friends Diane Jacquin, Joan Lalk, Charles and Virginia Moon, and Dr. and Mrs. Charles H. Sincox for their continued faith and trust.

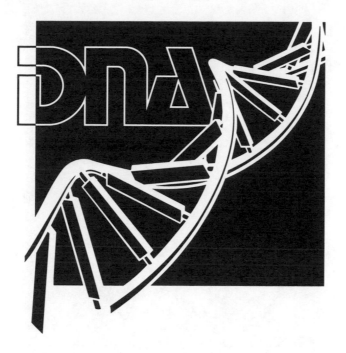

UNIT I

YOUR UNIQUENESS / YOUR HEALTH

WHY YOU NEED THIS BOOK

HOW TO USE THIS BOOK

KEEPING GENETIC INFORMATION CONFIDENTIAL AND AVOIDING DISCRIMINATION

CHAPTERS 1 THROUGH 5

This unit gives you a foundation for understanding the role that genetics plays in your life.

Chapters 1 through 5 contain information on genetic inheritance, as well as what takes place in the time from conception through birth and immediately following birth; how you acquired many of the physical attributes you have; and which lifestyle habits and practices can have an impact on your health. This information helps you create a complete health history, which lets your health-care provider plan and individualize your care.

As you answer the questions at the end of each chapter, fill out the related sections of your *HEALTH HISTORY FORM.* You will find this form in Appendix A at the end of this book. Later you will be escorted step by step through the process of constructing your family health pedigree.

Before you begin Chapter 1, read "How to Use This Book" on page 5.

WHY YOU NEED THIS BOOK

You are a unique, complex, multifaceted being, a product of your environment and the unique set of genes inherited from your parents. Despite your individual uniqueness, you are linked to your ancestors by genetically determined (inherited) traits that are passed from generation to generation. Some traits seem to jump or skip generations only to appear again in an offspring, a reminder that even though you may not exhibit or manifest the trait yourself, you can carry the gene and pass it to your children . . . and they to your grandchildren . . . and they to your great-grand-children . . . and so on.

Genetic science is the study of heredity, the study of how inherited traits, including disease, are determined and transmitted by genes. Genetic science has come a long way in the last 20 years, virtually exploding with new gene discoveries and technological advances that are read about or heard about almost daily. As researchers continue to uncover genetic connections (inherited links) associated with health and disease and the susceptibility or predisposition to developing disease, the importance of knowing your family health history becomes increasingly apparent. You can use a record of your family health information to identify your own health strengths and risks, thereby providing you with the opportunity to take action that may prevent or delay the development of disease. As technology continues to advance and more disease-causing genes are discovered, new techniques for diagnostic testing and treatment of genetic diseases will assuredly be developed.

GENETIC CONNECTIONS™—A GUIDE FOR DOCUMENTING YOUR INDIVIDUAL AND FAMILY HEALTH HISTORY was written to help you document your family's health history and prepare a family health pedigree—a one-page representation of your and your family's health history. Accomplishing this documentation may seem an enormous task, because it is. However, this book is a tool to help you accomplish this most important task. This book will help you understand DNA (deoxyribonucleic acid), genes, and chromosomes, and how they make you what you are. It will also help you understand the general principles of maintaining a healthful lifestyle, and the systems and structures of the body and their functions. In addition it gives you valuable reference information on selected diseases (both genetic and nongenetic in origin), including their causes, signs and symptoms, and established treatments.

The information you document about your and your family's health history is confidential and should be handled as such. So you and your family can fully benefit from the information you document, it is to be shared with your health-care provider(s), who may be a medical physician (M.D.), an osteopathic physician (D.O.), or a nurse practitioner (a nurse who has received additional schooling and clinical experience).

Your primary health-care provider is responsible for managing and overseeing your health care. In the past, families could have seen the same health-care provider all their lives, an advantage because that provider grew to know every family member and their health histories. Today, however, people frequently change health-care providers, either by choice, as the result of a move, or because the particular health insurance plan their employer is participating in at the time dictates what provider they see. This loss of continuity in the delivery of health care demonstrates why it has become increasingly important for you and your family to maintain your own health records.

Chances are that you, like many people, not only see a primary general practitioner for health care, but also receive care from various specialists. It is vital that for each individual practitioner, information from each of the other providers is shared. Such shared health histories can save you time and money by avoiding the duplication of tests and examinations, not to mention saving you unnecessary discomfort.

Although compiling a genealogical history of your family is important, taking the time to trace your family's health history can offer a lifesaving picture of your future. Your family health history and pedigree, which this book shows you how to compile, can reveal to you and your doctor or other health-care provider those diseases which have occurred repeatedly among family members. That information can provide insight as to whether a genetic predisposition is to blame, plus clues as to how these diseases have been transmitted generation to generation. Your health-care provider can then determine if you or future generations are at risk of developing these same diseases. Once your risk factors are identified, your health-care provider can customize your care accordingly, such as by scheduling more frequent checkups or tests, and recommending diet and/or lifestyle changes that may prevent or delay the onset of disease. By "living right," you may prevent or delay the development of a disease to which you are genetically predisposed; as a result, you do not necessarily have to suffer the same consequences as your ancestors. Therefore, we believe that documenting a complete family health history is the single most important act of preventive medicine in which you can participate.

This book will help you begin keeping family health files. You may wish to keep additional pertinent health information and documents with your family health and pedigree information, such as copies of birth certificates, immunization records, admission and discharge summaries of hospitalizations, other office and hospital records, laboratory and other diagnostic test results, and so on.

We have made this book as user-friendly as possible while guiding you through your process of compiling and recording your family health history. Compiling that history will take some effort on your part. It may challenge you, but as you work through the text, you will expand your knowledge of the human body and how it functions, discover ways in which you are personally prone to disease, and learn how you may minimize and prevent such disease.

At a time when health care is considered to be in a state of crisis, it is imperative that you educate yourself about your health-care risks and needs and also assume a degree of responsibility for your health. The information you absorb and compile using **GENETIC CONNECTIONS™** will be invaluable to you, your family members, and those family members yet to be.

Knowledge is empowering, and that power can be yours if you take the initiative to obtain it. This book was written not to help you make medical decisions, but to be a tool to help you compile the information your health-care provider can use to manage your and your family's health care. This tool also helps you organize your health information so it can be quickly and easily accessed and carried with you when needed in times of emergency. Knowledge of your family health history—your **GENETIC CONNECTIONS™**—can lead to prevention, early detection, and early treatment of disease. And that just may save your life.

HOW TO USE THIS BOOK

This book is presented in three units:

Unit I includes Chapters 1 through 5, which discuss genes, chromosomes, the inheritance of diseases and physical traits, the time periods from conception through birth, events that can affect health, and general principles for healthful living.

Unit II is made up of Chapters 6 through 18, which discuss the systems of the body chapter by chapter, with information on the *structures and functions* of each system. Also included is information on a select group of *structural defects* as well as *diseases and disorders* that can occur in each particular body system.

Unit III contains step-by-step instructions for creating your family health pedigree. In addition, information in this unit helps you begin the important task of keeping accurate, current health files for yourself and your immediate family, and it gets you started on becoming an educated participant in your own health care, thereby taking control of your health destiny.

These units help you achieve the following goals:

1. Documenting your personal health history information;

2. Acquiring a basic understanding of genetics and of the human body and how it functions;

3. Drawing your family health pedigree, which is a single-page graphic representation of you and your family members that includes pertinent health information; and

4. Becoming a proactive participant in your health care by keeping your own personal health files, thereby improving the communication between you and your health-care providers as you supply the health history information they need to help you live a healthier, longer life.

HOW TO BEGIN:

Remove the *GENETIC CONNECTIONS™ HEALTH HISTORY FORM* from the back of the book (see Appendix A). You may wish to make a photocopy of the form and replace the original so it will be there when you are ready to make additional copies for other family members' health histories. Or use the original for your own health record and use the order blank located in the back of this book for ordering additional health forms. (They are printed on acid-free paper.)

First read Chapter 1 in its entirety. When you are through, answer the questions presented at the end of Chapter 1 and document your answers in Section 1 of your *HEALTH HISTORY FORM.*

Note: In completing the *HEALTH HISTORY FORM*, use pencil, not ink. As long as you keep your papers protected, pencil will last for generations.

Next, keep your *HEALTH HISTORY FORM* handy as you explore each additional chapter in Units I and II. Answer the questions presented at the end of each chapter and document your answers in the corresponding section of your *HEALTH HISTORY FORM.*

By the time you reach the end of Unit II you will have completed your own health history.

The *HEALTH HISTORY FORM* enables you to record a wide variety of health-related information, including infectious illnesses, genetic diseases, hospitalizations, medications, immunizations, surgeries, accidents, and so on.

It is not necessary to read all the information in every chapter, although if you did so you would receive maximum benefit from the book. Check the title page to each chapter for its contents.

KEEPING GENETIC INFORMATION CONFIDENTIAL AND AVOIDING DISCRIMINATION

Carol Isaacson Barash, Ph.D.

The purpose of this foreword is to introduce you to the possibility that your awareness of your genetic inheritance may influence not only your personal medical decisions but also your life decisions, thereby having far-reaching effects on your life. Most of these will have a positive impact on your life; however, some have the potential to be negative, whether intended or accidental; specifically those negative consequences imposed upon people who have, or carry a gene for, a genetic disease or disorder. Being alert to the potential for misuse of your genetic information by others can help you prevent negative effects from occurring.

GENETIC INFORMATION

This term is used to describe a person's genetic makeup or genome, the unique set of DNA (deoxyribonucleic acid) that makes up the genes and chromosomes you inherited from your parents. Precise information about an individual's genetic status can be obtained by genetic tests, which are usually performed to identify (or rule out) the presence of specific gene or chromosome abnormalities. Calculated assumptions or probabilities concerning an individual's genetic status are sometimes based on family history and sometimes on medical tests about which a genetic diagnosis can be made. Sometimes personal genetic information is public knowledge because it is visible. For example, your eye color, hair color, shape of your eyes and nose, and so on, are physical features determined by your genes. Most genetic information, however, cannot be seen by others, unless an abnormality in one or more genes or chromosomes causes specific symptoms, features, or characteristics of a genetic disease or disorder to be apparent.

Discovering the *heritability*—the passing from generation to generation—of certain human traits and diseases is not a new science; classical genetics dates back to the mid-1800s. The myriad of genetic discoveries currently underway, such as the discovery of the gene causing Huntington disease and a gene responsible for some cases of familial breast cancer, are possible because of recent advances in technology and scientific techniques that provide a way to identify individual genes on a chromosome (both the healthy and the abnormal genes). In the summer of 1989, representatives of the National Institutes of Health and the Department of Energy drafted a plan for the "Human Genome Project," which is now an international endeavor involving researchers and scientists from Belgium, England, France, Japan, and Switzerland, to name a few of the many countries involved. The goal of the Human Genome Project is to identify and map every gene found on each human chromosome. Once a gene is identified, scientists can study how the gene functions and what it controls. The significance of the Human Genome Project is that once the entire human genome is identified and mapped, the capability of diagnosing both genetic diseases and genetic predispositions to diseases would then become possible, and research concentrating on finding treatments and/or cures for these diseases would be accelerated.

Media coverage of recent gene and gene marker discoveries spawned by the Human Genome Project, and the resulting development of genetic tests, have helped make "genetics" a household word. If you have little or no experience with genetic disease or genetic services, you may wonder whether genetics has any relevance to you or your family. The answer is yes, for you have (as everyone does) a unique set of genes—your personal genetic information—which among other things forecasts your inherited health strengths and risks and your future health status. Each of us carries roughly 5 to 20 mutant (altered or abnormal) genes which have the *potential* to cause diseases or abnormalities. This is a potential only; some of these genes require the interaction of environmental factors to cause disease while others are rendered inactive by stronger, dominant healthy genes. As of this writing, more than 5,000 genetic conditions have been identified, ranging from rare and obscure diseases to fairly common ones.

As researchers and scientists continue to discover disease-causing genes for common ailments once thought not to have genetic causes, it will become increasingly important to know and maintain the confidentiality of your personal genetic information. Your genetic status is valuable information that health-care professionals use in their efforts to identify your particular health-care needs. It can also be information to consider in making important personal life decisions, such as those concerning career moves, marriage, and childbearing. While being aware of your personal genetic information is clearly an asset to you, if you have a genetic disease or a family history of one, it is *possible* for this information to be used to impose limitations on you by third parties: outside individuals, groups, and organizations who are not directly involved in administering your health care, such as insurance companies, employers, adoption agencies, and other social institutions that gain access to your personal genetic information. The exclusion of individuals from certain social benefits or entitlements—such as insurance, employment, adoption, military service, health-care delivery, or educational opportunity—based on their genetic status has been termed genetic discrimination, a practice that is not only unfair and unjust, but illegal in some states. Although the benefits of knowing your genetic strengths and risks are tremendous, *especially* in regard to your health, it is in your best interest to be savvy to the importance of keeping genetic information confidential.

Whereas your personal and family genetic information is invaluable to your physician(s), your sharing that information with other individuals, groups, or organizations (third parties) should be carefully considered and evaluated for the possibility that your disclosure of this information may be used to generate negative consequences. Therefore, be cautious about releasing your genetic information to anyone other than your health-care provider, and consider the possibility that your confidentiality *may* be compromised. Some situations encourage unnecessary disclosure of personal genetic information.

MEDICAL VERSUS GENETIC INFORMATION

Knowing the difference between genetic and basic medical information and some of the more common sources of access to personal genetic information can help you protect against misuse of your genetic information.

Basic medical information includes a record of past illnesses and injuries, personal health-care habits, and routine information gathered by health-care providers such as doctors and dentists, plus facts such as your height, weight, blood pressure, and heart rate. Although this medical information provides a profile of your health status and the risk factors of your developing certain diseases, it does not represent predictive value about your future health status—whereas *genetic information can.* For example, your genetic makeup may be such that you do not carry the gene that causes Huntington disease. This means you have a genetic benefit, as you will not develop the disease. On the other hand, if you do have the gene for Huntington disease, it can be predicted with a high degree of certainty that you will develop the disease. Thus, the predictive value of genetic information is largely what distinguishes it from basic medical information.

However, many diseases—often called multifactorial diseases—are determined not only by specific genes but by the interaction of these genes with certain environmental factors. Although inheriting a genetic *predisposition* for a multifactorial disease (such as heart disease and many cancers) puts you at higher risk of developing that disease, this genetic predisposition does not necessarily predict that you will actually *develop* the disease. The development of a multifactorial disease to which you are genetically predisposed might be avoided or delayed (to varying degrees) by your complying with preventive strategies, such as eating foods believed to lower risk, exercising regularly, maintaining a healthy body weight, and taking specific medications.

A second important factor distinguishes basic medical information from genetic information: your genetic information can reveal or imply personal genetic information about your blood relatives because you share a certain percentage of common genes. For example, if you know that I am at risk for Huntington disease, and if you know that Huntington disease is inherited as an autosomal dominant disorder (a genetic disease caused by inheriting the gene from one parent who has the disorder), you can deduce that one of my parents has the gene for Huntington disease and has (or will have) developed the disease. Furthermore, if you know that I have four siblings, you can also deduce that each of them is equally at risk. Third parties can also make these same deductions and may impart limitations or exclusions, or charge higher fees for services, if they become aware of such genetic information.

To reemphasize a point, whether you do or do not have a genetic disease or carry a gene for one, your compiled health history and pedigree are confidential and should be treated as such, to be shared only in confidence with your health-care provider(s) and blood relatives.

COMMON SOURCES OF ACCESS TO PERSONAL GENETIC INFORMATION

SELF-DISCLOSURE, PUBLIC KNOWLEDGE, FAMILY HISTORY

Based on data from a 1994 Department of Energy study of genetic discrimination, the most common way that third parties gain access to personal genetic information is through the willing disclosure of individuals themselves. The individuals in the study tended to self-disclose their genetic status with apparently little awareness of the possibility of negative consequences. Voluntary self-disclosure to other people (that is, friends, neighbors, and casual acquain-

tances) is also a significant way that an individual's genetic status becomes public knowledge within a community.

Personal genetic information may become public knowledge involuntarily, as well. For example, while not always correct, the public may infer that you have a genetic risk of disease if (1) you have a blood relative with a genetic disorder; (2) public records such as obituaries have indicated a genetic disorder in a blood relative; and (3) common knowledge of a long-standing family history of a particular genetic disorder has been passed from generation to generation within your community. Public records and public knowledge can also provide access to inquiring third parties. Some people actually choose to receive health care out of town in an attempt to maintain privacy and bypass inadvertent public knowledge of their personal health status, whether or not they have a genetic disease or carry the gene for one.

MEDICAL RECORDS

Medical records contain basic medical information (described above) but may also contain personal genetic information; for example, test results for a particular genetic disease. Hospital, clinic, and office medical records are routinely accessed by health-care professionals so they can deliver safe, prompt, and effective health care. Other staff and employees of a hospital or clinic have access so they can promptly deliver services, such as insurance filing and maintaining hospital files and records in accordance with federal and state regulations. Access to your medical records by these people is both necessary and beneficial. However, it is important that the medical information within your record be accurate. If you have concerns about accuracy, ask your health-care provider (doctor) for a copy of your record so you can check the contents for accuracy.

Medical records are confidential; stringent rules governing the release of patient medical record information exist on both state and federal levels. However, intrusion into your privacy by people who have no real need to view your medical records but nevertheless do, or by those who indiscriminately converse about your medical information among hospital/clinic staff and employees, is hard to prevent. Talk to your doctor if you have concerns about the confidentiality of your medical records, especially in regard to personal and family *genetic information,* and instruct him or her to relay those concerns to all people who handle the medical records.

Some insurance companies require a review of an applicant's medical record before deciding to issue a policy. Similarly, employers in some situations may gain access to employee medical records during the course of employment (for example, if the company is self-insured). Institutions such as these, which have access to medical records, may decide to offer limited or restricted opportunities to individuals on the basis of their genetic information, especially if genetic disease or predisposition exists. While certainly unfair, these types of exclusions *may also* be illegal, depending on the laws and regulations in the particular state. It is unclear as of this writing the extent of federal protection afforded under the Americans with Disabilities Act to individuals who have a genetic disease or disorder or who carry the gene for one.

Hospitals, clinics, doctors' offices, and other health institutions cannot release information about your medical record to any individual or institution without your written consent or authorization. This includes their releasing the information to an insurance company for the purpose of your obtaining health or life insurance coverage or their seeking monetary reimbursement from your health insurance company for health care services you have received. Your consent for the release of your records is obtained usually in a broad-scoped permission statement you are asked to sign prior to purchasing an insurance policy or undergoing medical treatment or testing. Always read authorization permits thoroughly before signing. In some instances, you may want to specify or limit your authorization to the release of only the particular medical record information that is pertinent and relevant to the immediate care or testing you are receiving and not the release of your entire medical record. You may also want to specify which third party is to have access to your medical record information. Some people place a time limit (for example 30 days) on the medical record release authorization.

An individual's genetic status may be accessed by insurance companies through their review of medical records, as required by the application process

(assuming the individual has a genetic disease or predisposition that is documented in his or her medical record). Insurance companies that are members of the Medical Information Bureau (the MIB) report to it an applicant's medical record information obtained through medical record review and other information pertinent to health and longevity, such as height, weight, blood pressure, blood cholesterol level, present medical conditions, lifestyle habits such as smoking, the results of tests required as part of the insurance application process, and so on. The MIB is a nonprofit trade association made up of several hundred insurance companies formed to provide a way to record and exchange confidential underwriting information among member companies. Through the MIB, all member companies have access to applicants' MIB records (which contain the medical record review and insurance application and screening information).

The primary purpose of the MIB is to identify misrepresentation and/or omission of pertinent health data on an individual's insurance application to guard against insurance fraud and abuse. MIB information is purportedly used only to alert a member company to the need to investigate an insurance applicant further before it issues insurance coverage, and not to deny insurance coverage. The MIB does not have files on everyone. To request a copy of your MIB file (if one exists) contact MIB, P.O. Box 105 Essex Station, Boston, MA 02112, or call 617-426-3660. If you discover errors in your MIB file, get them corrected. If you are ever denied insurance, find out why, and act accordingly.

RESEARCH STUDIES

If you consider participating in medical research, make sure that any resulting genetic information will be retained separately from your general medical record, and that the information will be kept absolutely confidential. Such protection is required by federal human subject research regulations. Note that research records, though contained in computerized databases, are identified numerically to any researcher using the data, thereby guaranteeing participant anonymity.

EMPLOYERS

If your employer maintains health information files on its employees, ask who has access to those files and how your confidentiality is protected. Some employers separate employee health files from personnel files, code health files to guarantee employee anonymity, and limit who has access to health files in order to protect their employees' rights to confidentiality. Some employers, however, allow other personnel, such as managers, access to the health files of personnel.

Companies that are self-insured (and many mid- to large-sized companies are) receive copies of any and all insurance claims filed by their employees. If your employer is self-insured, ask who is allowed access to employee health files and health insurance claims. Some individuals in this type of employment situation, to protect their privacy, choose to pay cash for certain tests or procedures (especially when related to a genetic disease or disorder) to avoid having their insurance company and employer learn about a genetic condition. On the other hand, many people choose to use their deserved insurance coverage for all health-care services.

GENETIC TESTING

Genetic test results constitute the most basic source of personal genetic information. When scientists discover the gene(s) responsible for a disease or disorder, a test is ultimately developed that can identify whether people with a family history of that disorder have the disease-causing gene(s). Genetic test results should be used in a positive way: to begin early treatment, take precautionary measures, or make plans for future health-care needs. The main reasons for genetic testing include (1) identifying people at risk of genetic disease who are presently asymptomatic (without symptoms); (2) verifying diagnosis of genetic disease in symptomatic individuals; (3) identifying people who are carriers of a gene that could be transmitted to and cause genetic disease in an offspring; (4) identifying the fetus or newborn with a genetic disease; and (5) DNA profiling used in forensic cases to identify genetic "fingerprints" of crime victims and suspects.

Although most of the human genome as of this writing has not been identified, mapped, sequenced, and functionally understood, already more than 100 genetic tests are available. While this number may seem large, it is relatively small in comparison to what is anticipated once the entire human genome is revealed. Projected increases in the development and commercial availability of new genetic tests indicate a potential for subsequent increases in consumer use of those tests. Who should have access to your test results—and for what reasons and in what situations—is not exactly clear: should it be the spouse, blood relatives, employers, insurance companies, the military, people who see your medical record, day care providers, adoption agencies, others? With increasing commercial availability of genetic tests and a potential for increased commercial pressure on the consumer to utilize existing genetic technology (such as genetic testing and screening), there is some concern that people who do not need or do not want to have genetic testing will be pressured to do so, or that those who want to may not have access to services because of high cost or because of the distance between their homes and the medical facilities where testing is available. Moreover, there is some concern that this most basic form of genetic information may be misused or inappropriately handled without regard to confidentiality. Therefore, it is recommended that you receive counseling from a medical geneticist or trained genetic counselor before you agree to participate in genetic testing. Genetic testing may indeed be indicated to help plan your health care or that of your family, but there are times when testing is not indicated. A professional genetic counselor can give you information to help you make an educated decision about testing. Your primary health-care provider (doctor) may be able to assist you in finding a professional genetic counselor, or you can contact the National Society of Genetic Counselors, which provides assistance. Other questions may be directed to the Center for Genetics, Nutrition and Health, 202-462-5062; or the Genetics Institute, 301-571-9488.

Protecting the right of confidentiality in regard to genetic information (specifically genetic test results) is a concern for everyone. Remember, you have specific rights to protection under both federal and state law, but state laws vary. Many states have legislation in effect or pending that helps preserve the privacy (and confidentiality) of personal genetic information and protect against its unlawful misuse by third parties.

Appendix F includes a list of organizations, agencies, and commissions that provide information about your rights. Further resources are listed in the Bibiliography.

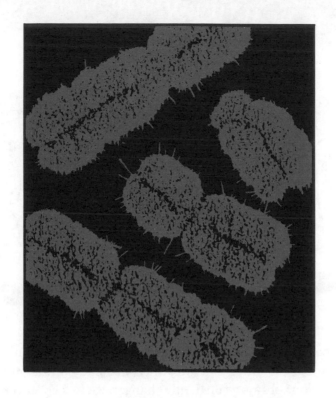

CHAPTER 1
GENETIC INHERITANCE

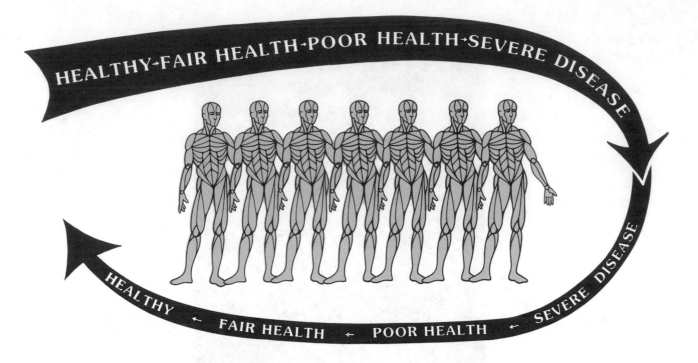

HEALTHY·FAIR HEALTH·POOR HEALTH·SEVERE DISEASE

HEALTHY ← FAIR HEALTH ← POOR HEALTH ← SEVERE DISEASE

Imagine a health continuum with the state of perfect health at one end and severe disease at the other. You are always at some point along this health continuum, but your position constantly changes. Factors contributing to your specific point at a specific time on this continuum include your ancestral heritage, your genetic inheritance, and your environment.

ANCESTRAL HERITAGE

Knowing the races and nationalities of your ancestors and from which countries or geographic regions they originated is important because many diseases occur at much higher rates in some populations than in others (see figure 1.1). Knowing your ancestry can help you identify your risk of developing

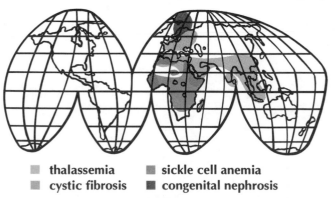

■ thalassemia   ■ sickle cell anemia
■ cystic fibrosis   ■ congenital nephrosis

Figure 1.1. Some geographic regions have a higher incidence of specific genetic diseases

certain diseases and your risk of transmitting those diseases to future generations.

Individuals who are adopted are too often disadvantaged by not knowing their biologic parents' health histories or their ancestral heritage. It is important that adoptees access this information so they and their health-care providers can fully understand their health strengths and risks.

GENETIC INHERITANCE

Your biologic and chemical makeup—and, to a great extent, your physical appearance—are determined by the combination of genetic traits inherited from your parents. These traits are determined by structures called genes. Altered, defective, or damaged genes function abnormally and are called gene mutations. A mutant gene can cause disease, protect you from disease, or make you susceptible or predisposed to certain diseases when you are placed in certain environments or exposed to certain environmental elements. Scientists and researchers are continuing efforts to identify gene mutations in the hope that genetic disease can be treated or prevented in the future. It is estimated that everyone carries from 5 to 10 mutant genes. Fortunately, these genes usually have no effect because healthy genes are able to override them. The complete, unique set of genes that you inherited from your parents comprises your genetic makeup, better described as your genetic inheritance or genome.

To help you understand your genetic inheritance, the following is a brief explanation of how genes are passed (transmitted) from generation to generation and how they shape you as an individual.

REPRODUCTIVE CELLS

You began as a single living cell that resulted from the union of the human reproductive cells from your mother and father, the egg (ovum) and the sperm (spermatozoa). Reproductive cells are produced by special glands in the body called gonads: the female ovaries and the male testes. The gonads also produce hormones that influence the physical development and maturation of the reproductive organs and specific gender characteristics.

THE EGG

The female infant is born with many thousands of immature egg cells (ova) in each ovary. They remain quiet, or latent, until she reaches puberty, usually between ages 9 and 17 years. At that time, interplay among hormones and the central nervous system triggers the female reproductive cycle into action, resulting in ovulation. Ovulation is the release of a mature egg from an ovary, an event that occurs approximately every 28 days. If the egg is not fertilized by a sperm, hormonal changes occur which in turn initiate menstruation, the shedding of the uterine lining that thickens each month in preparation for the implantation (attachment) of a fertilized egg.

egg

sperm

Even though females are born with many immature egg cells within their ovaries, only a small percentage of the eggs mature for release during ovulation. Egg cells that do not mature eventually

disintegrate. Female children hold within their ovaries the egg cells that will be released during their childbearing years. It is suspected that childhood exposure to infectious diseases, radiation, or other environmental hazards can damage these immature cells, resulting in gene mutation or chromosomal abnormalities. Therefore, the ovaries should be protected from these elements whenever possible. For example, if a young girl requires an x-ray procedure, her ovaries should be protected from the radiation with a lead shield when possible. Radiation cannot pass through lead.

THE SPERM

In the male, sperm production does not occur until the onset of puberty, usually between ages 10 and 19 years. Sperm are produced in the testes and stored in structures called epididymides (epididymis is the singular form) which are located near the testes. Semen, also called seminal fluid, is a combination of sperm and fluids produced by several glands (including the prostate and bulbourethral glands and the seminal vesicles). This fluid helps transport, protect, and nourish the sperm, which survives only a few weeks in the male reproductive system. After the sperm enter the female reproductive tract they survive only two to three days. The health and production of a man's sperm can be influenced by his body temperature, age, environment, and history of infectious diseases. Sperm are produced throughout a man's reproductive years, puberty through death.

GENES

Egg and sperm contain genetic information, sometimes referred to as genetic messages or codes within their DNA (deoxyribonucleic acid), a chemical compound found in most living things. DNA consists of four base elements that pair up and link together in various sequences to form long chains. The structure of the DNA chain looks like a spiral ladder or double-helix configuration. The specific arrangement of the DNA base elements creates units called genes, which determine and regulate specific traits and characteristics. Genes accomplish this by following the instructions contained in the DNA and dictating the production of the proteins and other molecules that make up virtually all body structural and chemical components,

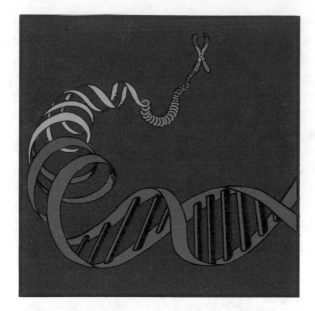

Figure 1.2. A single chain of DNA holds many genes; coiled tightly, it forms a chromosome

CHROMOSOMES

Each cell in the human body contains 23 pairs of chromosomes (46 individual chromosomes), with the exception of egg and sperm cells. The egg and sperm divide as they mature by a special process known as meiosis (see figure 1.3). This type of cell division results in egg and sperm cells that contain 23 single chromosomes, instead of 23 pairs. Thus, each of your parents contributed one of the chromosomes in each of your 23 chromosome pairs.

Meiosis allows the paired or "counterpart" chromosomes you inherited from your parents to exchange genes during a certain point of cell division. For example, the chromosome 14 that you inherited from your mother and the chromosome 14 you inherited from your father are counterpart chromosomes. During meiosis, they pair up and "exchange" genes (see figure 1.3b).

When an egg and sperm unite (conception), the sperm spills the genetic information contained within its 23 individual chromosomes into the 23 individual chromosomes of the egg. The result is a fertilized egg cell with 23 chromosome pairs. From the time of conception, the fertilized cell and all subsequent cells divide by a process called mitosis (see figure 1.4). This type of cell division creates two exact duplicates of the original dividing cell. The DNA in the cell (half of which is from the egg and half from the sperm) duplicates itself before the cell divides so that each new cell has an identical copy of the DNA and identical chromosomes with identical genes. This means that each of

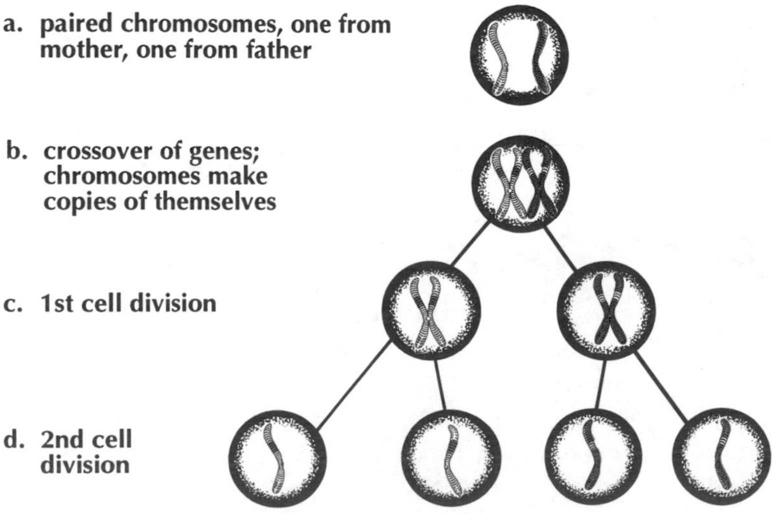

including the skin, muscle, organs and connective tissues, antibodies, enzymes, and some hormones. Each chain of DNA contains 1,000 or more genes which, when coiled tightly together, form a compact unit called a chromosome. DNA is the reason the body has so many types of cells with a multitude of differing functions—skin cells, bone cells, muscle cells, blood cells, and so on. The genetic messages or codes that DNA holds function as a blueprint or instruction manual for the construction of your entire body. This blueprint determines which genes within a cell will or will not be activated, thus creating the many different cell types and functions.

a. **paired chromosomes, one from mother, one from father**

b. **crossover of genes; chromosomes make copies of themselves**

c. **1st cell division**

d. **2nd cell division**

Figure 1.3. Meiosis: cell division of egg and sperm

a. **paired chromosomes, one from mother, one from father**

b. **chromosomes make exact copies of themselves**

c. **cell divides, leaving one copy of each chromosome in each new cell**

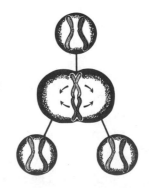

Figure 1.4. Mitosis: cell division of body cells

your body cells, which number 100 trillion, contains identical DNA, identical chromosomes, and identical genes.

The complete set of genetic material (DNA, genes, chromosomes) you inherited from your parents makes up your genetic inheritance or genome, the unique set of genes that make you genetically different from any other person, unless you are an identical twin. Identical twins have identical genetic makeups because they began life as a single fertilized egg that split shortly after conception, resulting in two individuals with exactly the same genome.

When scientists study chromosomes they photograph them, separate them into 23 matching pairs, and arrange them in numeric order according to specific characteristics such as size, length, and the number and location of light and dark bands that can be seen with the use of special laboratory stains and equipment (see figure 1.5). Each chromosome pair is unique and can be distinguished from the others. The first 22 chromosome pairs are called autosomes or nonsex chromosomes. The 23rd pair of chromosomes is called the sex chromosomes because they determine whether the person is male or female.

Chromosomal abnormalities and syndromes can result when too few or too many individual chromosomes are inherited or when there are mutations or alterations in the structure of individual chromosomes.

GENETIC TRAITS

A trait is an inherited (genetically determined) condition such as blood type or the shape of one's nose. Genes responsible for specific traits are located at similar points on counterpart chromosomes. For example, you inherited two genes for blood type, one located at a certain point on the chromosome you inherited from your mother and one at the same point on the counterpart chromosome you inherited from your father.

Some genes have a dominant effect over others and are called dominant genes. Nondominant genes are called recessive genes. If you inherited a dominant gene from one parent and a recessive gene from the other parent at the same location on counterpart chromosomes, the dominant gene would have caused the recessive gene to be ineffective or silent and the dominant trait to be expressed (that is, it would be present). (See autosomal dominant inheritance, page 16.) In that situation, however, you would still have the recessive gene on one chromosome, and it would have the same chance of being passed to your children as the dominant gene.

If you inherited recessive genes for a trait on both counterpart chromosomes, they work in the absence of a dominant gene to determine characteristics and traits; for this to occur, recessive genes must be inherited from both parents. (See autosomal recessive inheritance, page 16.)

Two parents who each exhibit a dominant trait (because they carry a specific dominant gene) could have a child who does not exhibit that same dominant trait—if both parents carry a recessive gene on their counterpart chromosomes and each passes the recessive gene to the child (see figure 1.6).

Some diseases are genetic, inherited through genes. Sometimes a single disease-causing (mutant)

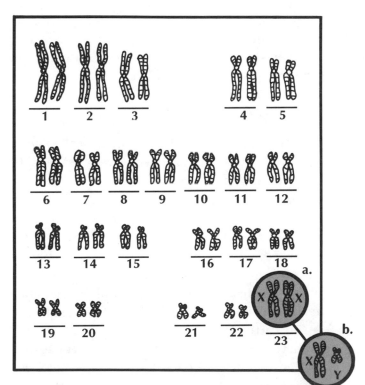

Figure 1.5. A photographic representation of a set of human chromosomes, known as a karyotype:
a. females have two X chromosomes at pair 23
b. males have one X and one Y chromosome at pair 23

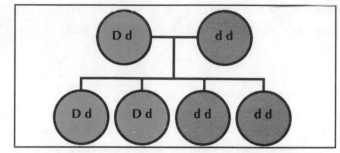

Figure 1.6. Dominant inheritance: possible gene combinations that can be transmitted to offspring

D dominant gene
d other gene

■ dominant gene and trait present

dominant gene is inherited from one parent; sometimes a pair of disease-causing (mutant) recessive genes are inherited, one from each parent. Genetic disease can also result when a combination of various genes are inherited, when genes or gene groups are missing or deleted from a chromosome, or when excess genes are present or duplicated on a chromosome. Many diseases appear to be caused by an interaction between genes and environmental factors, and are called multifactorial disorders.

PATTERNS OF INHERITANCE

Three major patterns of inheritance are recognized in the transmission and appearance of genetic traits, be it an inherited characteristic (physical feature) or genetic disease. The first pattern is called autosomal dominant inheritance.

AUTOSOMAL DOMINANT INHERITANCE

In an autosomal dominant inheritance pattern, only one gene is necessary to cause the trait or disease because the gene involved is a dominant gene. The parent who transmitted the dominant gene to the child also has that trait or disease. If only one parent carries this dominant gene (see figure 1.6), the child has a 50% chance of inheriting the gene. That's because the parent with this gene holds a pair of genes, one from each of his or her parents. One of those genes is the dominant gene being referred to, but the other gene on the parent's counterpart chromosome—which is most likely different—also has a 50% chance of being passed to the child. These percentages change if both parents carry the dominant gene (see figure 1.6).

Autosomal dominant traits and diseases can appear spontaneously as a result of new mutation, a situation in which a gene has been altered or damaged at some point in the egg or sperm. The cause of new mutations is usually not known, but once they occur, they can be passed to future generations.

Sometimes a dominant trait or disease appears to skip generations. This may be due to nonpenetrance of a dominant gene. Nonpenetrance occurs when a dominant gene is in fact inherited but the person does

a. if one parent carries the dominant gene, offspring have a 50% chance of inheriting the gene and a 50% chance of *not* inheriting the gene

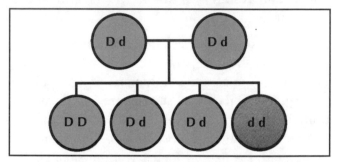

b. if both parents carry the dominant gene, offspring have a 25% chance of inheriting the gene from both parents, a 50% chance of inheriting the gene from one parent, and a 25% chance of *not* inheriting the gene

not show (manifest) the trait or disease or appear to have it, in spite of having the gene. Even though this dominant gene is not being expressed, it can be passed to future generations.

AUTOSOMAL RECESSIVE INHERITANCE

In the second inheritance pattern, called autosomal recessive inheritance, recessive genes must be inherited from each parent for the trait or disease to be expressed (see figure 1.7). In other words, the person has inherited a pair of recessive genes on counterpart chromosomes. The two recessive genes act in the absence of a dominant gene to express the trait or disease. Someone who inherits a recessive gene from only one parent is a carrier, as is (most likely) the parent who passed the recessive gene to that person. People who are carriers do not show the trait or disease, but they have the recessive gene and can pass it on to their children. Children of parents who are carriers of a recessive gene have (1) a 25% chance of inheriting the recessive gene from each parent and thereby possessing the trait or disease; (2) a 50% chance of inheriting the gene from only one parent and thereby being a carrier of the trait or disease; and (3) a 25% chance of

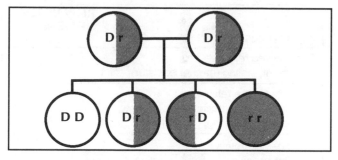

r   recessive gene   Dr carrier of recessive gene
rr recessive trait or disease present

Figure 1.7. Recessive inheritance: possible gene combinations that could be transmitted to offspring when both parents carry a recessive gene

not inheriting the gene from either parent. In the latter case, children are free of the trait or disease and cannot pass it on to future generations.

X-LINKED INHERITANCE

The third inheritance pattern, called X-linked inheritance, involves the 23rd pair of chromosomes (the pair that determines sex), primarily the X chromosome.

The egg (ovum) always carries an X chromosome because females have two X chromosomes (XX) at the 23rd pair. Reproductive cells (egg and sperm) carry only single chromosomes, so no matter which of her two X chromosomes a mother passes to her child, it is always an X.

A male, on the other hand, has one X chromosome and one Y chromosome (XY) at the 23rd pair. Thus, each sperm carries either an X or a Y chromosome, whichever the sperm ends up receiving after the cell divides (see meiosis, page 14). If a sperm carrying an X chromosome fertilizes an egg, the child will be female (XX), with two X chromosomes. If the sperm carries a Y chromosome, the child will be male (XY), with one X and one Y chromosome (see figure 1.8). The sperm determines the sex of the child.

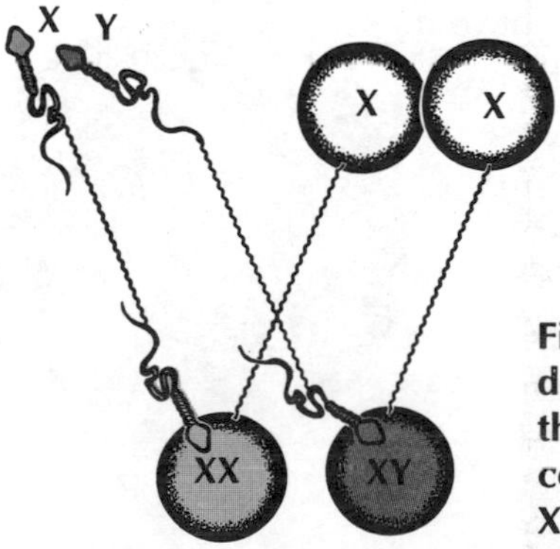

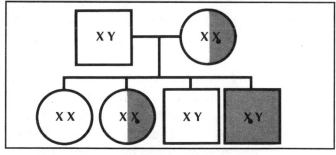

■ male   ■ female

Figure 1.8. The sperm determines the sex of the child by its contribution of either an X or a Y chromosome

In an X-linked inheritance pattern, the gene causing a trait or disease is located on an X chromosome. Women frequently are only carriers of X-linked traits and diseases because their second X chromosome most likely includes normal genes that can override any mutant genes of the first X chromosome. Men cannot be carriers because they have only one X chromosome. Boys and men who inherit a specific gene on their X chromosome will have the trait or disease.

A woman with a specific gene on one of her X chromosomes is a carrier. She has a 50% chance of passing this gene via an X chromosome to each of her children. If she passes the X chromosome with this specific gene to a daughter, the daughter will also be a carrier because the X chromosome the child inherits from her father is most likely not carrying this same gene. However, if the woman passes the X chromosome bearing the specific gene to a son, he will have the trait or disease because—in having received a Y chromosome from his father—he has no other X chromosome to override the gene on his X chromosome. Therefore, all of the woman's daughters have a 50% chance of inheriting the specific gene and thus being carriers of it; and all of her sons have a 50% chance of inheriting the specific gene and thus having the trait or disease (see figure 1.9).

These percentages of risk change when a man has the specific gene on his X chromosome. If the mother of his children has two normal X chromosomes that

XY male   XX female
X chromosome that carries the specific gene
XY male with the X-linked trait or disease
XX female carrier of the X-linked trait or disease

Figure 1.9. X-linked inheritance: possible gene combinations that could be transmitted to offspring when the mother has the specific gene on one of her X chromosomes

do not carry this same specific gene, all of his daughters will be carriers of the specific gene (a 100% chance), because he contributed his X chromosome, which bears the gene. None of his sons, however, will inherit the gene, nor will they have the trait or disease, because they will have inherited his Y chromosome and (most likely) a healthy chromosome from their mother (see figure 1.10).

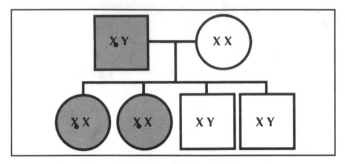

XY   male   XX female
X   chromosome that carries the specific gene
XY   male with the X-linked trait or disease
XX   female carrier of the X-linked trait or disease

Figure 1.10. X-linked inheritance: possible gene combinations that could be transmitted to offspring when the father has the specific gene on his X chromosome

SPONTANEOUS GENETIC DISEASE

Genetic diseases are inherited as a result of mutant genes being transmitted through the major patterns of inheritance, but sometimes genetic disease seems to appear with no family history of occurrence. This can happen for several reasons. First, a mutant recessive gene can be passed down for generations before it is finally paired with another mutant recessive gene on the counterpart chromosome, thereby resulting in expression of the disease. Children conceived by two blood relatives (a consanguineous marriage or relationship) have a higher risk of inheriting a recessive genetic disease than do children of unrelated parents, because they have a higher chance of having genes in common. The closer the blood relationship, the more genes two people will have in common (see table 1.1). Many recessive genetic disorders are also seen in

RELATIONSHIP	PROPORTION OF GENES IN COMMON
First-degree relatives Parent, sibling (brother or sister), child	½

Second-degree relatives
   Grandparent, uncle, aunt, nephew,
   niece, half-sibling, grandchild
	¼

Third-degree relatives First cousins	⅛

Table 1.1. The percentage of common genes found in blood relatives

higher incidences among certain ethnic or racial groups, especially those with common geographic ancestral heritages.

Spontaneous genetic disease may also result from new gene mutation (see page 16), and once it occurs the mutant gene can be passed to future generations through one of the major patterns of inheritance.

A third reason genetic disease seems to appear spontaneously is that in the past, genetic disease may have gone undiagnosed. Many old death certificates list cause of death simply as "natural causes." Thus, a family may have a history of genetic disease and not know it.

ENVIRONMENT

Another factor that influences your placement on the health continuum is your environment. Environmental factors include a person's geographic location, food resources and general nutritional state, personal health habits and practices, socioeconomic level, access to health care, and exposure to pollutants and chemical or infectious agents (such as bacteria, viruses, fungi, and parasites). These environmental factors, alone or in combination with inherited genetic predispositions, have an impact on your health and can increase or decrease your risk of developing disease.

INSTRUCTIONS: To be sure your health-care provider has all the information needed to plan and individualize your health care, answer the following questions after you read Chapter 1, Genetic Inheritance. Write your answers in Section 1 of the *GENETIC CONNECTIONS*™ *HEALTH HISTORY FORM,* which you will find at the back of this book. Use a separate *HEALTH HISTORY FORM* for each family member.

SECTION 1
GENETIC INHERITANCE

1.1 Full name. Include confirmation, maiden, and other names, if applicable. Indicate "A" if adopted; "DS" if conceived with donor sperm; "DO" if conceived with donor ovum.

1.2 Mother's full name, including her maiden name. Father's full name. List names of the biologic parents, if different from above, and if known.

1.3 Date of birth. Place of birth (the city, state, country, province, region, etc.). Attach a copy of the birth certificate, if desired.

1.4 Any countries immigrated to. Dates of immigration. Means of transportation.

1.5 Full name of spouse, if applicable. Date and place of marriage. List the same information for any previous marriages and the dates of divorce or widowhood. Full name of each child. Indicate for each child "AI" if adopted into the family; "AO" if put up for adoption; "DS" if conceived with donor sperm; "DO" if conceived with donor ovum.

1.6 All places of residence and the year(s) lived at each.

1.7 Education received, degrees earned, schools/ universities attended, and years of attendance. List any professional certification (e.g., CPA).

1.8 Occupations or trades, and the dates of service. Also list any known occupational hazards exposed to.

1.9 Dates and locations of military service, if applicable. Branch of service.

1.10 Political affiliation and religious denomination (include if desired).

1.11 Creative work accomplished; e.g., publications, patents, awards.

1.12 Avocations; i.e., hobbies, recreational interests, and activities.

1.13 If this form is being completed for a person who is deceased, list the date and place of death, age at death, and cause of death, if known. Retain a copy of the death certificate, if desired.

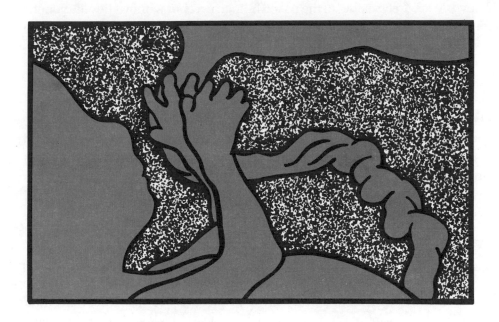

CHAPTER 2
PRENATAL HISTORY

The prenatal period is the time from conception to birth. The fertilized egg (ovum) is barely visible to the naked human eye, but within it lies the genetic potential of the resulting individual. A healthy and safe fetal environment (within the womb) is crucial in safeguarding that potential. If the fetal environment is unhealthy, some genetically given potential can be lost forever. Many factors influence fetal environment: the mother's overall general health; her physical environment; exposure to potentially damaging agents such as alcohol, drugs, and certain infections; and events of the pregnancy, labor, and delivery. It is the responsibility of both parents to provide as safe an environment as possible to give the child the best chance to be born with all the gifts and capabilities inherited from them.

PRECONCEPTIONAL AND GENETIC COUNSELING

A woman with a chronic health condition (such as diabetes, thyroid disease, seizure disorder, or high blood pressure), or a family history of genetic disease, chromosomal abnormalities, or failed pregnancies (miscarriage), benefits from receiving counseling before becoming pregnant. Preconceptional counseling from a health-care provider gives prospective parents information about pregnancy-associated risks, which are determined by the couple's health history and that of their families. They can also learn about available prenatal tests and screenings that they can utilize. Seeing a health-care provider prior to conception also allows a couple the opportunity to discuss possible outcomes of the pregnancy and receive answers to questions they may have concerning pregnancy. Today, even couples with no known risk factors are seeking preconceptional counseling to maximize their chances of having healthy pregnancies and babies. Couples with an individual or family history of genetic disease, chromosome abnormalities, birth defects, or repeated miscarriage can benefit from receiving genetic counseling from a medical geneticist or genetic counseling team. These professionals can calculate the couple's risk of transmitting a genetic disease or disorder to an offspring, and can provide information regarding available parental and prenatal (before birth) testing. Genetic counseling services can be obtained at most major hospitals and university medical complexes. Your doctor may also provide adequate counseling in some situations.

PREGNANCY

Gestation is the length of pregnancy; in human beings it is 9 calendar months, 10 lunar months, or 40 weeks from the start of the last menstrual period. This time is further divided into three blocks called trimesters, each of which consists of roughly three calendar months. Pregnancies that are delivered between 37 and 42 weeks from the start of the last

Others who may also benefit from genetic counseling include people who want to know:

- if they themselves have a genetic disease
- if they are carriers
- if they run the risk of having a child affected with a particular genetic disease
- what the implications are if they are planning parenthood and a genetic disease has already been diagnosed, and what the prognosis and treatment options are

- what help they can get in making a decision about the options of prenatal diagnosis, elective abortion, artificial insemination by donor, or adoption
- what kind of help is available for an already affected child and where it can be found.

Source: A. Milunski, "Genetic Counseling," in *Heredity and Your Family's Health* (1992), p. 223. Used with permission.

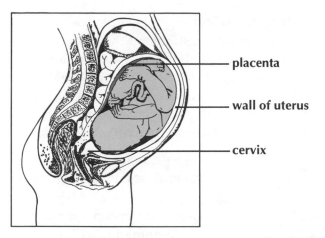

Figure 2.1. Pregnant uterus at term

placenta

wall of uterus

cervix

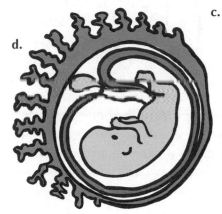

Figure 2.2. Embryo at different stages:
a. 2 weeks
b. 4 weeks
c. 6 weeks
d. 8 weeks

woman's blood to cross through to the fetus. These membranes also allow waste products from fetal blood to pass back into the woman's circulation so that they can be eliminated through her body systems. Unfortunately, certain chemicals and infectious agents that are harmful can cross the placental membrane as well. Medical disorders, infections, and chemical agents that interfere with the formation and function of the placenta can negatively affect the fetus.

Pregnancy can be divided into three stages of fetal development: preembryonic, embryonic, and fetal. The preembryonic stage lasts from conception to roughly 14 days postconception. The embryonic stage lasts from 14 days through 8 weeks. These two stages are times of very rapid growth as cells and tissues differentiate and begin to form essential organs and body structures. These are the most critical and sensitive times in fetal development. Exposure to damaging agents during these stages can result in severe birth defects. The fetal stage begins after week 8 and ends with delivery. By the time the fetal stage begins, all organs and organ systems are formed; they continue to mature throughout the remainder of pregnancy and into childhood.

PRENATAL CARE

A major factor that contributes to a healthy pregnancy and newborn is early and continuous prenatal care from a qualified health-care provider. Ideally, a couple planning to start a family visits their health-care provider before conceiving. During the initial prenatal visit, risk factors and maternal disorders that may require treatment or special care during the pregnancy are identified from the physical and laboratory evaluations of the woman and the health histories of the woman, her partner, and their families. With continuous prenatal care, couples have the opportunity to ask questions, receive educational information, and stay informed about the progress of the pregnancy. The health-care provider monitors both the woman and the fetus for complications and continually addresses the woman's physical, emotional, and educational needs.

menstrual period are classified as term pregnancies or term gestations. Infants born before week 37 are preterm or premature; infants delivered after week 42 are called post-term.

PLACENTAL AND FETAL DEVELOPMENT

Conception usually occurs in one of the two fallopian tubes that provide a passageway from the ovaries to the uterus. After conception, the fertilized egg completes its journey through the fallopian tube into the uterus and implants itself in the uterine wall, which has become thick and vascular in preparation for this very event.

At the site of implantation, the placenta begins to form. It attaches the fertilized egg securely to the wall of the uterus and is responsible for many functions that support the fetus. The placenta forms villi, thin membranes that allow oxygen and nutrients from the

Early identification and management of complications gives the best chance for a favorable pregnancy outcome—a healthy mother and baby.

NUTRITION

Good nutrition is essential in pregnancy. The placenta allows nutrients circulating in the woman's bloodstream to filter across the placental membrane to the fetus. Adequate nutrients must be available in the maternal blood supply to ensure the growth and development of a healthy baby. Research indicates that specific dietary deficiencies or excesses during pregnancy may cause or contribute to the development of some types of birth defects and may interfere with normal neurological development. For example, a deficiency of folic acid during pregnancy has been found to contribute to the occurrence of neural tube defects such as anencephaly and spina bifida.

A woman's caloric and nutritional needs increase during pregnancy because she now supports the growth of both the fetus and her own expanding body. The pregnant woman should follow a well-balanced diet throughout pregnancy, preferably three well-balanced meals a day and nutritious snacks such as fresh fruits, vegetables, and cheese between meals and at bedtime. Nutritional counseling can come from the woman's primary health-care provider, a nutritionist, or a dietician; this is especially important when there are special dietary considerations, such as with maternal diabetes. The pregnant woman needs approximately 300 additional calories a day to meet her and her baby's nutritional requirements. If she is underweight or a teenager she may be encouraged to add more. Vitamin supplements are often recommended early in pregnancy; some providers prescribe an additional iron supplement in month 5 or 6 of pregnancy.

Adequate fluid intake is important during pregnancy. The pregnant woman should drink 8 to 10 glasses of fluid per day. At least half of these should be water.

Caffeine intake during pregnancy should not be excessive. Caffeine is a stimulant that increases the heart rate, causes blood vessels to narrow, and acts as a diuretic resulting in body fluid loss. Health-care providers sometimes recommend that caffeine intake during pregnancy be limited to no more than two cups of coffee, for example, or two cans of soda per day.

A woman who is a vegetarian can achieve adequate nutrition during pregnancy if she gives special attention to the proper combination of foods she eats, especially in regard to specific amino acids (the basic units that form proteins). Because meat and animal products are major sources of complete proteins that provide the amino acids essential to the body, the woman who is a true vegetarian should know (or learn) how to combine foods to meet pregnancy protein requirements. Dietary guidelines can be obtained from health-care providers, nutritionists, or dieticians.

WEIGHT GAIN

The current acceptable weight gain during pregnancy is 20 to 30 pounds, but this may vary in specific instances. More important than the total weight gain is the pattern of weight gain. Deviation from the expected weight gain pattern—for example, gaining too little or too much weight within a week's time—may indicate complications such as fetal growth retardation or pregnancy-induced hypertension. A pregnant woman who exercises regularly should take in additional calories for use during exercise so that enough remain available for the fetus.

EXERCISE

Another factor contributing to a healthy pregnancy is exercise. Exercise tones muscles, strengthens the cardiovascular system, increases physical endurance, helps decrease stress, and promotes a sense of well-being. Guidelines for exercise during pregnancy should be discussed with the health-care provider because pregnancy-induced body changes alter the woman's physical tolerance to exercise. First, the woman's heart works harder even when she is at rest because of increases in blood volume that occur to support tissue growth during pregnancy. Second, hormonal changes relax muscles, ligaments, and tendons, making the woman more prone to joint and muscle injury. Third,

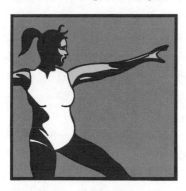

the enlarging uterus affects the curves of the spine, causing changes in posture and center of gravity, which affect the woman's balance and make her more prone to falls.

In consideration of these body changes, the American College of Obstetricians and Gynecologists developed safety guidelines for exercise during pregnancy that can be obtained from the prenatal health-care provider. Pregnant women should discuss these guidelines with their health-care provider during their first prenatal appointment. In general, women who exercise regularly before becoming pregnant can continue their routine through most of pregnancy, barring any complications. Routines may need modification during the last months or weeks of pregnancy. Women who do not routinely exercise before becoming pregnant should start very slowly and progress gradually as directed by the health-care provider.

TERATOGENS

A very important aspect of maintaining a healthy pregnancy is avoiding exposure to teratogens. A teratogen is an agent that can damage the developing fetus, causing birth defects. A teratogen may harm the fetus by disrupting organ development or by affecting the woman's health and thereby indirectly harming the fetus. Teratogenic agents are divided into three categories: physical, chemical, and infectious.

PHYSICAL AGENTS

Radiation exposure is a physical teratogenic agent. The degree of risk to the fetus depends on the age of the fetus (or embryo) at the time of exposure, the amount or strength of radiation, and the length of radiation exposure time. Most diagnostic tests that use radiation—for example, dental, chest, stomach, or abdominal x-rays—deliver radiation levels far below those associated with fetal damage. Although these "low-dose" radiation procedures are not associated with fetal defects that are evident at birth, some studies show these procedures to be linked with a higher risk of childhood cancers (including leukemia) that can appear years later. High-dose radiation—for example, doses used for cancer therapy or exposure to nuclear radiation—may be associated with physical and mental defects in the fetus.

Exposure to excessive heat, also a physical teratogenic agent, is a concern because persistent elevation of the pregnant woman's body temperature to above 100.4°F (38°C) has been associated with fetal central nervous system defects. As the woman's body temperature rises, so does the temperature of the fetus and the surrounding fluid; because the fetus has no mechanism to dissipate heat, this can be damaging to fetal tissue. A pregnant woman should avoid saunas and hot tubs, not only to avoid excessive body temperature, but because the heat can dilate her blood vessels and lower her blood pressure, which may potentially decrease blood flow through the placenta.

CHEMICAL AGENTS

Chemical agents include prescription and over-the-counter medication, recreational or illicit drugs, and occupational and household substances.

MEDICATION. Although most prescribed medications can be safely taken during pregnancy, some cannot. The health-care provider weighs the benefits to the woman against the risks to the fetus when prescribing medicine. If medicine is necessary to the woman's health, it will be prescribed under close supervision. Pregnant women should not use home remedies and over-the-counter medications until they check with their health-care provider.

TOBACCO. Women who smoke cigarettes have smaller babies on average than women who do not smoke. This may occur because

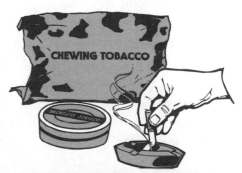

nicotine causes blood vessels to constrict (narrow), decreasing blood flow through the placenta. That decreases the delivery of oxygen and nutrients to the fetus. Also, carbon monoxide inhaled from cigarette smoke competes with oxygen for transportation sites on red blood cells, decreasing the amount of oxygen available to the fetus.

Smoking has also been implicated as a possible factor in stillbirths, sudden infant death syndrome (SIDS), and growth and development deficits such as low intelligence, hyperactivity, and attention span disorders. Therefore, the best advice is not to smoke during pregnancy. A health-care provider can help a smoker quit.

ALCOHOL. Alcohol use during pregnancy not only affects the woman's health but can have devastating effects on the fetus. Alcohol freely crosses the placental membrane, causing fetal blood-alcohol levels to 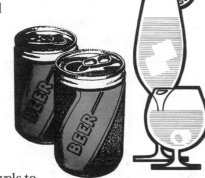 be comparable to the woman's levels. Women who drink excessively during pregnancy have a greater risk of miscarriage, stillbirth, bleeding complications, and early infant death.

Alcohol use by pregnant women has been cited as one of the western world's leading known causes of mental retardation (Abel and Sokol, 1986). Continued exposure to high levels of alcohol can cause fetal alcohol syndrome (FAS). FAS was first described in the late 1970s and is characterized by both physical and mental defects. Mental retardation (in varying degrees) and growth retardation (low birth weight) are very common. Birth defects, including malformations of the heart, brain, or skull, and abnormal facial features, can also occur with FAS. The March of Dimes states that the incidence of FAS in the United States is comparable to the incidence of Down syndrome.

FAS occurs in all socioeconomic groups and in most major countries. Some studies suggest that affected infants have inherited a genetic susceptibility to the effects of alcohol, which would partially explain why the severity of FAS does not always correlate with the amount of alcohol their mothers consumed, and why some ethnic populations have higher incidences of FAS than others.

The amount of alcohol needed to cause FAS is not known. It is known, however, that a woman need not be an alcoholic for her baby to have FAS. Fetal alcohol effects have occurred in the infants of women who drank moderate to heavy amounts throughout their pregnancies and in those who drank only intermittently. This makes it difficult to set a safe limit for alcohol consumption. Therefore, the best advice is to not consume alcohol during pregnancy.

COCAINE. Cocaine is a short-acting central nervous system stimulant that produces a state of euphoria. It stimulates the heart and causes constriction of the blood vessels, resulting in rapid heart rate and increased blood pressure. High fever, stroke, heart attack, and fatal disturbances in heart rhythm (dysrhythmia) have occurred after its use.

Cocaine reaches the brain and affects the central nervous system within minutes after being inhaled through the nose (snorted) and within seconds after being injected or smoked. Unfortunately, cocaine quickly crosses the placental membrane and exposes the fetus to the same risks. Cocaine can also be passed to a child through breast milk or by inhalation of second-hand cocaine smoke.

The increase in the pregnant woman's heart rate, blood pressure, and body temperature following the use of cocaine interferes with placental function by decreasing the oxygen and nutrients passed to the fetus, and can thereby cause fetal growth retardation. Cocaine stresses the fetus by increasing its heart rate, blood pressure, and temperature. Bleeding into the brain (stroke) has occurred in infants whose mothers ingested cocaine close to the time of delivery; this can cause permanent brain damage and death of the fetus.

Infants of women who use cocaine are often born prematurely and exhibit irritability of the central nervous system and withdrawal-like symptoms. These infants are jittery, easily disturbed but not easily consoled, and difficult to feed; often they exhibit disturbed sleep patterns. Their ability to interact with their environments is limited, and they often have behavioral, developmental, and intellectual problems that become increasingly apparent with age.

Women who use cocaine during pregnancy have been shown to have more miscarriages (spontaneous abortion) and other bleeding complications during pregnancy, including abruptio placentae (a premature separation of the placenta from the uterus). Because the placenta is responsible for transferring oxygen, nutrients, and waste products between the woman and fetus, abruptio placentae can cause fetal death; maternal death can occur as a result of extreme blood loss in a matter of minutes.

In conclusion, cocaine is not the only illicit drug that is harmful to the fetus. Other drugs, such as heroin, are also damaging and sometimes fatal, but are not discussed here. For the well-being of both the woman and her baby, the safest behavior is simply not to take any type of medication or drug during pregnancy unless directed by a physician.

INFECTIOUS AGENTS

Infection from bacterial, fungal, viral, and parasitic microorganisms can cause a wide range of defects in the fetus.

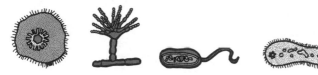

The following infections have the potential to cross the placental membrane and cause fetal injury or death. Infection during the first trimester (the first three months of pregnancy) usually causes the most severe damage, although exposure at any point may be harmful to the fetus. These infections can be medically diagnosed, but are not always treatable.

VIRAL INFECTIONS
CYTOMEGALOVIRUS (CMV)

Cytomegalovirus is a member of the herpes virus group. CMV is spread by sneezing, coughing, poor handwashing, and person-to-person contact such as kissing, sexual intercourse, or breastfeeding. The virus is carried in many body fluids, including saliva, respiratory mucus, breast milk, urine, feces, cervical mucus, semen, and blood. The fetus can be infected when the virus crosses the placental membrane. Newborns can be infected after exposure to their mother's infected body fluids during birth. Women with CMV infection usually have no symptoms; the occasional occurrence of symptoms may be similar to those of infectious mononucleosis, liver inflammation, or respiratory infection. After the initial CMV infection, a person may continue to shed the live virus in body secretions for months to years.

While many infants with CMV infection suffer no ill effects, some are born with intrauterine growth retardation, hearing and/or eye defects, mental retardation, brain abnormalities, and liver and bone disease. Fetal death can occur. CMV is a major cause of hearing impairment in children. The full degree of associated hearing and mental impairment may not become evident until the child is older.

CMV has no treatment or vaccine. Condom use during sexual intercourse can help prevent transmission from person to person and therefore help prevent fetal infection.

HEPATITIS B

Commonly referred to as serum hepatitis, hepatitis B is caused by the hepatitis B virus (HBV), which is found in all body fluids (blood, saliva, semen, urine, vaginal secretions) of infected people and of those who are chronic carriers. Hepatitis B is transmitted primarily through sexual contact or exposure to contaminated blood or blood products. Pregnant women who contract the disease have the same symptoms as the general population; usually the disease does not affect the course of the pregnancy. Symptoms can range from flu-like symptoms to full-blown liver failure.

An infant can become infected with the hepatitis B virus following exposure to the mother's blood and other body fluids at the time of delivery or, rarely, if the virus crosses the placental membrane. Infected infants risk becoming hepatitis B carriers, which means that active hepatitis B virus continues to reside in their bodies, and they are infectious to others. The child who is a carrier has a significant risk of developing fatal liver disease and liver cancer in young adulthood.

There is no known cure for hepatitis B, but there is a vaccine to prevent infection. Many women are tested for hepatitis B early in their pregnancies, because the newborn can be treated with agents to prevent infection. Newborns can now receive the hepatitis B vaccine as part of their routine immunization protocols regardless of their mother's status. The vaccine gives the child long-lasting protection against hepatitis B infection.

HERPES

Herpes is caused by the herpes simplex virus (HSV) and is classified into two types. Type I infections are usually associated with lesions on the skin, lips, mouth, and nose, and are commonly referred to as cold sores or fever blisters. Type II infections are associated with genital infection. As many as 10% of type I infections cause genital herpes, and vice versa, as a result of oral-genital contact.

Genital herpes infection is usually spread by physical contact (usually sexual) with someone who has active herpetic lesions. The virus can also be spread by touching an active lesion and then touching another body area that the virus can invade, such as the eye, lip, mouth, genital area, or any break in the skin. The eye is especially vulnerable to the virus, and infection can result in blindness.

In adults, symptoms of genital herpes infection usually begin with genital itching, burning, or a prickling sensation. A rash appears consisting of small, itchy, and/or painful bumps, which become clusters of small blisters that break open and turn into painful ulcers. The ulcers eventually scab over and heal; primary (initial) infections may take a month to heal, while recurrent (subsequent) infections may heal within 7 to 10 days. Fever, swollen glands in the groin, and muscle tenderness and pain also occur with the infection.

The first outbreak of a genital herpes infection, referred to as the primary infection, can be extremely painful and require hospitalization. After the first outbreak has healed, the virus retreats into nearby nerve cells and becomes inactive or dormant. Weeks, months, or even years later, the virus can become active again and cause a much milder recurrence of the same symptoms. Recurrences can be triggered by fever, stress, menstruation, and exposure to sunlight; however, the exact cause of recurrences is unknown. Rates of recurrence vary from person to person. Topical and oral medication can decrease the frequency and severity of outbreaks. For pregnant women, these medications may need to be temporarily discontinued.

Herpes infection of the fetus by direct transfer of the virus across the placental membrane is rare, but the risk is highest if the woman's first genital infection occurs during the pregnancy. Some sources believe there may be some immunity against placental transfer if the woman was exposed to either type of HSV before becoming pregnant. If early fetal infection does occur, the incidence of miscarriage, severe birth defects, and fetal death is 50% to 70%.

The major route of herpes transmission to a newborn infant is delivery through an infected vaginal canal. In newborns who are exposed to active herpes infection in this manner, less than 50% will develop symptoms of infection. Of those infants, however, 60% to 70% may die. A large number of infants who survive infection will have some degree of mental deficit. Symptoms of infection in the infant may include elevated or decreased body temperature, jaundice (yellow skin), seizures, poor feeding, and a blister-like skin rash.

Women who have genital herpes should notify their health-care provider immediately. If an active herpes infection is present at delivery, birth by cesarean section is indicated. A woman with a history of genital herpes whose bag of waters either breaks or begins to leak should see her health-care provider immediately, because if an active virus is present it can infect the fetus.

HSV infection is a lifelong disorder for which there is no known cure. As with all sexually transmitted diseases, it is the responsibility of each infected person to prevent its spread. Routine condom use, good hand-washing habits, and abstinence from intercourse during active outbreaks reduce the risk of transmission.

HUMAN IMMUNODEFICIENCY VIRUS (HIV)

HIV is the virus associated with acquired immune deficiency syndrome (AIDS). HIV is found in all body fluids, including the blood, semen, breast milk, and vaginal secretions of infected people. In a large percentage of cases, the virus is spread through sexual contact. It also can be contracted through infected blood and blood products and can cross the placental membrane to the fetus.

The risk of transmission through breast milk is unclear, so women who test positive for HIV are usually advised against breastfeeding. AIDS is not contracted from casual contact such as hugging or kissing, or by sharing eating utensils, classrooms, or living quarters.

When HIV enters the bloodstream it attacks the immune system, the body's natural defense against infection. After exposure to the virus, the body develops specific antibodies that can be detected by certain tests. People who test HIV-positive have been infected by the virus and have developed these specific antibodies. Antibodies formed by the body's immune system in response to an infection usually destroy the causative microorganisms, but unfortunately these specific antibodies are not effective in destroying the HIV. It may be weeks or months after the original infection before the antibodies show up on testing. During this in-between time, referred to as the window period, HIV tests indicate negative results; however, infected people who have not yet developed antibodies can transmit the virus to others. People who are HIV-positive are at risk of developing AIDS, although it may be years before this occurs. AIDS results as the body loses its ability to fight even mild infections or to differentiate its own cells from invading micro-organisms. Susceptibility to cancer greatly increases, and microorganisms that do not usually cause disease can result in life-threatening infection.

Symptoms of AIDS include fever, loss of appetite, weight loss, fatigue, swollen lymph nodes, diarrhea, skin rash, night sweats, and susceptibility to infection. Much is still not known about AIDS. Certain groups have a higher risk of infection than the general population: intravenous drug users, prostitutes, homosexual or heterosexual men with multiple partners, and the sexual partners of members of these groups. Hetero-sexual transmission (male to female or female to male) has been increasing in the United States; in some countries this is the primary method of transmission. The number of women infected with HIV is increasing, resulting in an increase in the number of newborn infants with HIV infection.

Pregnant women in a high-risk category or who have been sexually active with a high-risk partner should notify their health-care provider as early as possible so that counseling and testing can be done. Even with no symptoms present, a person can be HIV-positive. The rate of placental transmission (from mother to fetus) may be as high as 30% (Nair, 1992). An infant can also become infected at birth with direct exposure to the mother's blood and other body fluids. Cesarean delivery would not protect the newborn from exposure to the mother's body fluids, nor is it used as a means of prevention. Most infants born with HIV die by the age of 3 or 4, many within the first year.

HUMAN PARVOVIRUS

This virus, called human parvovirus B19, is the agent that causes human parvovirus infection, also known as erythema infectiosum, fifth disease, and B19 infection. As many as 50% of women living in U.S. cities are suspected to have immunity against the virus as the result of previous exposure. It is thought that the virus is spread through respiratory droplets of infected persons, and possibly through infected blood and blood products. Human parvovirus infection is one of the common communicable diseases associated with rash formation among children. Symptoms of infection in adults include headache, sore throat, and reddish rash. Human parvovirus can spread from an infected woman to her fetus through the placenta. Infection during pregnancy usually has no effect on the fetus; however, it may cause severe fetal anemia, congestive heart failure, and fetal death. Maternal infection has not been associated with structural birth defects. Infection early in the first half of pregnancy carries the greatest threat to the fetus. Fetal death and spontaneous abortion (miscarriage) may occur. Infection later in pregnancy may be reflected by anemia present in the infant at birth. There is no treatment or vaccine for human parvovirus infection other than treatments to relieve symptoms. Intra-uterine fetal blood transfusion may be attempted in some situations when life-threatening fetal anemia is occurring.

RUBELLA

Rubella, commonly referred to as the German or three-day measles, is caused by the rubella virus. It is spread by small water droplets from the lungs, throat, mouth, and nose of an infected person or by direct contact with infected people. Symptoms are generally mild: fever, sore throat, muscle and joint pain, and a raised red rash that usually fades after a few days. The disease is usually self-limiting and rarely causes complications in adults, but fetal infection can be deadly.

Pregnancies exposed to rubella in the first trimester have an extremely high miscarriage rate of 30% or higher. Studies indicate that 50% to 80% of fetuses exposed to rubella early in pregnancy have some degree of defect as a result of the infection, including cataracts, deafness, mental retardation, heart defects, and intrauterine growth retardation. Fetal death can occur. Infants born with rubella infection may continue to shed live rubella virus in urine and other body fluids for months, posing a risk to others who are not immune.

The first step in preventing rubella and its profound fetal effects is to identify the woman who is at risk of contracting the disease. People who have had rubella are usually immune to it for life. One of the first screenings a pregnant woman receives determines her level of immunity against rubella. If she is not immune (susceptible) to the rubella virus, she is encouraged to avoid crowds and children or young adults who are ill, especially those known to have rubella. Once a non-immune woman has delivered her baby, she is given the rubella vaccine to protect both her and future pregnancies. Because the vaccine itself is made with live (but deactivated) rubella virus, women should not become pregnant for at least three months after receiving the rubella vaccine.

The second step in preventing rubella infection is to immunize all children against it. Recent outbreaks of rubella in young adults imply that one rubella vaccine given in infancy may not achieve lifelong immunity. Current recommendations are that a second rubella vaccine, or booster, be given to all school-aged children. Unfortunately, a significant number of women of childbearing age (possibly as high as 20% in some urban areas of the United States) remain unprotected against rubella.

TOXOPLASMOSIS

Toxoplasmosis is caused by a single-cell parasite called *Toxoplasma gondii*. Toxoplasmosis is contracted by coming in contact with cat litter or soil that is contaminated with infected cat feces or by eating infected rare or undercooked meat. The infected woman often has no symptoms or may have general symptoms of illness such as muscle soreness, fatigue, and swollen lymph nodes in the neck. Fetal infection can result in defects of the eyes and in central nervous system disorders such as seizures and hydrocephalus. Miscarriage, premature delivery, stillbirth, and early infant death occur in a significant percentage of pregnancies that are exposed early to toxoplasmosis infection.

Infants who survive prenatal (before birth) infection may be born blind, deaf, or mentally retarded.

A pregnant woman with known toxoplasmosis infection can be treated with medication. Although fetal infection cannot be prevented, treating the woman may lessen injury to the fetus. The best treatment is prevention. Pregnant women should avoid handling cat litter unless they wear gloves and a mask or filter device over the mouth and nose (to prevent inhaling airborne toxoplasmosis spores) and wash their hands thoroughly after handling. They should also wear gloves when gardening or landscaping and should cook all meat thoroughly.

VARICELLA-ZOSTER

Varicella-zoster virus causes chickenpox; the virus is a member of the herpes virus group. It is spread through respiratory secretions and contact with fluid from the skin lesions (see page 72 for symptoms).

Most people have chickenpox during childhood and as a result have immunity against the virus. Therefore, it is not a common infection among pregnant women. In the few adults who have not had chickenpox (and thus are not immune), the infection can be serious and complicated by life-threatening pneumonia or inflammation of the blood and lymphatic vessels. Complications can become more severe in the non-immune pregnant woman.

The fetus can become infected through the placenta if the non-immune woman contracts chickenpox during the pregnancy. Congenital varicella syndrome can occur, but fortunately is rare; it is associated with severe birth defects including limb deformities, small head, infection and inflammation of the retinas, cataracts, hearing loss, mental retardation, and fetal death. Infants born to women who show symptoms of chickenpox infection four to five days before childbirth can be critically ill at birth if they too are infected with the varicella virus. These infants are given immune globulin (protective antibody proteins) in an effort to contain the infection. Infants whose mothers showed signs of infection within the first two days following childbirth receive gamma globulin as well, even if the infants are showing no signs of infection.

If there is doubt whether or not a pregnant woman who has been exposed to the varicella-zoster virus has ever had chickenpox, she will be tested to determine if she has immunity to this virus. If she is found to have no immunity, she will be given immune globulin specific for the varicella-zoster virus to prevent infection. Otherwise, there are no drugs to treat the infection. A chickenpox vaccine is to come, but is not available to the general population at this time.

SEXUALLY TRANSMITTED DISEASES

CMV, hepatitis B, HIV, and herpes are also classified as sexually transmitted diseases (STDs), which means they can be spread, although not exclusively, through sexual contact. Other STDs harmful to the fetus or newborn are chlamydia, gonorrhea, and syphilis.

Screening (testing) for many of the major STDs is usually done on the first prenatal visit. This screening is essential because women may have no symptoms and therefore be unaware they are infected with a disease that could potentially harm their babies. If treatment is available and received early, harmful effects can be prevented. It is equally important for sexual partners of infected women to receive treatment to prevent reinfection and further spread of the disease.

Women with incurable STDs, such as herpes, hepatitis B, or HIV infection, should be under close medical supervision, which makes possible the early recognition of pregnancy complications and the start of appropriate health-care intervention.

CHLAMYDIA

Chlamydia trachomatis is a microorganism found frequently in association with gonorrheal infections. It is spread by sexual or other direct contact. In women, chlamydia infection can cause genital burning, itching, and pain in the lower abdomen that may be accompanied by a thick grayish or yellowish-white vaginal discharge. Most women, however, have no symptoms. If untreated, infection can lead to pelvic inflammatory disease and scarring of the fallopian tubes, which can cause infertility or increase risk of tubal pregnancy. Symptoms in men may be mild or severe; they include pain on urination and a mucus discharge from the urethra. If untreated, infection can spread to the testes and/or other glands of the male reproductive system and result in sterility.

Infection in the newborn occurs with delivery through an infected vaginal canal. Infection of the eyes, ears, and/or lungs may result. Treatment is possible with antibiotics. Chlamydia is highly contagious, and some sources say it is the number one sexually transmitted disease in the United States.

GONORRHEA

Gonorrhea is caused by a bacteria named *Neisseria gonorrhoeae,* which invades the mucous membranes of the genital and urinary tracts of both males and females. Men usually have a pus-like discharge from the urethra (the opening at the end of the penis) that may persist for weeks and can be accompanied by painful burning on urination. Approximately 80% of infected women have no symptoms, while some develop vaginal discharge and/or painful urination. In both males and females, infection can spread to other internal organs and may result in sterility.

Gonorrhea can be successfully treated with penicillin or other antibiotics if it is diagnosed early. However, treatment cannot erase tissue scarring of internal organs or sterility that may have already occurred from advanced, untreated disease.

A newborn can become infected with gonorrhea if delivered through an infected vaginal canal. Gonorrheal infection of the eyes was once a leading cause of newborn blindness. However, all states now require that every infant receive preventive eye drops within one hour after delivery, a practice that has greatly reduced newborn blindness.

SYPHILIS

Caused by the bacteria *Treponema pallidum,* syphilis is transmitted by direct contact. It can cross the placental membrane to cause infection in the fetus. Once this bacteria enters the blood, it spreads throughout the body.

If untreated, syphilis progresses through stages. In the primary stage, a blister-like sore called a chancre develops where the bacteria entered the body, typically the genital area. This lesion may be painless. Women can be totally unaware of the infection if a lesion is located in the vagina and is not visible. These lesions "weep" a fluid that contains more of the highly contagious bacteria. The chancres heal with or without treatment in several weeks, but if untreated the infection progresses to the second stage.

In secondary syphilis, symptoms of general illness, usually accompanied by a rash, occur. The rash may cover the entire body, including the palms of the hands and the soles of the feet. This secondary stage can occur weeks or months after the first stage and may recur more than once.

Syphilis infection can lapse into an inactive or latent state for months or years between any of its stages, giving the false impression that the disease has gone away by itself. Infected people are not infectious to others at this time, but an infected pregnant woman can nevertheless infect her fetus through the placenta. Syphilis is still treatable during the secondary stage or latent periods.

If syphilis is not treated, tertiary syphilis infection (the third stage) develops years after the first infection. In this final stage, destructive lesions develop within body organs, resulting in blindness, deafness, crippling, skin and bone destruction, and disease and/or dysfunction of the liver, lungs, spinal cord, and brain. Syphilis in this final stage is still treatable, but existing organ and tissue damage cannot be reversed.

Pregnancies exposed to syphilis through the placenta have a high rate of miscarriage and stillbirth. Infected fetuses that survive can have physical deformities, skin lesions, deafness, blindness, and mental retardation. Early treatment of the pregnant woman with antibiotics can sometimes prevent the infection from damaging her baby.

In conclusion, sexually transmitted diseases are a concern during pregnancy and for society in general. Although abstinence from any kind of genital-to-skin contact is the surest method of protection against STDs, risk can also be reduced by limiting sexual activity to monogamous relationships and using condoms.

OCCUPATIONAL EXPOSURE TO TERATOGENS

A pregnant woman's work environment should be evaluated by her health-care provider for the presence of chemicals or other agents that could pose a risk to pregnancy outcome. It is also important that her employer be aware of the pregnancy so that protection can be provided as necessary. Additional information about occupational hazards and safety can be obtained from the Occupational Safety and Health Administration (OSHA) and the National Institute for Occupational Safety and Health (NIOSH).

MEDICAL CONDITIONS AND PREGNANCY

Heart disease, chronic hypertension (high blood pressure), pregnancy-induced hypertension, thyroid disease, kidney disease, anemia, and other medical conditions all require close medical supervision during pregnancy to ensure the good health of both the pregnant woman and the fetus.

CHRONIC HYPERTENSION

Chronic hypertension is a consistent blood pressure of 140/90 or higher. A woman with high blood pressure can be treated safely with medication during pregnancy; she and her fetus will be monitored closely. High blood pressure can decrease or diminish blood flow through the placenta and can result in intrauterine growth retardation and/or fetal distress. Even if high blood pressure is successfully treated during pregnancy, the fetus can still be affected by it; however, the outcome is usually worse if hypertension is untreated.

PREGNANCY-INDUCED HYPERTENSION (PIH)

PIH is high blood pressure that develops during pregnancy. Most at risk for developing PIH are women with chronic high blood pressure, women having their first pregnancy, teenagers, women over age 35, multiple-gestation pregnancies (more than one baby at a time), pregnancies with Rh incompatibility, women with a family history of PIH, and women who have diabetes, heart disease, or kidney disease.

PIH can develop during the last half of pregnancy, during labor and delivery, or during the first few days after delivery. Its classic features are elevated blood pressure, swelling of the entire body (including the face and hands), and protein in the urine. Its cause is unknown, but PIH has been associated with poor nutrition, lack of prenatal care, and genetic factors. In the past, PIH was referred to as toxemia. Today the terms preeclampsia and eclampsia are used to describe different degrees of PIH. Although PIH occurs in fewer than 10% of pregnancies, it is a major health problem that even today can result in maternal and fetal death.

A pregnant woman's body contains at least 30% more blood than a nonpregnant woman's. During pregnancy, her blood vessels become less responsive to body chemicals that normally cause them to constrict and increase blood pressure. This resistance to constricting chemicals allows her blood vessels to become more relaxed and elastic. Hormones produced during pregnancy most likely contribute to this elasticity. The woman's blood vessels simply expand, or dilate, to handle the increased blood volume, causing a slight decrease in her blood pressure and better blood flow through the placenta. This allows optimum levels of oxygen and nutrients to be transferred to the fetus.

In PIH, resistance to those constricting chemicals seems to be lost and the pregnant woman's blood vessels spasm and narrow (vasospasm), causing her blood pressure to rise. This vasospasm interferes with her kidney function, leading to fluid retention, decreased urine output, and loss of blood proteins into the urine. This loss of protein causes fluid to leave the blood vessels and accumulate in the woman's body tissues, causing generalized swelling (edema) and increased weight gain. Vasospasm also causes a marked reduction of blood flow through the placenta, decreasing the transfer of oxygen and nutrients to the fetus.

If symptoms of PIH are mild, the woman can be treated initially with bed rest at home under close medical supervision. If her symptoms worsen, however, hospitalization is required. The term pre-eclampsia is used to describe PIH at these levels. Preeclampsia can, however, progress very quickly to eclampsia, the most severe form of PIH. In eclampsia, the high blood pressure and swelling become so severe that seizures and coma result. The woman is also at risk for stroke, retinal detachment of the eye, or premature separation of the placenta from the uterus (abruptio placentae). Severe preeclampsia and eclampsia are medical emergencies that require immediate intensive care.

Although medications are used to decrease the symptoms of PIH, the only cure is delivery of the fetus. The optimal treatment is to safely control PIH as long as needed to prevent the birth of a severely premature infant. However, if PIH continues to advance, preterm delivery may be the safest choice for both mother and baby.

DIABETES MELLITUS (DM)

Diabetes, like high blood pressure, may be present before pregnancy or occur during pregnancy.

In diabetes mellitus, the body is unable to use carbohydrates for energy because of poor or absent production of insulin by specialized cells within the pancreas. Blood sugar (glucose) levels become abnormally elevated because of this lack of insulin, and the body is forced to break down fat and muscle for energy. Long-term complications of diabetes include atherosclerosis (the deposition of fat along blood vessel walls), kidney disease, heart disease (including high blood pressure, stroke, and poor peripheral circulation), damage to the retina of the eye, and nerve damage within the extremities.

Diabetes can affect pregnancy outcome and fetal health. If severe, diabetes can affect the vascular formation and function of the placenta, resulting in decreased blood flow to the fetus and intrauterine growth retardation; also, persistent uncontrolled elevation of the woman's blood sugar can cause the infant to grow very large for its gestational age, increasing the risk of birth trauma to both infant and mother with vaginal delivery. Infants born to diabetic women are also at risk for complications such as premature birth, hypoglycemia (low blood sugar), respiratory distress, seizures, and jaundice (yellow skin) shortly after birth, and have a higher incidence of birth defects.

Diabetes in pregnancy is associated with an increased incidence of stillbirths, pregnancy-induced hypertension, maternal infection, and hemorrhage after delivery. Not long ago, women with severe diabetes were discouraged from becoming pregnant because of the high risk of poor outcome for both the woman and her baby. Since then, health-care providers have learned a great deal about how to successfully manage diabetes during pregnancy by keeping the woman's blood sugar within normal limits at all times and closely supervising both her and the fetus throughout the pregnancy.

Women who have diabetes should receive pre-conceptional counseling. The goal is to have their diabetes controlled at least three months before the onset of pregnancy. Oral medications used to treat diabetes are not recommended during pregnancy because they may damage the fetus. Instead, diabetes is controlled with insulin. Pregnancy affects insulin needs in various ways, so that even women with previously well-controlled diabetes require intensive monitoring.

GESTATIONAL DIABETES

Gestational diabetes occurs only during pregnancy. Because gestational diabetic pregnancies have some of the same risks as other diabetic pregnancies, all pregnant women have their urine checked at every prenatal visit for sugar (glucose) spillage, which could indicate a high blood sugar level and the development of gestational diabetes. Additionally, testing for gestational diabetes is typically performed on all women between months 5 and 7 of pregnancy, when symptoms of gestational diabetes usually begin. Because women who have gestational diabetes are more likely to develop diabetes mellitus later in life, they should be screened for diabetes during annual routine checkups throughout their lives.

Rh INCOMPATIBILITY (ISOIMMUNIZATION)

The rhesus (Rh) factor is located on the surface of red blood cells. People with the factor are considered to be Rh positive; people without it are Rh negative. If Rh positive blood is given to a person who is Rh negative, the Rh negative person's immune system produces antibodies that destroy the Rh positive red blood cells. When an Rh negative woman develops these antibodies, they can cross the placental mem-

brane during pregnancy and attack the red blood cells of an Rh positive fetus.

In a pregnancy with an Rh negative mother and an Rh positive father, the fetus has a high likelihood of also being Rh positive. If this is the woman's first pregnancy and the infant is indeed Rh positive, the fetus is usually not harmed. However, during delivery, some of the Rh positive fetal blood cells can enter the woman's system and cause her body to produce the antibodies against Rh positive blood cells. (When these antibodies are found in a woman's blood, she is said to have been sensitized.) During a subsequent pregnancy with an Rh positive fetus, the woman's antibodies can cross the placental membrane, enter the fetal bloodstream, and begin to destroy the fetus's red blood cells, a condition called hemolytic disease (see figure 2.3). This disorder can cause severe fetal anemia and death. No harm occurs to the woman from Rh incompatibility.

In past years, fetal hemolytic disease was a significant problem. Today, however, the woman is tested for Rh status at the first prenatal examination. A pregnant woman at risk for Rh incompatibility is monitored for the development of antibodies throughout pregnancy.

The biggest advancement in prevention of hemolytic disease was the introduction of Rh immune globulin (RhIG or RhoGAM) in 1968. When given to an Rh negative woman within 72 hours after delivery of an Rh positive child, Rh immune globulin prevents the formation of antibodies in the woman's blood, thereby protecting future Rh positive pregnancies.

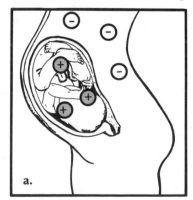 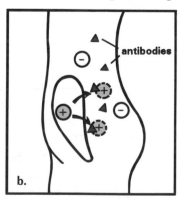 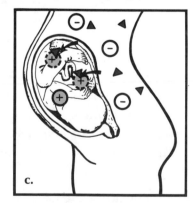

a. Rh negative woman during first pregnancy with an Rh positive fetus

b. after delivery some Rh positive fetal blood cells enter the woman's system and stimulate production of antibodies against Rh positive cells

c. destruction of red blood cells by the woman's antibodies in a subsequent pregnancy with an Rh positive fetus

Figure 2.3. Rh incompatibility and the development of fetal hemolytic disease

Rh immune globulin must be given after each Rh positive pregnancy to be effective. Rh immune globulin should also be given to Rh negative women after the following: spontaneous, therapeutic, or elective abortion; ectopic pregnancy; abdominal injury; episodes of vaginal bleeding; amniocentesis or chorionic villus sampling; and after any pregnancy in which the fetal blood type cannot be determined, such as long-standing fetal death. Rh negative women should be given a dose of Rh immune globulin at 28 to 32 weeks of pregnancy to prevent early antibody formation. However, if the baby is determined to be Rh negative after birth, there is no need for the woman to receive Rh immune globulin. If the woman has already developed antibodies, Rh immune globulin is of no use because it does not destroy existing antibodies.

Even though Rh immune globulin prevents Rh antibody formation, some women fail to receive it, are already sensitized, or receive an inadequate dose if more than usual fetal blood enters the mother's bloodstream during childbirth. That may explain why hemolytic disease still affects several thousand newborn infants each year. It is important for pregnant women to know their Rh factor and that of their partner, and to receive early, continuous health care throughout pregnancy.

VAGINAL BLEEDING DURING PREGNANCY

Bleeding complications can affect pregnancy outcome and threaten the lives of both woman and fetus.

MISCARRIAGE (SPONTANEOUS ABORTION)

The most common cause of bleeding during the first three months of pregnancy is miscarriage, referred to medically as spontaneous abortion. Miscarriage is divided into different categories. Threatened abortion occurs when the woman has unexplained bleeding and perhaps some cramping, but the opening (cervix) into the uterus is still closed. Ultrasound imaging can be used to confirm that the fetus is still alive. Most vaginal bleeding that occurs in the first three months of pregnancy stops by itself, and the pregnancy continues to term. Inevitable or imminent abortion is diagnosed if the cervix begins to dilate. If the fetus, placenta, and membranes are expelled from the uterus, complete

abortion has occurred. If all the tissue is not expelled from the uterus, incomplete abortion is diagnosed. The retained tissue in incomplete abortion is most commonly the placenta or some of its fragments, which must be removed by a surgical procedure called dilation and curettage, also known as D and C.

Missed abortion is a situation in which the fetus dies in the uterus, but the woman's body does not recognize this. The cervix remains closed, preventing expulsion of the uterine contents. Discomfort associated with pregnancy, such as morning sickness and breast tenderness, suddenly disappear, and the woman simply may not "feel pregnant" anymore. Once fetal death has been verified with ultrasound imaging, the uterus must eventually be emptied. If, after a short period of time, spontaneous expulsion fails to occur, a D and C or induction of labor may be necessary.

Miscarriage has been estimated to occur in at least 15% of pregnancies. Many speculate, however, that the true rate is much higher because miscarriage can occur before a woman even realizes she is pregnant, and therefore, it is not reported. A large percentage of miscarriages are associated with chromosome abnormalities; other causes include exposure to teratogens, structural malformations of the woman's reproductive tract, or chronic maternal medical disorders.

RECURRENT MISCARRIAGE

Three or more miscarriages in a row are referred to as recurrent spontaneous abortion. Women and their partners can be evaluated for metabolic, infectious, hormonal, or genetic causes for these pregnancy losses. If either parent has a chromosome rearrangement (translocation) that contributes to or causes fetal death and/or miscarriage, pregnancy losses will not necessarily be consecutive. With medical guidance and persistence, many couples can be successful in having children.

INCOMPETENT CERVIX

Women who have recurrent or repeated miscarriages in the second trimester (the second three months of pregnancy) may have a condition called incompetent cervix. For unknown reasons, the cervix (the opening to the uterus) begins to dilate prematurely. The cervix simply cannot stay closed (remain competent) against increasing pressure created by the growth of both the uterus and fetus. Abnormalities in the structure of the cervix or previous injury to the cervix may predispose a woman to having an incompetent cervix. Women whose mothers took the drug diethylstilbestrol (DES) during pregnancy are at higher risk of incompetent cervix, and they can be tested to evaluate their cervical competency before becoming pregnant.

A surgical procedure called a cerclage, in which the cervical opening is stitched closed, can be done at the start of the second trimester to keep the cervix from dilating prematurely. Cerclage is successful in maintaining pregnancy 80% to 90% of the time.

ECTOPIC PREGNANCY

Ectopic pregnancy occurs when the fertilized egg implants outside the uterus. An ectopic pregnancy can implant in the abdomen, on an ovary, or on the cervix, but the majority of such pregnancies implant within the fallopian tubes that lead from the ovaries to the uterus (see figure 2.4). This explains why ectopic pregnancies are frequently referred to as tubal pregnancies. When the fertilized egg attaches to the inner wall of the fallopian tube (or other ectopic site outside the uterus), it begins to grow. Hormones that occur normally during pregnancy are produced, causing the woman to feel pregnant and have common symptoms of pregnancy such as morning sickness, breast tenderness, and cessation of menstrual periods. Within a short period of time, however, the embryo outgrows the space within the fallopian tube, causing the tube to rupture and bleed into the woman's abdominal cavity. This rupture causes the woman severe

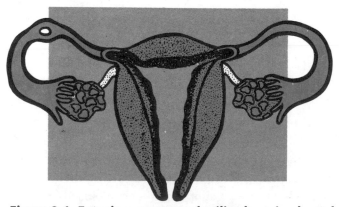

Figure 2.4. Ectopic pregnancy: fertilized egg implanted in a fallopian tube

abdominal pain (and frequently shoulder discomfort) and the death of the embryo/fetus. Vaginal bleeding may or may not be present, but internal bleeding can rapidly lead to shock and even death if not treated immediately. This situation is a medical emergency that requires surgery to remove the tissues of pregnancy and stop the bleeding.

The cause of ectopic pregnancy is often unknown, but disorders or procedures that scar the fallopian tube(s) can increase a woman's risk. Although the incidence of ectopic pregnancy has increased in recent years, early diagnosis and treatment have decreased the number of maternal deaths significantly.

GESTATIONAL TROPHOBLASTIC DISEASE

Also called molar pregnancy or hydatidiform mole, gestational trophoblastic disease is another cause of bleeding during pregnancy. With gestational trophoblastic disease, the fertilized egg or embryo dies

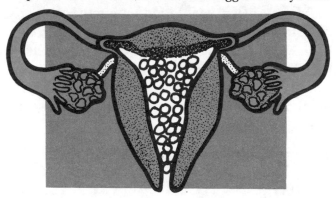

Figure 2.5. Gestational trophoblastic disease: proliferation of trophoblastic clusters within the uterus

early in the pregnancy because of severe chromosomal abnormalities. The tissues that would normally have developed into the placenta become fluid-filled clusters that spread very rapidly throughout the uterus (see figure 2.5). The woman experiences discomfort commonly associated with pregnancy, although nausea and vomiting may be severe. The size of the uterus may increase much faster than expected because of the rapidly proliferating clusters, and the woman may have symptoms of pregnancy-induced hypertension earlier in pregnancy than is usually seen. Vaginal bleeding—often a brownish liquid discharge —may contain some of the fluid-filled clusters (sometimes described as small and grape-like in appearance).

Molar pregnancies are classified as partial or complete, depending on whether any normal placental tissue is present within the uterus. If complete, there is a risk that a cancer called choriocarcinoma may develop in which the proliferating clusters become malignant and spread throughout the body. Any woman who has a molar pregnancy is closely monitored for one year for increasing levels of the pregnancy hormone human gonadotropin. This particular hormone increases in pregnancy as well as with choriocarcinoma; therefore, it is critical that the woman not become pregnant again during this time. If choriocarcinoma develops, the woman is treated with chemotherapy; in a few cases, surgery is necessary. If hormone levels remain negative throughout the year, it is safe for the woman to become pregnant again. The risk of gestational trophoblastic disease recurring in subsequent pregnancies is low in the majority of cases but should be discussed with a health-care provider.

Vaginal bleeding that occurs in the last half of pregnancy is primarily related to placental abnormalities, specifically placenta previa and abruptio placentae. Even though these two disorders can cause bleeding at any time during a pregnancy, they typically become evident in the third trimester (the last three months).

PLACENTA PREVIA

Placenta previa is a condition in which the placenta develops abnormally low in the uterus, covering part or all of the cervical opening (see figure 2.6). Bleeding can occur in association with physical activity, including sexual intercourse, or it can occur abruptly when at rest or at the beginning of labor. During labor, as the cervix begins to dilate, the placenta is torn away and bleeding begins. Fetal distress and

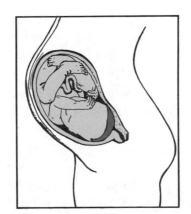

Figure 2.6. Placenta previa: the placenta is low in the uterus, covering the opening of the cervix

death can result from blood loss or lack of oxygen. Maternal death can also result from the excessive blood loss. If the placenta completely covers the cervix, delivery by cesarean section is indicated.

ABRUPTIO PLACENTAE

Abruptio placentae is a premature separation of the placenta from the wall of the uterus (see figure 2.7). As the placenta tears away and separates, bleeding occurs within the uterine cavity. This is a serious complication that can lead to premature delivery, fetal death, and maternal death, even with immediate emergency medical care. Many times the cause of placental abruption is unknown, but it occurs more

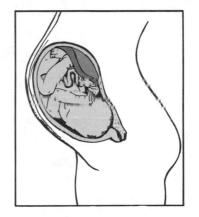

Figure 2.7. Abruptio placentae: the placenta is tearing away from the uterus

frequently in women who have high blood pressure, pregnancy-induced hypertension (especially if eclampsia develops), or abdominal trauma, and in women who use cocaine.

PREMATURE RUPTURE OF MEMBRANES (PROM)

PROM is the rupture of the amniotic sac or membrane (bag of waters) and subsequent loss of fluid surrounding the fetus before the onset of labor. The cause is not usually known. Suspected risk factors are maternal infection or infection within the uterus and the membrane, structural abnormalities in the membrane or of the cervix, and preterm labor (labor before week 37 of pregnancy).

PROM increases the woman's risk of infection and can result in prolonged hospitalization if the pregnancy is preterm. PROM increases the fetus's risk of infection, premature birth, compression of the umbilical cord (or its prolapse through the cervix into the birth canal), an abnormal birth presentation, and death.

If infection develops, it is treated with intravenous antibiotics, and the fetus is delivered vaginally or by cesarean section even if the infant is premature. Medication may be given to stimulate fetal lung maturity if preterm delivery is imminent. If there is no infection or other complication and the pregnancy is preterm, the woman may be closely monitored in the hospital as the pregnancy progresses. If the woman is close to term and the fetal lungs are mature, labor may be induced. If PROM occurs extremely early in pregnancy (before week 20 of pregnancy), miscarriage (spontaneous abortion) may occur.

OTHER COMPLICATIONS OF LABOR AND DELIVERY

Conditions that complicate labor and delivery can be attributed to uterine, pelvic, and fetal factors.

UTERINE FACTORS

The uterus is an extremely muscular organ; the rhythmic contractions of its muscles during labor move the fetus through the birth canal. Conditions that result in the overdistention of the uterus—such as multiple pregnancy, excess fluid around the fetus, or a very large fetus—or labor that continues for an extended period of time can make the muscle contractions less effective. The uterine muscles can simply tire out, prolonging labor even further. Without strong uterine contractions, the descent or progression of the fetus through the birth canal is slowed, causing stress to both the fetus and the woman. Medication that strengthens uterine muscle contractions can sometimes be used to help labor progress.

PELVIC FACTORS

The size and shape of the woman's pelvic bones determine the dimensions of the birth canal. If the passage is not large enough for the fetus, labor will be prolonged and very difficult, like trying to force a square peg through a round hole. Cesarean section in this instance is indicated.

FETAL FACTORS

Sometimes the fetus is too big to pass through the birth canal of a pelvis that would ordinarily be considered adequate for vaginal delivery. Genetic factors certainly influence fetal size, but medical disorders such as maternal diabetes can also cause large fetal size. In some instances birth defects may make delivery difficult, especially protruding defects, such as some types of spinal column abnormalities, or defects that result in fetal head enlargement.

Another fetal factor that can complicate labor and delivery is an abnormal fetal position or presentation (see figure 2.8). In a transverse presentation the baby lies side-to-side instead of in the usual head-down position, with the fetal back or abdomen trying to come through the birth canal first. In a shoulder presentation, a shoulder tries to come through first. In breech presentation, the buttocks (with or without feet) are the first to deliver through the birth canal. In face presentation, although the head is presenting, the neck is hyperextended so that the widest (instead of the smallest) diameter of the fetal face is coming through the birth canal first. And in compound presentation, more than one body part of the fetus, such as an arm (or arms) and head, tries to come through the birth canal at the same time.

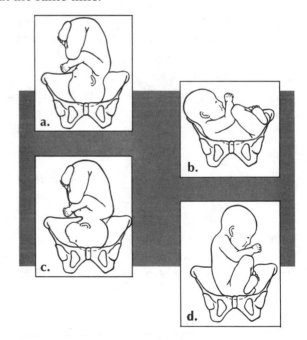

Figure 2.8. Birth presentations:
  a. vertex (head down)   b. transverse
  c. face   d. breech

Even with good uterine contractions and a favorably shaped pelvis, vaginal delivery of an abnormally presenting infant may not be possible. In transverse and shoulder presentations, the infant must be delivered by cesarean section. Rotating the fetus into the head-down position within the uterus may allow for vaginal delivery but cannot always be accomplished. In face presentation, a vaginal delivery may be possible, but often a cesarean section is necessary. Breech-presenting infants can be delivered vaginally, but only in specific instances and under close medical supervision in well-managed hospital delivery units. Attempts to rotate the breech-presenting infant into a head-down position are sometimes successful, allowing for vaginal delivery.

FETAL DISTRESS

Fetal distress is an indication that the fetus may not tolerate the stress of labor and delivery without negative consequences. It has many causes, but all are warnings that the fetal environment is not optimal. Conditions that cause a lack of oxygen to the fetus, such as a poorly functioning placenta, compression of the umbilical cord, infection, or maternal disease, can result in fetal distress. Changes in the fetal heart rate are indicators of fetal distress. Use of a fetal heart rate monitor during labor and delivery provides a continuous printout of fetal heart rate activity, allowing opportunity for immediate recognition and treatment of fetal distress.

In conclusion, many complications can occur during pregnancy; some are avoidable, some are treatable, and some are not. Most have lifelong ramifications for women and their infants. Women who have genetic risk factors, health disorders, or diseases that may affect their pregnancies should see a health-care provider before they become pregnant for preconceptional and/or genetic counseling as indicated. All pregnant women, risk factors or no risk factors, deserve continuous prenatal health care not only to ensure their health, but also to ensure the best possible start for their children.

SECTION 2
PRENATAL HISTORY

2.1 List whether your mother took any of the following substances during her pregnancy with you:

- Prescription medications. If so, list the medications, and document whether they were taken during the first trimester (first 3 months), second trimester (second 3 months), or third trimester (last 3 months) of pregnancy.

- Tobacco. Indicate whether cigarettes or smokeless tobacco. If cigarettes, indicate how many packs per day. Indicate whether tobacco was used in the first trimester (first 3 months), second trimester (second 3 months), or third trimester (last 3 months) of pregnancy.

- Alcohol. Describe use as seldom, occasional, or daily. Document whether alcohol was used in the first trimester (first 3 months), second trimester (second 3 months), or third trimester (last 3 months) of pregnancy.

- Illicit drugs. List specific drug(s) used and whether they were used in the first trimester (first 3 months), second trimester (second 3 months), or third trimester (last 3 months) of pregnancy.

2.2 Indicate whether your mother was exposed to any infections during her pregnancy with you. If so, document the specific infection, if known. Indicate whether the infection occurred during the first trimester (first 3 months), second trimester (second 3 months), or third trimester (last 3 months) of pregnancy.

2.3 Indicate whether your mother had any of the following medical complications during her pregnancy with you:

- Chronic hypertension

- Pregnancy-induced hypertension

- Diabetes mellitus

- Gestational diabetes

- Rh incompatibility

2.4 Indicate whether your mother had any of the following bleeding complications during her pregnancy with you:

- Threatened miscarriage

- Incompetent cervix

- Placenta previa

- Abruptio placentae

2.5 Document whether your mother experienced premature rupture of membranes.

2.6 Document any other complications of labor and delivery.

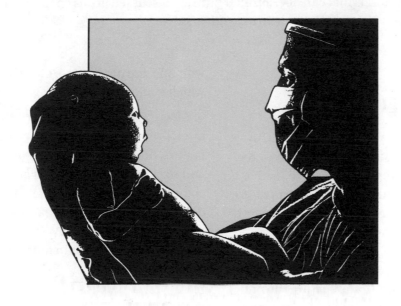

CHAPTER 3
BIRTH HISTORY

A birth history reveals information on the type of delivery and the health status of the individual at birth and shortly after birth. Chromosomal abnormalities and complications that can develop after birth are discussed in this chapter. These are important points to include in a health history.

BIRTH
METHODS OF DELIVERY

Natural delivery is birth via the vaginal (birth) canal. In a broader scope, natural delivery refers to childbirth in which the mother is an awake, active participant in the labor and delivery process. If complications occur during pregnancy or during the labor and delivery periods, the probability of surgical birth by cesarean section (C section) increases because delivery of the infant can be achieved in a short, controlled period of time. Complications do not always result in cesarean section, however, because vaginal birth can sometimes still be accomplished safely under close medical supervision.

GESTATIONAL AGE

The gestational age of a newborn infant is the number of weeks since the first day of the mother's last menstrual period; in other words, the length of the pregnancy. A human pregnancy lasts approximately 40 weeks. Infants delivered between 37 and 42 weeks of pregnancy (gestation) are technically classified as term infants. Infants born before 37 weeks of pregnancy are classified as premature (preterm) infants; those born after 42 weeks of pregnancy are classified as post-mature (post-term) infants. An infant born 8 weeks early would have a gestational age of 32 weeks (40 weeks minus 8 weeks = 32 weeks). Gestational age is confirmed by examining specific physical and neurologic characteristics of the infant rather than by depending solely on the

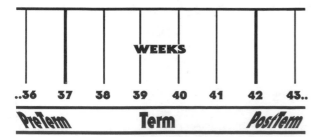

woman's due date or date of her last menstrual period, which could be in error.

It is medically important to record gestational age at birth because infants who are premature, post-mature, or who fall above or below the expected weight and size for their gestational age are at higher risk for complications than other newborns. Also, premature deliveries tend to run in families; you would find it helpful to know if they ran in your family since prematurity can result in long-term health problems.

BIRTH WEIGHT AND LENGTH

Standard ranges for expected or "normal" weight, length, and head circumference have been established for newborn infants in relation to their gestational age

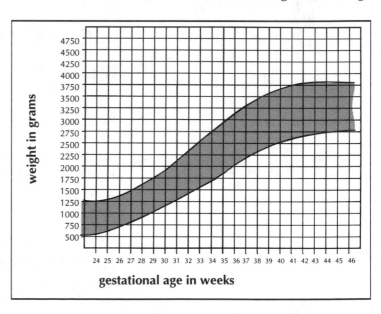

Figure 3.1. Birth weights for gestational age, with shaded area (10th to 90th percentile) indicating appropriate birth weights

(see figure 3.1). Variations from these standard ranges are seen among different populations and races because of genetic, environmental, and nutritional differences. At birth, an infant's weight, length, and head circumference measurements are compared to the standard ranges expected for the gestational age to see if the infant's size and growth are normal. Infants whose measurements fall within the standard ranges are considered appropriate for gestational age (AGA). Infants whose measurements fall below the 10th percentile are considered small for gestational age (SGA), and infants whose measurements fall above the 90th percentile are considered large for gestational age (LGA).

Infants may be SGA or LGA because of their genetic inheritance; some families typically have large or small babies. But infant size may also reflect some other occurrence or disorder. For example, women who have diabetes during pregnancy may have either SGA or LGA infants. Women with high blood pressure may have SGA infants. Infection, environmental insults, and some genetic disorders can also affect infant growth. Infants who are LGA or SGA at birth have higher morbidity and mortality rates than do AGA infants.

BLOOD TYPES

Blood types are checked at birth to determine whether incompatibilities exist between the mother's and infant's blood types. There are four blood groups: A, B, AB, and O. The Rh factor classification of positive or negative is an equally important part of the blood type. If the blood type is B negative (B-), the blood group is B and the Rh factor is negative. Blood type is a genetically determined trait.

BIRTH DEFECTS AND GENETIC DISEASE

Birth defects are the abnormal formation, growth, and/or function of fetal structures. The majority of birth defects are evident at birth, but some are not diagnosed until later. In most cases the cause of the birth defect is unknown, although some causes have been identified.

The term *birth defect* can be used broadly to encompass chromosomal abnormalities and genetic disorders and diseases. Some birth defects are classified as multifactorial or polygenic because they do not follow a normal inheritance pattern; it is not known exactly why they occur. Multifactorial defects may be caused by a single gene or a combination of genes that

show up only when certain environmental influences exist. Certain agents have been proven to cause defects in varying degrees and should be avoided during pregnancy. These damaging agents, called teratogens, fall into three basic categories: physical, chemical, and infectious agents (see page 25). Specific structural birth defects and genetic diseases are listed in the chapter covering the appropriate body system (see the index for page numbers). Selected chromosomal abnormalities are listed below.

CHROMOSOMAL DEFECTS

Chromosomal defects or syndromes occur when an abnormal number of chromosomes is present or the structure of one or more chromosomes is altered. Classic Down syndrome, for example, is called trisomy 21 because there are three number 21 chromosomes instead of two in each body cell, resulting in a total chromosome count of 47.

Many times the cause of chromosomal abnormalities is not clear. Abnormalities in the total number of chromosomes increase in relation to the advancing age of the pregnant woman, especially women aged 35 and over. In some chromosomal abnormalities a complete extra chromosome has been inherited or is missing from one of the reproductive cells (the egg or sperm). This is thought to occur because of a failure of the egg or sperm to split evenly during cell division (meiosis), causing some eggs and sperm to contain duplicate chromosomes and others to be missing chromosomes. In some chromosomal defects only a portion of a chromosome is extra or missing. In others, pieces of two chromosomes break off and switch places, causing a translocation. Some people have a mosaic chromosome pattern: some of their cells contain the normal number of chromosomes (23 pairs, for a total of 46), and other cells contain an abnormal number.

Considerable research on chromosomal abnormalities continues. Most chromosomal disorders do not follow a specific inheritance pattern and occur sporadically; however, a few specific types are inherited. Chromosomal abnormalities can occur in any of the chromosomes. Most cause death. Statistically, chromosomal abnormalities (defects) occur in 0.7% of all live births, in 2% of pregnancies of women over age 35, and in 50% of all spontaneous first trimester abortions (miscarriages).

NONSEX CHROMOSOMAL (AUTOSOMAL) DISORDERS

CRI DU CHAT

Also known as cat cry syndrome and 5p- syndrome.

The incidence is approximately 1 in 50,000 live births, and it occurs in females almost twice as often as in males. In as many as 15% of cases, the chance of recurrence in siblings is high. Part of one chromosome 5 is missing. As a rule, the greater the amount of missing genetic material, the more severe the syndrome.

SIGNS AND SYMPTOMS. Infants usually have a very distinctive cry for at least the first weeks of life. It sounds like a cat, high pitched and shrill. These children typically have low birth weight, growth delays, and characteristic facial features, such as a head that is small relative to body size, a round face with widely spaced eyes that slant, a broad-based nose, low-set ears, and a small chin. These children may also have eye abnormalities and other congenital defects, such as heart defects. Mental retardation is present in varying degrees.

TREATMENT. There is no treatment to correct or reverse chromosome abnormalities. All attempts are made to help these children reach their maximum level of independence and achievement. Special education services should be provided as early as possible. Health-care management includes a team approach by various specialties involving regular health-care evaluations, speech and language therapy, physical therapy, behavior modification techniques, and family counseling and support.

DOWN SYNDROME

Also called trisomy 21; was formerly referred to as mongolism.

The incidence is approximately 1 in 700 to 1,000 live births. It occurs in all races and both sexes. The risk of occurrence increases in relation to advancing age of the pregnant woman and somewhat with advancing age of the father. Down syndrome is the most frequent genetic cause of mental retardation.

Down syndrome occurs when a fetus inherits three number 21 chromosomes instead of two. This is called trisomy 21. Ninety-five percent of all people with Down syndrome have classic trisomy 21, with every body cell containing an extra chromosome 21. Roughly 4% of all people with Down syndrome have a translocation, which means that the extra chromosome 21 is actually attached to one of the other chromosomes. A few people with Down syndrome have a mosaic chromosome pattern, which means that some body cells have the normal number of 46 chromosomes, whereas other cells have 47 because of the extra chromosome 21. If a hereditary translocation is the cause (the translocated or "combination" chromosome was inherited from a parent), the risk of recurrence in subsequent children can be from 3% to 15%. Chromosomes of both parents must be examined to determine whether the translocation is hereditary. Risk of classic trisomy 21 recurring in subsequent births is 1% to 2%.

SIGNS AND SYMPTOMS. Unique physical characteristics are usually identifiable at birth and include a flat facial profile; up-slanting eyes; a flat nasal bridge; small ears; a relatively small mouth with large, protruding tongue; short neck with skin folds; "floppy" muscle tone with loose joints; and short, broad hands and feet with a larger than normal space between the first and second toes and a single crease on the palms of the hands. In addition to these evident physical features, congenital heart defects and other congen-

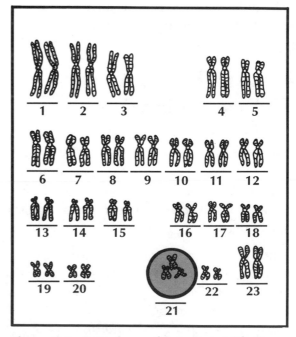

Figure 3.2. Karyotype of a person with Down syndrome

ital birth defects occur in a significant number of people with Down syndrome. Mental retardation is present, but the severity varies widely. Behavior and physical development also vary. People with Down syndrome are prone to ear and respiratory infections and have leukemia about 20 times more often than the general population.

TREATMENT. There is no treatment to correct or reverse chromosomal abnormalities. A supportive team approach from various health-care specialties, with surgery to correct associated birth defects and antibiotics to treat infections, has considerably increased the life expectancy of people with Down syndrome. Early intervention with routine health care and special education is important to help affected people achieve their fullest potential.

EDWARDS SYNDROME
Also called trisomy 18 syndrome

The incidence is 1 in 6,600 live births, of which almost 80% are female. The risk of occurrence increases in relation to the age of the pregnant woman. In 95% of cases, Edwards syndrome occurs when three number 18 chromosomes are inherited instead of two. In the remaining 5% of cases, Edwards syndrome is caused by a translocation in which an extra number 18 chromosome is attached to another chromosome. If the translocation is hereditary (that is, the translocated or combination chromosome was inherited from a parent), the risk of recurrence of Edwards syndrome in subsequent offspring may be significant. Chromosomes of both parents must be examined to determine whether the translocation is hereditary.

SIGNS AND SYMPTOMS. Children with Edwards syndrome are typically born postmature but very growth retarded and small for their gestational age. Physical characteristics of Edwards syndrome include an elongated head with a prominent protrusion at the base of the skull, small but wide-set eyes, small mouth and chin, low-set and/or malformed ears, and a short breastbone (sternum). Perhaps the most distinctive physical feature in the infant is clenched fists, with the index finger overlapping the other fingers; the thumbs may be malformed or missing, and the fingernails and toenails may be underdeveloped. Other congenital defects (anomalies) that frequently occur with Edwards syndrome are heart and kidney defects, abnormalities of the lungs and diaphragm, and hernias.

Mental retardation is usually profound. A significant number of children do not survive beyond the first few months of life, and the majority do not survive past one year. A few have survived to adolescence.

TREATMENT. No treatment corrects or reverses chromosomal abnormalities. A supportive team approach includes various health-care specialties that provide regular health-care evaluations, and family support.

PATAU SYNDROME
Also called trisomy 13 syndrome.

The incidence is approximately 1 in 25,000 live births. Risk increases with advancing age of the pregnant woman. In 75% of cases, Patau syndrome occurs when the fetus inherits three number 13 chromosomes instead of two. About 20% of cases are due to a translocation (the attachment of an extra number 13 chromosome to another chromosome), which may indicate an increased risk in subsequent offspring if it is a hereditary translocation (inherited from one of the parents). Chromosomes of both parents must be examined to determine whether the translocation is hereditary.

SIGNS AND SYMPTOMS. Children with Patau syndrome usually have similar physical characteristics, including a small head, sloping forehead, small eyes, sores or open areas on the scalp, abnormal ears, cleft lip and palate, and extra fingers and/or toes (polydactyly), with the fists usually held in a characteristic clenched position. The majority of children with Patau syndrome also have congenital heart and urogenital defects.

The majority of children die within the first year, and few survive beyond the age of two. Those who survive are mentally and growth retarded, and often have seizure disorders.

TREATMENT. No treatment corrects or reverses chromosomal abnormalities. A supportive team approach includes various health-care specialties that provide regular health-care evaluations, and family support.

SEX CHROMOSOME DISORDERS
FRAGILE X SYNDROME (FXS)

FXS is the most common cause of inherited mental retardation; it has a high risk of recurrence in subsequent offspring. Incidence in males is approximately 1 in 1,000 to 1,250 live births and in females approximately 1 in 2,000 live births. FXS occurs when a mutant gene on the X chromosome is inherited, causing the X chromosome (under certain laboratory conditions) to appear as though the bottom tip is about to break off, thus the term fragile X syndrome.

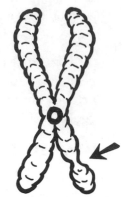

Figure 3.3. Chromosome with fragile X abnormality

SIGNS AND SYMPTOMS. Usually, children born with FXS are large at birth and throughout childhood, and may have loose muscle tone and joints. As they grow they develop distinctive facial features that include a large head, long and narrow face, prominent brow and chin, and large ears. At puberty males may also have enlarged testicles that were not evident before puberty. Other defects, such as deformed heart valves and eye disorders, occur frequently. Some children may have only learning disabilities with normal intelligence quotients, but a great number have mental retardation, some severe.

Females are usually affected to a lesser degree than males, but not always. The carrier rate for FXS is estimated at approximately 1 in 1,000 live male births and 1 in 700 live female births. Female carriers may show no indication of FXS or may have some degree of mental impairment. The transmission of FXS from generation to generation seems to be more complex than in many other genetic disorders. For example, a male who has the FXS gene on his X chromosome may be of normal intelligence and unknowingly pass it to his daughters, who may subsequently bear severely affected sons of their own.

TREATMENT. No treatment corrects or reverses chromosomal abnormalities. Various health-care specialties—including special education, speech and language therapy, occupational therapy, and regular medical examinations—are combined to construct a program of care for the individual with FXS.

DNA testing is available to identify people who have the fragile X chromosome and those who are carriers without symptoms.

KLINEFELTER SYNDROME
Also called 47,XXY syndrome.

The incidence is 1 in 1,000 live male births. Klinefelter syndrome occurs when a male inherits one extra X chromosome, giving him 47 chromosomes rather than the normal 46. Instead of the normal XY combination of sex chromosomes that make a male, he has two Xs and a Y (XXY). A few males may have mosaic chromosome patterns.

SIGNS AND SYMPTOMS. At puberty, the physical changes usually noted in males do not occur. Their breasts usually enlarge (gynecomastia), and body hair is sparse and thin. Men are typically tall and slender with disproportionately long legs. They have a more female pattern of body fat distribution, with narrow shoulders and wide hips. One of the most characteristic features is the frequent failure of the testicles to produce sperm, causing sterility. In fact, some men with Klinefelter syndrome are not diagnosed until they seek infertility counseling as adults. Although some males have varying degrees of mental retardation, some have normal or near-normal intelligence. Two-thirds of people with Klinefelter syndrome have associated learning disabilities and behavioral or personality problems.

TREATMENT. Male hormones are given to masculinize physical features, and surgery can reduce breast tissue. Counseling to assist with the psychological and emotional impact of the syndrome and regular health-care follow-ups are recommended. The risk of breast cancer for men with Klinefelter syndrome is more than 65 times the risk of males without Klinefelter syndrome.

TURNER SYNDROME
Also called 45,X or XO syndrome and monosomy X.

The incidence is approximately 1 in 5,000 live female births. Turner syndrome occurs when a female inherits only one X chromosome instead of the normal two, causing her to have only 45 chromosomes per cell instead of the normal 46.

SIGNS AND SYMPTOMS. Turner syndrome is usually evident at birth by the swelling of the hands and feet and a webbed appearance of the skin of the neck. Other associated findings include heart defects, kidney abnormalities, short fingers and toes, and hearing problems. Growth is usually normal until around three years of age, at which time growth begins to slow. At puberty girls are short in stature, do not have the growth spurt usually seen in adolescence, do not start menstrual periods, and lack breast development. The ovaries of affected females are underdeveloped, making them basically infertile. Although some individuals have learning disabilities, particularly in the area of spatial perception, or they appear to be immature in social interaction, intelligence is usually normal.

TREATMENT. Growth hormone is given in early childhood to stimulate growth in stature (height). At adolescence, hormones are given to initiate breast development and stimulate menstruation and are continued until age 40 or 50.

COMPLICATIONS AFTER BIRTH

Despite every effort by pregnant women to maintain good health during pregnancy, complications such as premature birth, infections, and bleeding disorders can occur. These complications may lead to extended hospitalization for the infant and may require life-saving treatments or procedures that can themselves cause permanent disability or injury. For example, the birth of a premature infant may require the use of a mechanical ventilator to perform "breathing" functions and to deliver high levels of oxygen. Although this treatment may save the baby's life, it increases the infant's risk of chronic lung disease. Be sure to record any complications as part of each family member's health history.

Newborns considered to be high risk include those who were preterm or post-term, had low birth weight, and/or were subjected to some type of distress during pregnancy, labor, or delivery.

APNEA

Apnea is the cessation of breathing. Although newborns frequently have short pauses in their breathing patterns, true apnea can be life threatening. Preterm infants frequently have problems with apnea. This is thought to be due to the immaturity of the respiratory center in the brain. Preterm infants even-

tually outgrow this "apnea of prematurity." Other causes of apnea in newborns include central nervous system disorders or defects, chemical imbalances or disorders, and infection.

SIGNS AND SYMPTOMS. Apnea is present if the nonbreathing episode persists for 10 to 20 seconds or more, if the episode causes the infant to become pale or cyanotic (a bluish discoloration of the skin), or if the episode causes the heart rate to drop below normal levels (bradycardia).

TREATMENT. All infants who have repeated apnea require apnea monitoring to alert parents and caregivers when the apnea occurs. Physical stimulation is often all that is needed to restore breathing. If apnea is caused by something other than prematurity, the underlying cause is treated and corrected when possible. Apnea can sometimes be treated with medication. Parents, babysitters, and others who care for infants who have apnea should learn *infant* CPR from qualified instructors.

BRONCHOPULMONARY DYSPLASIA (BPD)

This lung disease is primarily seen in premature infants who have had hyaline membrane disease (see next page) and have required mechanical ventilation with high levels of oxygen for an extended time to maintain adequate blood oxygen levels. These events are thought to lead to the thickening and scarring of the air passage walls that constitute bronchopulmonary dysplasia (BPD).

SIGNS AND SYMPTOMS. The clinical picture of an infant with BPD is similar to that of an adult with chronic lung disease. The infant has persistent respiratory distress and impaired gas exchange within the lungs. That is, the thickened and scarred air passages make it difficult for carbon dioxide waste to pass from the blood into the lungs, or for oxygen to pass from the lungs into the blood. Therefore, blood analysis reveals high levels of carbon dioxide and low levels of oxygen, necessitating continued use of mechanical ventilation and oxygen. Changes in the infant's lungs that occur with BPD can be detected with chest x-ray.

TREATMENT. Because of the tissue damage and scarring within the lungs, oxygen is usually required for an extended period of time, possibly a year or more, in children with BPD. Medications, including bronchodilators, steroids, and diuretics, may also be used. Although 25% to 35% of infants who develop BPD die, the lungs of survivors heal and can function normally within a few years. Preventing premature delivery is the best method of preventing BPD.

HYALINE MEMBRANE DISEASE (HMD)

Also known as respiratory distress syndrome.

HMD is primarily seen in premature infants and infants of low birth weights. Special cells in the walls of the alveoli (small sac-like structures in the lungs where gas exchange occurs) are too immature to produce enough surfactant, a substance that in normal amounts prevents the alveoli from collapsing each time the infant exhales.

SIGNS AND SYMPTOMS. To maintain normal blood oxygen levels, infants born without enough surfactant may need help breathing from a mechanical ventilator (a respirator) and extra or supplemental oxygen. The lack of surfactant results in damage to the alveoli and triggers the formation of a thin membrane (a hyaline membrane) along the inner surface of the alveoli. This membrane makes the gas exchange of oxygen and carbon dioxide through the alveoli difficult despite help from the mechanical ventilation and supplemental oxygen. The infant's condition usually deteriorates in the first 72 hours after birth but then begins to improve steadily as surfactant production within the lungs gradually increases and the hyaline membrane dissolves. HMD causes a significant number of neonatal deaths.

TREATMENT. Surfactant has been successfully placed directly into infant lungs, but studies of this treatment are incomplete. Preventing preterm delivery is the best way to prevent HMD. Administering steroid medication to a woman who is about to deliver prematurely has proved to help stimulate fetal surfactant production, thus decreasing the risk or severity of HMD.

INFECTION/SEPSIS

Infection of the newborn can be caused by a variety of microorganisms (germs) that would not usually cause infection in an older infant. Newborns are susceptible to such infection because they have left the protective, sealed environment of the uterus and suddenly entered a world filled with germs, and their immune systems are not ready or mature enough to produce antibodies that could protect them from infection.

Term newborns have some protection (although incomplete) against infection because they receive antibodies from their mother during the last weeks of pregnancy. Although these antibodies last only a few months, they help protect a newborn from infection while the newborn's own immune system matures enough to begin producing antibodies. Preterm newborns, however, are often born before receiving these protective antibodies, increasing their risk of infection. Preterm infants also frequently require invasive lifesaving procedures that can inadvertently expose them to infection-causing microorganisms. Preterm and term newborns receive protective antibodies against infection when they are breast fed.

Newborns can be exposed to infectious microorganisms in various ways. Prenatal exposure (exposure during the pregnancy across the placental membrane) can be devastating, even fatal. A group of infections called the TORCH group, which stands for toxoplasmosis, rubella, cytomegalovirus, herpes simplex virus, hepatitis B virus, and human immunodeficiency virus, are among those known to be damaging to prenatally exposed fetuses. Newborns can be infected during birth if the birth canal contains infectious microorganisms, including many of the sexually transmitted diseases (see page 31).

A major cause of newborn infection is the group B streptococcus bacterium. These bacteria live within the vaginal canal and/or the cervix without causing symptoms or illness. Women with this condition are called "carriers." As many as 20% of all pregnant women may be carriers. Infection of the newborn can also occur if the mother-to-be has a urinary tract infection or sexually transmitted disease at the time of labor and delivery, if her bag of waters (amniotic membranes) was ruptured more than 24 hours before birth, or if her labor was more than 24 hours or traumatic.

SIGNS AND SYMPTOMS. Infection can produce irritability, jitteriness, floppy muscle tone, poor feeding ability, difficulty keeping a normal body temperature, jaundice (yellow discoloration of the skin), vomiting, diarrhea, skin rash, respiratory distress (difficulty in breathing), and apnea (periods of nonbreathing).

TREATMENT. Newborn infection is treated aggressively because it can easily spread throughout the body, a condition known as sepsis, and can be fatal. After initial specimens of the infant's blood and other body fluids are collected and sent for examination, antibiotics and/or other antimicrobial medications are begun, along with other intensive care treatments such as mechanical ventilation and intravenous fluids.

Because of the high mortality rate associated with neonatal infection, its prevention is a major priority. Women are screened for infections during pregnancy, labor, and delivery. This is yet another reason prenatal care is so important to the health of newborns.

JAUNDICE

Also called hyperbilirubinemia.

Jaundice is the discoloration of the skin caused by the deposit of bilirubin, a pigment found in red blood cells (RBCs) that is released into the bloodstream as the cells break down (die naturally) or are destroyed. Bilirubin is normally converted within the liver into a water-soluble form and becomes one of the elements present in bile. The bilirubin-laden bile is then released into the small intestine through the bile duct and eliminated from the body with the stool. Red blood cells are constantly "dying" and being replaced with new cells produced within the body. Fetal red blood cells, which are present in newborns, have a shorter-than-normal lifespan, and the level of bilirubin in infants increases over the first several days of life. The newborn's liver, however, is relatively immature at birth and cannot always handle the extra bilirubin that accumulates in the blood. As a result, this buildup of nonsoluble or unconverted bilirubin becomes deposited within the skin, giving it jaundice.

- **PHYSIOLOGIC JAUNDICE.** This normal and expected jaundice usually occurs from the third to the fifth day in term infants (a little later if preterm), and then reverts to normal within several days.

- **PATHOLOGIC JAUNDICE.** Jaundice in a newborn that occurs within the first 24 hours of life is considered "pathologic," meaning it is caused by an abnormal condition such as Rh or blood group incompatibility, infection, or by genetic diseases that cause massive red blood cell destruction or enzyme deficiencies that interfere with the breakdown of bilirubin. Pathologic jaundice is a concern because high levels of bilirubin that accumulate within brain cells can cause permanent damage, a condition known as kernicterus.

- **BREAST-MILK JAUNDICE.** This occurs in a small percentage of breast-fed infants. The exact cause is unknown. Breast-milk jaundice does not become noticeable (evident) until several days after the mother's mature breast milk comes in. Although bilirubin levels get quite high, breast-milk jaundice has not been associated with kernicterus. The infant may be taken off breast milk for a day or two while other causes for the jaundice are ruled out. Usually the infant's bilirubin levels drop during this period, confirming the cause to be breast milk. Breastfeeding is usually resumed, and the infant's health-care provider monitors bilirubin levels frequently and may start phototherapy.

SIGNS AND SYMPTOMS. Jaundice, more a symptom than a disease entity itself, is the yellow discoloration of the skin and other body tissues, such as the whites of the eyes (the sclera), palms of the hands and soles of the feet, gums, and internal organs.

TREATMENT. Treatment is aimed at preventing kernicterus and is frequently initiated even when no real threat of kernicterus is thought to be present. It is not known how high the bilirubin level has to be for kernicterus to occur; however, general danger levels are known and are used as guides in determining treatment.

The infant with jaundice is given plenty of fluids and adequate nutrition to guarantee bilirubin elimination through the stool. Phototherapy uses fluorescent lights (referred to as "bili-lites") to convert bilirubin within the skin to a water-soluble form that can then be eliminated from the infant's body through both bile and urine. Phototherapy can sometimes be performed in the home. An exchange transfusion, a procedure in which small increments of the infant's blood are removed and replaced by donor blood, is performed primarily in infants with severe pathologic jaundice who are at risk for kernicterus.

MECONIUM ASPIRATION SYNDROME (MAS)

MAS can occur in infants who are stressed before birth, resulting in a drop in fetal blood oxygen levels. This decrease in oxygen causes the fetus to have a bowel movement while still in the uterus. This initial stool, called meconium (which is a black, tarry, "sticky" substance) floats in the amniotic fluid that surrounds the fetus and is breathed into the fetal lungs. Meconium is passed in response to stress, but also in mature (term) infants without identifiable stress. MAS occurs when this material is inhaled into the lungs before or after birth, especially with the infant's first breath. Attempts to remove meconium from the airway (throat) before the first breath may reduce the risk of this disease.

SIGNS AND SYMPTOMS. Meconium lodged within the air passages blocks air flow both in and out of the lungs and irritates lung tissue, resulting in serious respiratory distress. Bacteria may begin to grow in the meconium, resulting in infection that worsens the infant's condition.

TREATMENT. MAS can be fatal. Surviving infants may require prolonged hospitalization until normal lung function returns. The outcome (prognosis) depends a great deal on the amount and thickness of the meconium the infant has inhaled (aspirated).

NECROTIZING ENTEROCOLITIS (NEC)

This severe disorder is seen most often in premature and low-birth-weight infants. Dying and/or dead (necrotic) patches of tissue within the mucosal lining of the bowel interfere with the digestive and absorption functions of the bowel and can result in life-threatening complications, including complete erosion and perforation through the bowel wall, spread of the infection into the abdominal cavity (peritonitis), or the halting (cessation) of bowel motion.

The cause is thought to be related to episodes of decreased blood flow to the bowel that occur during episodes of low oxygen or shock. During such events, the body automatically decreases the blood flow to the bowel to increase the blood flow to more vital organs such as the brain and heart. This lack of blood flow and subsequent oxygen deprivation is thought to cause the areas of mucosal damage within the bowel wall that are seen in NEC; these areas are then invaded by bacteria that are normally present within the bowel.

Breast-fed infants have a lower incidence of NEC than formula-fed infants. NEC sometimes occurs as a complication of serious infection or after blood exchange transfusions in newborns.

SIGNS AND SYMPTOMS. Lethargy, poor feeding, slowed gastric emptying, vomiting, increasing abdominal circumference, blood in the stool, apnea, and unstable body temperature occur. Late complications include bowel narrowing and blockage in approximately 20% to 25% of infants.

TREATMENT. Mouth (oral) feedings are halted; intravenous fluids allow the bowel to rest; and antibiotics prevent further infection. The necrotic bowel segments may need to be surgically removed.

RETINOPATHY OF PREMATURITY (ROP)
Previously known as retrolental fibroplasia.

This disorder of the retina of the eye is almost exclusively seen in preterm infants with low birth weight; the lower the birth weight, the higher the risk of ROP. The vessels of the retina proliferate, or overgrow, and lead to fluid accumulation and scarring within the retina. These changes can result in permanent loss of vision. Although prolonged use of oxygen and the use of oxygen in high concentrations has been associated with the occurrence of ROP, research indicates that the biggest factor is the immaturity of retinal blood vessels present in preterm infants. The exact cause remains unknown.

SIGNS AND SYMPTOMS. Evidence of developing (and progressing) ROP can be detected by means of an eye examination by an eye specialist. As the child ages, evidence of vision loss (if present) becomes increasingly apparent.

TREATMENT. Infants at risk are examined periodically by an eye specialist to check the retina, and oxygen therapy is closely monitored by health-care personnel. ROP can sometimes be treated using freezing techniques (cryosurgery) or laser therapy to halt or control the overgrowth of retinal blood vessels and scarring, which may save some degree of vision. Infants at risk should receive long-term follow-up to detect further vision complications.

SECTION 3
BIRTH HISTORY

3.1 Indicate if you were delivered vaginally (V) or by cesarean section (C/S).

3.2 Indicate if you were a term, preterm, or post-term infant. List approximate gestational age in weeks or months, if known.

3.3 Indicate your weight at birth, using kilograms and grams or pounds and ounces (see conversion chart, table 3.1).

3.4 Indicate your length at birth, using centimeters or inches (see conversion chart, table 3.2).

3.5 Record your blood type: A, B, AB, or O, and if you are Rh negative or positive.

3.6 Indicate whether you have ever received blood or blood product transfusions. If so, list the date(s) and the type of blood product(s) received (i.e., whole blood, plasma, platelets, packed red blood cells, clotting factors, etc.). List the reasons you received the blood or blood product(s), if known.

3.7 List any chromosomal abnormalities or syndromes you have, such as cri du chat syndrome (5p- syndrome); Down syndrome; Edwards syndrome; Patau syndrome; fragile X syndrome (FXS); Klinefelter syndrome (47,XXY); Turner syndrome (45,XO); or others.

3.8 Indicate whether you had any of the following complications at or shortly after birth: apnea; hyaline membrane disease (HMD); broncho-pulmonary dysplasia (BPD); meconium aspiration syndrome (MAS); retinopathy of prematurity (ROP), also called retrolental fibroplasia (RLF); necrotizing enterocolitis (NEC); jaundice; infection (sepsis); or others.

CONVERSION OF POUNDS AND OUNCES TO KILOGRAMS FOR PEDIATRIC WEIGHTS

pounds	kilograms	ounces	kilograms
1	0.454	1	0.028
2	0.907	2	0.057
3	1.361	3	0.085
4	1.814	4	0.113
5	2.268	5	0.142
6	2.722	6	0.170
7	3.175	7	0.198
8	3.629	8	0.227
9	4.082	9	0.255
10	4.536	10	0.283
11	4.990	11	0.312
12	5.443	12	0.340
13	5.897	13	0.369
		14	0.397
		15	0.425

Table 3.1.

CONVERSION OF INCHES TO CENTIMETERS FOR PEDIATRIC HEIGHTS

inches	centimeters	inches	centimeters
12.0	30.5	18.0	45.7
12.5	31.8	18.5	47.0
13.0	33.0	19.0	48.3
13.5	34.3	19.5	49.5
14.0	35.6	20.0	50.8
14.5	36.8	20.5	52.1
15.0	38.1	21.0	53.3
15.5	39.4	21.5	54.6
16.0	40.6	22.0	55.9
16.5	41.9	22.5	57.2
17.0	43.2	23.0	58.4
17.5	44.5	23.5	59.7

Table 3.2.

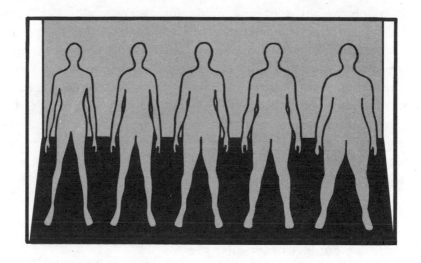

CHAPTER 4
PHYSICAL ATTRIBUTES

Physical attributes are the characteristics of your appearance, such as height, body frame, weight, skin tone, hair color, and eye color. Other physical attributes include such characteristics as attached ear lobes, hairy ears, long eyelashes, curly hair, baldness, facial dimples, a folding or curlable tongue, and the shape of your nose, and whether your great toe or your second toe is the longest toe of your foot. All these are inherited traits, but some, such as height and skin color, are strongly influenced by environmental factors as well. Some genetic disorders and syndromes are associated with one or more unique physical attributes. Therefore, recording the physical attributes of your ancestors can yield important information and may be helpful in identifying family members with undiagnosed genetic disorders.

HEIGHT

Your height is believed to be determined by several genes; some are tall genes and some are short genes. The combination of the tall and short genes that you inherited from your parents determines your potential for height, but environmental factors can influence whether or not you actually attain that height. For example, long-term malnutrition or chronic illness (both considered environmental factors) can impede growth and keep you from reaching your genetically predetermined height.

HEALTHY BODY WEIGHT

Maintaining an "ideal" body weight or—more accurately—a "healthy" body weight is one of the most important factors related to good health that you can control to some extent, and that will improve your position on the health continuum. Maintaining healthy body weight is important for children as well as for adults.

1. Calculate "ideal" body weight based on height
   • FEMALES: Allow 100 lbs. for the first 5 feet
     Add 5 lbs. for each inch over 5 feet
   • MALES: Allow 106 lbs. for the first 5 feet
     Add 6 lbs. for each inch over 5 feet
2. Assess weight status

Underweight	Ideal Weight Range	Overweight	Obese
>10% under ideal	± 10% of ideal depending on size of body frame	10%–20% over ideal	>20% over ideal

Table 4.1. Calculate your healthy weight

Source: Susan G. Dudek, R.D., B.S., *Nutrition Handbook for Nursing Practice*, 2nd ed. (1993). Used with permission.

You can calculate your ideal or healthy body weight in various ways (see tables 4.1 and 4.2). Keep in mind that these are approximate guides to what would be considered healthy weights for you. Check with your health-care provider for exact guidance as to what your weight should be, because you may have special health considerations. Here is what the U.S. Department of Agriculture and U.S. Department of Health and Human Services have to say about maintaining a healthy weight:

What is an exact healthy weight for you? There is no exact answer right now. Researchers are trying to describe healthy weight more precisely. In the meantime, use the guidelines here to see whether your weight is within the range suggested for persons of your age, sex, and height. The weight ranges in Table 4.2 (page 55) are likely to change as research continues. In the table, weights are given in ranges because people of the same height may have equal amounts of body fat but different amounts of muscle and bone. The higher weights in the ranges are healthy for people who have more muscle and bone. Weights above the range are believed to be unhealthy for most people; weights slightly below the range may be healthy for some small-boned people, but low weight is sometimes linked to health problems, especially if it is the result of sudden weight loss.

Table 4.2 shows higher weights for people 35 years and above than for younger adults. This is because recent research suggests that people can be a little heavier as they grow older without added risk to health. Just how much heavier is not yet clear.

Source: U.S. Dept. of Agriculture and U.S. Dept. of Health and Human Services, *Nutrition and Your Health: Dietary Guidelines for Americans*.

DEVIATIONS FROM HEALTHY WEIGHT

LOW BODY WEIGHT

Low body weight can result from poor nutrition, chronic or long-term disease, or eating disorders. Two major eating disorders are anorexia nervosa and bulimia nervosa (see pages 111-12). These disorders are not fully understood, but researchers are beginning to identify some of their complex emotional and physical causes.

OBESITY

For a person who has a normal fat-to-muscle ratio, obesity is defined as having a body weight 20% to 30% greater than ideal body weight. Obesity is a major health problem in the United States. Many times poor eating habits combined with a lack of exercise result in obesity. Other factors contributing to obesity are environmental, social, and cultural influences and genetic predisposition. If both parents are obese, a child has as much as an 80% chance of being obese as

SUGGESTED WEIGHTS FOR ADULTS

| Height* | Weight in pounds** | |
	19 to 34 years	35 years and over
5'0"	97-128	108-138
5'1"	101-132	111-143
5'2"	104-137	115-148
5'3"	107-141	119-152
5'4"	111-146	122-157
5'5"	114-150	126-162
5'6"	118-155	130-167
5'7"	121-160	134-172
5'8"	125-164	138-178
5'9"	129-169	142-183
5'10"	132-174	146-188
5'11"	136-179	151-194
6'0"	140-184	155-199
6'1"	144-189	159-205
6'2"	148-195	164-210
6'3"	152-200	168-216
6'4"	156-205	173-222
6'5"	160-211	177-228
6'6"	164-216	182-234

*Without shoes. **Without clothes.

The higher weights in the ranges generally apply to men, who tend to have more muscle and bone; the lower weights more often apply to women, who have less muscle and bone.

Source: Derived from National Research Council, 1989.

Table 4.2. Suggested weights for adults

well. Obesity contributes to the development of other health disorders such as atherosclerosis, heart disease, high blood pressure, diabetes, low back strain, degeneration of weight-bearing joints, and other types of illness. Obesity can be psychologically harmful as well. People who are obese often have poor self-esteem and associated problems such as depression, in part due to the general view in many societies that people should be able to control their weight regardless of other factors, and that everyone "should" be thin.

Obesity is also a concern for children. Overeating and a lack of exercise in young children cause an increased number of fat cells to form within the body. (Fat cells are formed in the first few years of life only.) As the child ages, fat is stored within these same cells. As adults, these fat cells do not increase in number but increase in size as fat is deposited into them. This means that an overweight child (who forms more fat cells than a normal weight child) is more likely to be an overweight adult. Feeding children a healthful diet, teaching them healthful eating habits, and encouraging routine physical exercise reduce the risk of obesity and its associated disorders. However, you should consult your health-care provider before putting your children on a weight-loss or calorie-reducing program, because children need sufficient nutrients and calories for physical, mental, and emotional growth and well-being. Your health-care provider can guide you concerning your child's nutritional needs and appropriate body weight.

BALDING

The amount of hair you have is also a physical attribute. Male pattern and premature balding are traits apparently determined by a dominant gene on a nonsex chromosome (autosome). Although the gene can be present in males and females, usually it is expressed only in males because of the influence of male hormones. Females can carry the gene and pass it to offspring, but females rarely become bald, although with age their hair may thin dramatically.

PIGMENTATION

The pigmentation (color) of your skin, hair, and eyes is genetically determined. The pigment that gives color, called melanin, is produced by special cells called melanocytes. Melanocytes are located in the skin, hair, and the iris (the colored ring) of the eye.

Your actual skin tone is probably influenced by a combination of genes interacting with environmental factors. Skin tones vary greatly among races, within races, and among people. Races with darker skin tones have melanocytes that produce more melanin.

Melanin protects the skin and eyes from the damaging ultraviolet rays that come from the sun and other sources. In people of all races, melanin production increases when the skin is exposed to ultraviolet rays, causing the skin to darken or tan. This increased production of melanin is a way the body works to provide extra protection from damaging ultraviolet rays.

Some genetic disorders involve a lack of melanin in the body. Albinism, for example, is a disorder in which there is decreased melanin and therefore decreased pigment or color in the skin, hair, and eyes.

INSTRUCTIONS: To be sure your health-care provider has all the information needed to plan and individualize your health care, answer the following questions after you read Chapter 4, Physical Attributes. Write your answers in Section 4 of the *GENETIC CONNECTIONS™ HEALTH HISTORY FORM,* which you will find at the back of this book. Use a separate *HEALTH HISTORY FORM* for each family member.

NOTE: Do not limit yourself to documenting only the traits that are asked for. Document other prevalent, outstanding, or peculiar physical attributes that are or were present.

SECTION 4
PHYSICAL ATTRIBUTES

4.1 List maximum adult height in either meters and centimeters or in feet and inches. (1 meter = 39.371 inches.)

4.2 List average adult weight in either kilograms or in pounds and ounces. (1 kilogram = 2.2 pounds.)

4.3 Describe skin tone for ethnicity; for example: fair, medium, or dark.

4.4 Describe eye color; for example: blue, brown, gray, green, or hazel. Other?

4.5 Describe hair color; for example: blond, brunette, auburn, red, or black. Other? If graying, list the approximate age that graying began.

4.6 If balding or significant hair thinning, list the approximate age when hair loss began.

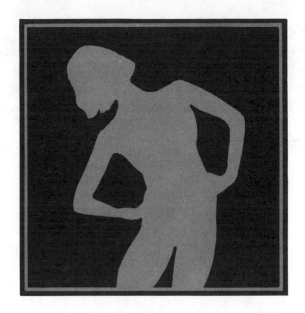

CHAPTER 5

GENERAL HEALTH INFORMATION

The personal lifestyle and health practices you follow throughout your life definitely affect your position on the health continuum. The best position possible—despite inherited predispositions to disease—comes from living a healthful lifestyle. Good health practices include maintaining a healthy body weight; following good nutrition practices; exercising regularly; avoiding the use of chemical substances such as alcohol, tobacco, and illicit drugs; getting enough quality sleep each day; preventing accidents and communicable diseases when possible; and seeking health care on a regular basis.

LIFESTYLE PRACTICES
BODY WEIGHT

Read the information about healthy body weight on page 54. Maintaining this weight is paramount to good health. Discuss with your health-care provider your ideal weight and how you can achieve it.

NUTRITION

It is important for everyone—infants to elders—to maintain good nutrition. Nutritional needs change over time; healthful nutrition habits help you maintain an optimal position on the health continuum. Adhering to a highly nutritious diet from childhood through adulthood decreases your risk of heart disease, high blood pressure, diabetes, and some cancers.

So how do you maintain a healthful, nutritious diet? The U.S. Departments of Agriculture and Health and Human Services have published easy-to-follow guidelines in *Nutrition and Your Health: Dietary Guidelines for Americans*. Below are excerpts.

√ Eat a variety of foods. People need more than 40 different nutrients, including vitamins, minerals, amino acids from protein, certain fatty acids from fat, and calories from protein, carbohydrates, and fat. These nutrients should come from a variety of foods, not from a few highly fortified foods or supplements.

Any food that supplies calories and nutrients can be part of a nutritious diet. The content of the total diet over a day or more is what counts. Many foods are good sources of several nutrients. For example, vegetables and fruits are important for vitamins A and C, folic acid, minerals, and fiber. Breads and cereals supply B vitamins, iron, and protein; whole-grain breads and cereals are also good sources of fiber. Milk provides protein, B vitamins, vitamins A and D, calcium, and phosphorus. Meat, poultry, and fish provide protein, B vitamins, iron, and zinc. No single food can supply all the nutrients in the amounts you need. For example, milk supplies calcium but little iron; meat supplies iron but little calcium. Therefore, a nutritious diet can come only from eating a variety of foods.

The U.S. Department of Agriculture's recently revised food pyramid (see figure 5.1) replaces the basic-four-food-group system that was first taught in the 1950s. It is designed to guide people to achieve balanced nutrition by eating a variety of foods.

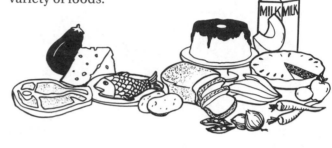

Foods on the pyramid are divided into six groups. The foods that form the lower portion or base of the pyramid should be consumed in larger quantities than those at the top. The base of the pyramid contains the bread, cereal, grain, and pasta groups; the next level contains the fruit and vegetable groups; the third level contains the milk and milk-products group and the meat and meat-substitute group. At the top of the pyramid is the fat, oil, and sweets group. Food items in this last group have the least mineral and iron content and the most calories and fat per ounce. These foods are the least healthful and, although fats and sweets play important roles in diet, they should be consumed in small amounts. The American Dietetic Association, in its *Eating Right America*, says, "Remember the basics. Eating right means having a wide variety of foods in moderation every day. There are no good or bad foods. There are only bad eating habits."

√ Maintain a healthy weight. Refer to the information on ideal/healthy body weight on page 54.

√ Choose a diet that is low in fat, saturated fat, and cholesterol. Most health authorities recommend that Americans consume less fat, saturated fat, and cholesterol than they now do.

Excessive dietary fat intake and high blood cholesterol and triglyceride levels are associated with the development of disease, including heart disease and some cancers; therefore, no more than 30% of your

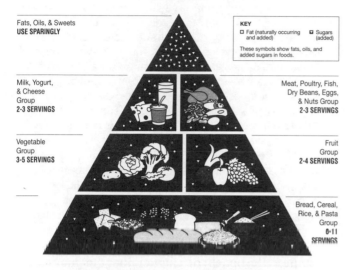

A Guide to Daily Food Choices

Fats, Oils, & Sweets
USE SPARINGLY

KEY
□ Fat (naturally occurring and added) ▨ Sugars (added)
These symbols show fats, oils, and added sugars in foods.

Milk, Yogurt, & Cheese Group
2-3 SERVINGS

Meat, Poultry, Fish, Dry Beans, Eggs, & Nuts Group
2-3 SERVINGS

Vegetable Group
3-5 SERVINGS

Fruit Group
2-4 SERVINGS

Bread, Cereal, Rice, & Pasta Group
6-11 SERVINGS

Figure 5.1. The food pyramid from the U.S. Department of Agriculture

daily calories should come from fat, and you should limit your intake of cholesterol and saturated fats. About 95% of consumed fats (also called lipids) are in the form of triglycerides; and cholesterol is part of the remaining 5%. Some fat is obvious or visible, such as butter and oils, but other fat is concealed, hidden in foods such as egg yolks, milk, milk products, and baked foods. Cholesterol is found in animal products, including eggs and milk products, whereas vegetables and fruits (except for avocados) are practically fat free.

TRIGLYCERIDES

Triglycerides contain fatty acids (fats). Fatty acids are important elements for the body, especially in energy production, but excesses are unhealthy. Fatty acids can be saturated fats, which are considered to be bad and associated with disease, or unsaturated fats, which are considered to be somewhat less harmful. Both monounsaturated fats and polyunsaturated fats are types of unsaturated fat, with polyunsaturated fats being the better of the two. When reading food labels, notice the number and size of servings in the package and the type and amount of fats in each serving. The liver converts saturated fats into cholesterol. So increasing your intake of fats, especially saturated fats,

elevates not only your blood triglyceride levels, **but** your cholesterol levels as well. Note: If unsaturated fats have been hydrogenated (chemically changed to increase the product's shelf life), they have become more saturated than the original fat.

To limit the fat calories in your diet to the recommended amount of 30% or less of your total caloric intake, multiply the number of calories you need per day (check with your health-care provider) by 0.30. This gives you the number of "fat calories" you are allowed each day. Since 1 gram of fat has 9 calories, divide this number by 9 to get the total allowable grams of fat you can consume each day.

Example:

Total daily calories for weight maintenance:

2000 calories

Multiplied by 0.30

600 fat calories allowed per day

600 divided by 9 = 67 grams of fat per day allowed.

To help you maintain a diet that contains no more than 30% of calories from fat, use the following formula for calculating the percentage of fat calories in a particular serving of food:

Figure the total number of calories per serving and the total grams of fat per serving (all fats, saturated and unsaturated) on the package label. Then take the following steps:

Step 1 - Multiply the grams of fat per serving by 9 for the total fat calories.

Step 2 - Divide the total fat calories by the total calories per serving.

Step 3 - Multiply your answer by 100. This is the percentage of fat calories provided by the food item per serving.

Example A:

Saltine cracker labeled "no cholesterol, low saturated fat." Total calories per serving = 60 calories; total grams fat per serving = 2 grams.

Step 1 - 2 grams x 9 = 18 fat calories.

Step 2 - 18 divided by 60 = 0.3.

Step 3 - 0.3 x 100 = 30%.

This product's total fat calories per serving are 30%. If all the foods you eat qualify as 30% or less in fat calories, your overall daily intake of fat calories would also be 30% or less.

Example B:

> Butter-flavored microwave popcorn labeled "no cholesterol." Total calories per serving = 90 calories; total grams of fat per serving = 5 grams (includes 1 gram of saturated fat that your liver converts to cholesterol).
>
> Step 1 - 5 grams x 9 = 45 fat calories.
>
> Step 2 - 45 divided by 90 = 0.5.
>
> Step 3 - 0.5 x 100 = 50%.
>
> This product's total fat calories per serving are 50%. If all the food you eat contains this percentage of fat calories, you are consuming too much dietary fat.

CHOLESTEROL

Cholesterol is an essential element needed by the body to perform several important functions. However, cholesterol need not be consumed through diet because it is produced by your liver from blood sugar (glucose) and saturated fats. That is why a diet low in saturated fats helps reduce your blood cholesterol levels more than a low cholesterol diet does. Dietary cholesterol is found in animal food products.

LIPOPROTEINS

Triglycerides and cholesterol (the lipids or fats) are carried through the blood by proteins; together, they form lipoproteins (fat + protein). Your blood cholesterol level, your triglyceride level, your specific lipoprotein levels, and their relation to one another can help your health-care provider establish your risk of developing heart disease. Here are the three different types of lipoproteins:

• High-density lipoprotein (HDL) is known as "good" cholesterol. Having high levels of HDL is thought to lower your risk of heart disease. HDL consists mainly of protein attached to small amounts of cholesterol and triglycerides. HDL is thought to be helpful in ridding excess cholesterol from the body by transporting it from body tissues to the liver, which gets rid of it as waste.

• Low-density lipoprotein (LDL) is known as the "bad" cholesterol. Having high levels of LDL is thought to increase your risk of heart disease. LDL consists mainly of cholesterol and is thought to transport cholesterol from the liver and dump it within other body tissues, including the arteries. As cholesterol collects and builds within the arteries, atherosclerosis develops, causing many types of cardiovascular disease.

• Very low-density lipoprotein (VLDL) consists mainly of triglycerides with small amounts of cholesterol and protein. VLDL transports and dumps triglycerides produced in the liver into body tissues. High levels may increase your risk of heart disease.

> √ Choose a diet with plenty of vegetables, fruits, and grains (all generally low in fat) to increase carbohydrates and decrease fats in your diet and add more dietary fiber. Complex carbohydrates, such as starches, are found in breads, cereals, pasta, rice, dry beans and peas, and other vegetables, such as potatoes and corn. Dietary fiber—a part of plant foods—is found in whole-grain breads and cereals, dry beans and peas, vegetables, and fruits. It is best to eat a variety of these fiber-rich foods because they differ in the kind of fiber they contain. Foods with fiber are important for proper bowel function and can reduce symptoms of chronic constipation, diverticular disease, and hemorrhoids. People with diets low in dietary fiber and complex carbohydrates but high in fat, especially saturated fat, tend to have more heart disease, obesity, and some cancers. Just how dietary fiber is involved is not yet clear.

Some of the benefit of a higher fiber diet may come from the food that provides the fiber, not from the fiber alone. For this reason, it is best to get fiber from food rather than from supplements. In addition, overusing fiber supplements can cause intestinal problems and interfere with the absorption of some minerals.

A high-fiber diet also helps your body rid itself of excess cholesterol. Because cholesterol is an element of bile, and bile is deposited into the intestines and eliminated from the body with body waste (feces), ensuring regular bowel functions is thought to assist the clearance of bile from the body.

> √ Use sugars in moderation. Sugars provide calories and flavor and are used as natural preservatives, thickeners, and baking aids in foods. But be careful not to eat sugars in large amounts or to snack frequently on foods containing sugars and starches. Sugars and many foods that contain them in large amounts supply many calories, but are limited in nutrients. Thus, sugars should be used in moderation by most healthy people and sparingly by people with low calorie needs. For very active people with high calorie needs, sugars can be an additional source of calories. Both sugars and starches, which break down into sugars, can contribute to tooth decay. Sugars and starches are found in many foods that also supply nutrients—milk, fruits, some vegetables, breads, cereals, and other foods. The more often you eat these foods—even in small amounts—and the longer they are in your mouth before you brush your teeth, the greater your risk for tooth decay. Thus, eating such foods as frequent between-meal snacks may be more harmful to your teeth than including them at meals.

WATER

Water is a most important nutrient—it is vital for many, many body functions. You should drink 6 to 8 cups of water each day. Juices, milk, and other beverages without caffeine can substitute for water, but caffeinated beverages (like coffee, tea, and some sodas) and alcoholic beverages cannot because they can cause the body to actually lose water. That, of course, defeats the purpose of drinking liquids.

In the United States, municipal water suppliers have to notify you if their water does not meet federal safety standards. Water supplies most likely to be contaminated are shallow wells, especially in areas where farming is or was a big industry.

Lead in water is a concern, especially for young children, because it is toxic to the brain, nerve tissue, gastrointestinal tract, and blood. Lead pipe fixtures and the use of lead solder were outlawed in 1986, but they were used and still exist in many old homes and are a continuing source for lead contamination.

One way to avoid ingesting lead when drinking tap water from plumbing pipes is to run the cold water faucet for several seconds before filling your glass. Lead dissolves more easily in hot water than in cold, so by using only cold water for cooking and drinking you can reduce the amount of lead you might otherwise consume.

If you are concerned about the quality of your water or the presence of contaminants (including lead), have your water analyzed *before* paying for a water filtration/purifying system. If you have city water, request a copy of your city's Municipal Drinking Water Analysis Report. If you have a private well, ask your county health department about the common water contaminants in your area and find out which water-testing lab(s) the health department uses. Independent laboratories are listed in the Yellow Pages as well. The U.S. Environmental Protection Agency's (EPA) Safe Drinking Water Hotline (800 426 4791) can give you the phone number of the certification office for your state, from which you can get a list of certified local testing labs.

You may need help from an expert to analyze your test results; someone who sells water purifiers/filters is not necessarily an expert. Then investigate the pros and cons of the various filtration/purification systems available. For information on water treatment devices and guidelines for determining your water quality, contact: NSF International, P.O. Box 130140, Ann Arbor, MI 48113 0140, phone: 313 769 8010.

EXERCISE

Exercise is an integral part of health that benefits you in countless ways. Some types of exercise build strength and endurance, some build muscle mass, and some increase the flexibility of your joints and muscles. Different types of exercise (isotonic, isometric, anaerobic, and aerobic) benefit you in a combination of ways, and all can be beneficial. For example, aerobic exercise is any activity that increases your heart rate and increases oxygen use by the body. When performed on a regular basis, aerobic exercise builds your endurance, improves your body's ability to process and use oxygen effectively and efficiently, and helps you to maintain a healthy heart. Aerobic dance, swimming, brisk walking, jogging, bicycling, and cross-country skiing are types of aerobic exercise.

Incorporate a time for exercise into your schedule at least three times a week and enjoy the following benefits of exercise:

For the musculoskeletal system (muscles and bones), exercise:

- increases muscle strength, tone, and mass;
- increases muscle endurance;
- increases coordination and balance;
- increases joint movement and flexibility;
- maintains bone density and strength.

For the cardiovascular system (heart and blood vessels), exercise:

- improves the strength of and blood supply to the heart;
- improves blood circulation to body tissues;
- conditions the heart so that daily activities can be performed without marked increases in your heart rate or blood pressure.

For your respiratory system (lungs), exercise:

- improves the exchange of oxygen and waste products within the lungs;
- improves lung capacity.

For metabolic and nutritional needs, exercise:

- lowers your blood triglyceride and cholesterol levels;
- helps blood sugar move into cells for energy use, lowering high blood sugar;
- lowers the amount of body fat and helps you achieve and maintain a healthy body weight;
- encourages movement within your gastrointestinal tract to maintain normal bowel function.

Exercise also:

- helps lower stress and nervous tension;
- promotes the production of endorphins (chemicals produced within the body that help to control pain);
- provides you with a sense of well-being;
- increases your energy level;
- improves the quality of your rest/sleep.

Now that you know its benefits, how can you afford not to participate in routine exercise? Your body is a truly wondrous and intricate piece of machinery. If you fuel it with a nutritious diet, it performs efficiently and cleanly. If you work it on a regular basis with routine exercise, its parts remain flexible, strong, and in sync with one another. Even Hippocrates, the great Greek physician (460–377 B.C.), realized the benefits of exercise when he said, "Walking is man's best medicine."

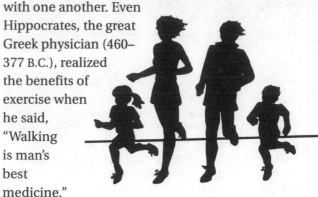

For more information on weight control, nutrition, and exercise, contact the American Dietetic Association, the National Center for Nutrition and Dietetics, the American Heart Association, and your health-care provider.

SUBSTANCE USE

Substance use includes the use/abuse of agents known to be harmful to health, such as tobacco, alcohol, and recreational or illicit drugs. Substance use can also include the indiscriminate use of prescription medication.

TOBACCO

Tobacco is derived from the plant *Nicotiana tabacum*. In the United States tobacco use is a major preventable cause of death from cardiovascular and lung disease. Of the different types of tobacco use, cigarette smoking has the highest mortality rate, but pipes, cigars, and smokeless forms of tobacco cause significant numbers of deaths as well. The American Cancer Society reports that 30% of all cancers can be attributed to tobacco use.

The diseases associated with tobacco smoke are caused by the many toxic substances it contains. Carbon monoxide, nicotine, and tar are just a few. Carbon monoxide is harmful because it is toxic to the body and because it competes with oxygen for the carrying sites on red blood cells. This means less oxygen is available to body tissues, including the heart muscle. The nicotine in tobacco smoke causes vasoconstriction (narrowing of the arteries), which decreases blood flow to the heart and to other body organs and tissues. Nicotine also has a stimulating effect on the heart, increasing its rate and therefore increasing its workload and its demand for oxygen. Tar is a known cancer-causing agent (carcinogen). Smoking also contributes to body-wide atherosclerosis formation, increases the risk of blood clot formation, and lowers the amount of good cholesterol (HDL) in the blood. Some diseases associated with tobacco use include cardiovascular diseases (coronary artery disease, peripheral vascular disease, high blood pressure, and stroke); peptic ulcer disease; lung diseases (chronic bronchitis, emphysema, chronic obstructive lung disease, asthma, and lung cancer); and cancers of the lip, mouth, larynx (vocal cords), stomach, kidney, bladder, and pancreas.

Tobacco smoke is also harmful to those who do not use tobacco themselves but inhale it second hand from someone else's cigarette, pipe, or cigar. Studies show that nonsmokers who are repeatedly exposed to second-hand smoke have an increased risk of developing tobacco-related diseases. Children who live in households among smokers have a higher risk of developing respiratory infections, chronic bronchitis, and asthma.

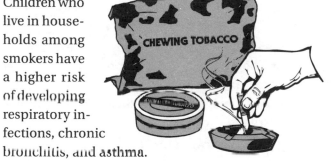

In the United States, cigarette smoking has declined considerably over the past 20 years. It is hoped that this trend will continue as more people become aware of the hazards of tobacco use and their responsibility to maintain their own health.

Although snuff and chewing tobacco do not subject others to second-hand smoke, their use is associated with most of the same diseases as smoking tobacco, because many of the toxic substances found in tobacco are easily absorbed through the tissues of the mouth or nose and enter the bloodstream. Even though lung diseases may not be as likely, cancers of the lip, mouth, throat, and gum are real possibilities for smokeless tobacco users. Ulcers of the stomach or small bowel and cardiovascular disease can also occur.

ALCOHOL

Alcohol is a drug found in alcoholic beverages. Its chemical name is *ethanol* or *ethyl alcohol*. Alcohol freely crosses into the brain and acts as a central nervous system depressant, slowing both the ability of the brain to function and the body functions controlled by the brain. The severity of central nervous system depression depends on the amount of alcohol in the blood. A blood-alcohol level of 0.1% is considered in most states to be the limit for legal intoxication; in some states it is even lower.

Alcohol is broken down or detoxified by the liver, but the liver is able to detoxify only small amounts of alcohol per hour. Drinking a lot of alcohol at once or having several drinks in a short period of time leads to elevated blood-alcohol levels, which result in intoxication or drunkenness. At very high blood-alcohol levels, a person can enter a state of general anesthesia and lose consciousness. At this point the body's protective reflexes (like the ability to gag, swallow, or clear the throat) and breathing are depressed. Breathing may completely stop. The loss of protective reflexes or the cessation of breathing can result in death.

Tolerance to alcohol and the rate at which the body detoxifies alcohol vary from person to person. For example, children of alcoholics have been noted to have an increased tolerance to alcohol. However, although continued use of alcohol can cause a person to develop a higher tolerance, the body's sensitivity to lethal blood-alcohol levels does not change. The effects of long-term and excessive alcohol use involve many body systems and can severely diminish health status. The effects of chronic alcohol consumption include:

- permanent damage to the brain and nerve pathways (nervous system);
- increased risk of high blood pressure and heart failure (cardiovascular system);
- increased risk of cancer of the mouth and esophagus, gastritis, ulcers, and malnutrition (gastrointestinal system);
- decreased ability to fight disease (immune system).

The American Psychiatric Association has established the following patterns of drinking that indicate unhealthy use:

- drinking every day or drinking large amounts of alcohol on a regular basis;

- drinking heavily only on the weekends;

- going for long periods of time without drinking at all and then drinking heavily, sometimes for weeks or months at a time.

Unhealthy drinking patterns may lead to alcoholism, a progressive, chronic, and potentially fatal disease. Alcoholism is a major health problem in many western societies. It disrupts the physical, mental, spiritual, and social well-being of the individual, and it disrupts society as a whole. It is very costly in terms of health, mortality rate, family disruption, and productivity.

Alcoholism occurs more frequently in people who have a family history of alcoholism. This and other evidence supports the theory of a genetic susceptibility to alcoholism. A specific gene pattern has been found in large numbers of people who are alcoholic. Many researchers feel that alcoholism is related to the interaction of one or more genes with environmental factors. People who inherit the susceptibility to alcoholism do not automatically have alcoholism. If they never drink alcohol, they will never develop alcoholism, although sometimes these individuals become dependent on other chemical substances.

Other factors that increase the risk of alcoholism are social pressure to drink and psychological stressors or disorders. During times of stress or emotional turmoil, people sometimes turn to alcohol instead of dealing with their problems in a constructive way or by seeking appropriate help.

ILLICIT DRUG USE

Other drugs besides tobacco and alcohol are abused in our society. This includes the illicit (illegal) use of controlled substances—drugs whose prescribing or dispensing are regulated by federal law and can legally be taken only under the direction (and prescription) of a physician. Many times this abuse results in psychological and/or physical addiction. The Drug Enforcement Administration of the U.S. Department of Justice divides these drugs into five categories:

- **NARCOTICS.** Legally, the term narcotic refers to any habit-forming drug. Medically, the term refers to drugs such as morphine, codeine, opium, and heroin that depress the brain and nerve pathways. Cocaine is also included in this group under the Controlled Substances Act.

- **DEPRESSANTS.** Depressants are sedative/hypnotic drugs such as barbiturates, Valium, and Quaaludes, which diminish the function and activity of the brain and nerve pathways.

- **STIMULANTS.** Stimulants such as amphetamines are drugs that cause increased activity and function of the brain and nerve pathways. Cocaine is also a stimulant that is designated as a narcotic under the Controlled Substance Act.

- **HALLUCINOGENS.** Also known as psychedelics, these drugs have consciousness-expanding effects. They increase sense perception (sight, smell, taste, touch, and hearing), and heighten the sense of awareness and/or unity with the environment. They can also cause hallucinations, psychotic-like behavior, and flashbacks. Examples are LSD (lysergic acid diethylamide), mescaline, and psilocybin.

- **CANNABIS.** This group includes derivatives of the Indian hemp plant *Cannabis sativa*, which has psychoactive properties capable of producing euphoria, sedation, and hallucination. Examples are marijuana and hashish.

CHEMICAL DEPENDENCE

Drug abuse is any use of drugs that deviates from medically approved or socially acceptable uses. Chemical dependence, or drug addiction, is a complication of the use/abuse of many illicit drugs—even prescription drugs. Behavioral patterns that indicate a chemical dependence include:

- the compulsive use of a drug;

- a preoccupation with securing a supply of a drug;

- a tendency to relapse after withdrawal from a drug.

The negative impact of alcohol and other chemicals of abuse and dependency can be seen in the physical, emotional, social, financial, and legal well-being of people who use or become dependent on drugs. This impact spreads to the user's family and community in the form of increased family problems, violent crimes, and health-care costs.

Suspected risk factors include family history, chemical imbalance in the brain, peer pressure to use, difficulty coping with stress, low self-esteem, dependence on other people, history of depression, and ready availability of the abused substance.

Substance abuse and dependence occur in males and females of all ages, from all socioeconomic classes. Abused substances may have depressing or stimulating effects on the body, and may or may not be prescribed by a physician.

Depending on the abused substance(s) involved, complications can include respiratory and cardiac arrest (the cessation of breathing and of heartbeat), gastrointestinal ulcers, decreased resistance to infection, cancer, and circulatory problems, and elevated cholesterol and triglyceride (blood fat) levels. In addition to physical problems, substance-dependent people may have relationship, job, school, and legal problems.

Alcohol dependence involves episodes of drinking to the point of drunkenness; drinking increasingly larger amounts of alcohol; lacking the desire to stop or decrease amount of alcohol intake; devoting a great deal of time to getting alcohol or recovering from its effects; continuing to drink despite the negative impact it has on job, school, relationships, and legal standing; having physical and emotional discomfort or withdrawal (such as nervousness and abdominal pain) when alcohol intake is stopped; drinking alone; drinking to relieve stresses or insomnia; having episodes of memory loss when drinking; and behaving in an intoxicated manner.

Dependence on substances other than alcohol can involve behaviors such as taking larger amounts of a medication than was prescribed or using the substance (medication) for a longer period of time than prescribed; spending considerable time getting, using, and recovering from the use of a substance; continuing use despite its negative impact on job, school, relationships, and legal standing; having physical and emotional discomfort when substance intake is stopped; using the substance when feeling stressed or to relieve insomnia; being restless or aggressive, showing symptoms of overdose or withdrawal; having impaired judgment; and experiencing changes in state of consciousness or changes in pulse, respiration, and blood pressure.

Regardless of the type of substance, treatment for substance abuse (chemical dependency) requires professional help, which frequently involves individual, group, and/or family therapy; support groups such as Alcoholics Anonymous (AA), Al-Anon, or Narcotics Anonymous (NA); medication; and temporary hospitalization.

SLEEP

You must have sleep to maintain well-being. Some people require more sleep than others, but everyone needs some sleep. Practically everyone has had some degree of sleep deprivation at some point in their lives; it impairs the ability to concentrate, think clearly, and perform well physically. Although researchers have documented the importance of sleep for our physical and mental well-being, they have not been able to identify exactly why sleep is so important.

Getting an adequate amount of sleep—6 to 9 hours a day for most people—seems to have a recuperative effect on human beings, allowing body tissues to rest and restore themselves from the day's activities. Some researchers say that sleep is an important factor in strengthening the immune system's ability to fight disease, and that sleep and the process of dreaming help to clear and organize mental circuits so the mind functions more effectively the next day.

For years researchers thought the brain itself rested and shut down during sleep. They now know the brain is very active during sleep. By studying brain activity, researchers have identified two different types of sleep: non–rapid eye movement (non-REM) and rapid eye movement (REM) sleep. Sleep occurs in a cyclic pattern, alternating between these two sleep types.

Non-REM sleep occurs in four stages (I–IV), beginning with very light sleep (stage I) and progressing to deep sleep (stage IV).

REM sleep is named after the actual rapid eye movements that can be observed through the closed eyelids of the sleeping person. The sleeper loses muscle tone and dreams during this stage. REM sleep occurs between the various stages of non-REM sleep, and is seen more frequently at the end of the night's sleep than at the beginning.

Both types of sleep are important for good health and well-being, and it is important that sleep be uninterrupted through these stages. If you took 8 one-hour naps throughout a 24-hour time span, you would not reach each level of sleep and would have some degree of sleep deprivation despite your having slept for 8 of the 24 hours.

The amount of sleep a person requires changes with age. Infants spend the majority of their time sleeping, with a greater amount of time spent in REM sleep. Adults need fewer total hours of sleep.

Sleep disorders (dyssomnias) interfere with sleep, making it difficult or even impossible to achieve an adequate amount of quality sleep. Sleep disorders include problems of sleeping and staying awake and odd behavior that occurs during sleep.

INSOMNIA

Difficulty in falling asleep and, once asleep, difficulty remaining asleep for long periods are symptoms of insomnia. Causes of insomnia are numerous and can be physical, psychological, related to caffeine or other drugs, or related to other sleep disorders.

NARCOLEPSY

People with narcolepsy have repeated, uncontrolled short episodes of sleep occurring during waking hours, lasting from a few minutes to an hour. This poses a great threat to the person's safety and ability to perform well during daily activities. There is evidence that narcolepsy has a genetic component; both mild and severe forms have occurred repeatedly within some families. The child of a parent with narcolepsy has a greater risk than the general population does of having the disorder. Narcolepsy affects males more often than females, and can appear any time from childhood to mid-adulthood (one's fifties). The incidence of narcolepsy in the general population is quite common, possibly as high as 1 in 2,500 people.

Two or more of the following five symptoms must be present for a diagnosis of narcolepsy to be made:

- experiencing drowsiness and sleep episodes during waking hours;
- reaching REM sleep within the first few minutes of sleep (normally REM sleep is not achieved until a person has been asleep for over one hour);
- experiencing muscle weakness or complete loss of muscle tone that is triggered by stress, emotional stimulation, or unpleasant memories;
- experiencing hallucinations on falling asleep or awakening;
- experiencing episodes of paralysis on falling asleep or awakening, including being unable to speak or to move, which persist for several minutes despite the fact that the person's mind is awake.

SLEEP APNEA SYNDROME

Sleep apnea syndrome is characterized by periods of nonbreathing (apnea) during sleep that frequently cause the sleeper to wake up repeatedly throughout the night. These interruptions cause varying degrees of sleep deprivation and daytime sleepiness. Sleep deprivation may cause problems in memory, concentration, or general performance during waking hours, which can increase the risk of accidents. The changes that can occur in blood oxygen and carbon dioxide levels, blood pressure, and in heart rhythm during periods of apnea can pose a serious health threat. The cause of sleep apnea is unknown but genetic influences may contribute to its occurrence. Other suspected contributing factors include obesity and a structurally small or occluded (blocked) airway passage of the throat (the pharynx).

SLEEPWALKING OR SLEEP-EATING

These sleep disorders may or may not be hazardous but can certainly be frightening and disruptive. Sleepwalking and sleep-eating may stem from emotional stress, but their exact cause is frequently unknown. Sleepwalking is not uncommon among children; however, most children outgrow sleepwalking by age 10. Sleepwalking is not normal sleep behavior in adults and can be hazardous.

In addition to weight gain, concerns with sleep-eating include the risk of injury from the use of knives and other utensils or the accidental ingestion of toxic and/or caustic substances such as household cleansers. People with sleep-eating disorder consume large quantities of food, and often very odd foods (e.g., cigarettes dipped in peanut butter) during sleep periods. Uncontrolled binge eating that occurs during sleep may sometimes be related to anorexia, but not always.

If you think you have a sleep disorder, talk to your health-care provider or contact a local sleep disorder center. Frequently, treatment is available to help control the disorder.

ACCIDENT AND TRAUMA

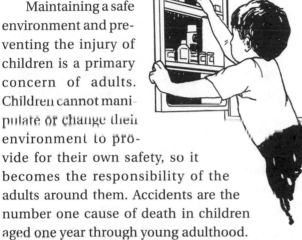

Maintaining a safe environment and preventing the injury of children is a primary concern of adults. Children cannot manipulate or change their environment to provide for their own safety, so it becomes the responsibility of the adults around them. Accidents are the number one cause of death in children aged one year through young adulthood.

A safe environment requires different interventions depending on the child's age and level of development. For example, keeping medications and toxic cleaning substances out of reach or in a locked cabinet is not as important to the safety of a newborn as it is to the safety of a toddler who is physically able to climb and open containers.

Major child safety concerns include preventing suffocation and asphyxiation, falls, burns, motor vehicle accidents, bodily damage, poisoning, choking, and drowning.

Talk to your child's health-care provider for specific age-appropriate measures you can take to protect your child from accidental injury.

IMMUNIZATION AND COMMUNICABLE DISEASE

Extremely important to safety is protection from communicable disease through immunization—the only way to prevent a person from contracting a disease that can have life-threatening or disabling effects.

COMMUNICABLE DISEASE PREVENTABLE BY IMMUNIZATION
DIPHTHERIA

Diphtheria is an infection caused by the bacteria *Corynebacterium diphtheriae*. It is spread by direct or indirect contact with an infected person. Diphtheria was once one of the more common fatal childhood illnesses, but thanks to immunization it has practically been eradicated in the United States.

A "patchy" membrane forms in the back of the throat; it can eventually fuse together and totally obstruct the airway. Other symptoms include a sore throat, swelling glands in the neck, fever, headache, and nausea. The diphtheria bacteria also releases a toxin that attacks body tissue, especially of the nerves and heart. Permanent damage to these tissues can result in death.

If begun early, treatment with antibiotics and antitoxin medication can be successful. Survivors of the disease have lasting immunity; however, immunity can be achieved with the diphtheria vaccine.

HAEMOPHILUS INFLUENZA TYPE B

The bacteria *Haemophilus influenzae* type B was once thought, incorrectly, to cause influenza. It is one of the major causes of serious illness in children five years old and younger. In this age group the bacteria is much more powerful and is spread easily by direct or indirect contact with respiratory secretions or droplets. The risk of exposure to this bacteria becomes greater as the infant or young child's contact with other children increases, such as occurs in child care settings.

The bacteria *Haemophilus influenzae* type B can cause severe throat and lung infection, ear infection, and inflammation and infection of the brain and spinal cord (meningitis).

Antibiotics can treat the infection, but it still has a significant death rate. In 1990 safe vaccines for infants were approved by the Food and Drug Administration and formally recommended by the Immunization Practices Advisory Committee. Immunization during infancy protects children when they are most vulnerable to the bacteria. By the time children are five years or older, they usually do not require the vaccine because they have developed enough antibodies against the bacteria to prevent serious disease.

HEPATITIS B

Hepatitis B infection is caused by the hepatitis B virus, referred to as HBV. It is still frequently called serum hepatitis because it was traditionally thought to be spread only through contaminated blood. Now it is known that the infection can also be spread through contact with other body fluids, including saliva, semen, and cervical mucus. Because of this, hepatitis B is now classified as a sexually transmitted disease, although this is not the only route of transmission (see page 27 concerning transplacental transmission).

Hepatitis B infection usually has a very slow onset. Symptoms take up to several months to occur. Hepatitis B affects the liver, causing inflammation and reduced liver function. Sometimes the infection is so mild it is not recognized as an illness. More common symptoms include mild fever, jaundice (yellowish skin), joint pain, stomach complaints, and a rash that may or may not cause itching.

Hepatitis B infection causes the greatest problems with people who become "carriers" of the hepatitis B virus (about 10%). They cannot rid themselves of the hepatitis virus and continue to be infectious to others. They usually have no symptoms unless they develop chronic hepatitis. With chronic hepatitis, symptoms may progressively worsen as the liver becomes more and more debilitated. The liver is responsible for many vital functions; permanent liver damage can cause death. Carriers also have a much greater risk of developing chronic liver damage (cirrhosis) and liver cancer. Increasingly, hepatitis B is being seen in children, contributing significantly to childhood morbidity and mortality.

Symptoms of hepatitis B infection can be treated by taking medication to reduce fever or decrease joint pain, for example; however, there are no specific medications to treat or cure the hepatitis B infection itself. The body does produce antibodies that prevent future reinfection.

A vaccine that provides immunity against hepatitis B infection is available. Although the vaccine was originally offered mainly to people who were at risk of coming in contact with infected blood products or infected people, it is now available to the general population, including newborn infants.

MEASLES

Measles, also called rubeola, the black measles, or seven-day measles, is caused by the measles virus. This virus is highly contagious and is spread by direct or indirect contact with respiratory droplets. The virus is also found in the blood and urine of infected persons. Worldwide, measles is estimated to cause over one million deaths a year. In the United States, a large portion of cases are seen in college-aged young adults, the population that received the original type of vaccine administered in the early 1960s, which was later found not to provide long-lasting immunity.

Initial symptoms of measles infection include flu-like complaints such as fever, muscle soreness, cough, runny nose, and eyes that are sensitive to light. By day 3 or 4, a reddish rash begins, typically on the head and face area, that works its way down the body within three days. Once the rash has spread, the fever usually drops and the rash turns a brownish color. Fine peeling or flaking of the skin may occur in areas where the rash was concentrated.

Complications of measles infection include pneumonia, which is responsible for a large number of measles-related deaths, and encephalitis (inflammation and swelling of the brain), which can result in permanent brain damage or death.

Because measles is a viral infection, antibiotics are not effective against it. Treatment is aimed at keeping the person as comfortable as possible while the disease runs its course. Active measles infection should build lifelong immunity; however, immunity can be achieved with the measles vaccine.

MUMPS

Mumps infection is caused by the paramyxovirus. It is spread by direct contact with infected saliva or by respiratory droplet.

Early signs of infection include headache, poor appetite, fatigue, and fever. Within a short period of time the person develops an earache that is typically aggravated by chewing. The ear pain is caused by swelling of the parotid glands (the saliva glands located in front of the ears). The viral infection may affect the parotid glands on both sides or only one side. The amount of swelling increases during the first few days and lasts about a week.

Complications of mumps infection, while not common, can include permanent deafness or inflammation of the heart, liver, or central nervous system. Approximately one third of men who have mumps after puberty develop *orchitis* (inflammation of the testes), which usually resolves without damage, but in some men results in sterility.

While the disease runs its course, the symptoms of mumps infection are treated (i.e., acetaminophen for fever and pain). Mumps infection usually builds lifelong immunity; however, immunity can be achieved with the mumps vaccine.

PERTUSSIS

Pertussis, also known as whooping cough, is caused by the extremely contagious bacteria *Bordetella pertussis*. It is spread by direct or indirect contact with secretions from the respiratory tract of infected persons.

Initially, the child with pertussis may appear to have the flu or a respiratory infection with congestion, coughing, sneezing, watering eyes, and a slight fever. In a few weeks the cough becomes more severe and comes in episodes that begin suddenly, occurring as often as 40 times or more a day. Vomiting may frequently accompany these coughing episodes. In the last stage of the disease the fever and other symptoms are gone, but the cough remains. Episodes of severe explosive coughing continue to occur, more often at night. The child coughs as many as 8 to 10 times without being able to take a breath, and then finally breathes in, making a distinct, high-pitched singing or "whoop" sound. This stage can go on for weeks, but eventually the coughing episodes begin to subside. The child may have recurrences of the coughing episodes during other respiratory illnesses for the next few years.

Pneumonia can be a life-threatening complication of pertussis. The force generated during coughing and the increased pressure that it produces within the body can cause hernias, prolapse of the rectum, and bleeding into the brain that can cause seizures and possible brain damage.

Pertussis can be treated with antibiotics. People at high risk (such as infants or children with suppressed immune systems) who are exposed to pertussis can be treated with pertussis-immune globulin, a natural protein antibody that can help destroy invading pertussis microorganisms and possibly prevent infection.

Survivors of pertussis infection have lasting immunity; however, immunity can be achieved with the pertussis vaccine.

Several hundred thousand cases of pertussis are reported each year in the United States, and it is still a serious worldwide disease. The pertussis vaccine is often given with the diphtheria and tetanus vaccines (DTP) in children under seven years of age. In children seven and older, the pertussis portion of the combined vaccine is not given because the disease is less severe in older children.

POLIOMYELITIS

Poliomyelitis, also known as polio or infantile paralysis, is caused by three types of related viral microorganisms (polio viruses) that are spread by direct contact with respiratory droplets, oral secretions, or feces of an infected person. In recent years a phenomenon called postpolio weakness or postpoliomyelitis muscular atrophy syndrome has developed in some adult survivors of childhood polio. In this phenomenon, new muscle weakness and deterioration develop either in the same muscles that were originally affected or in new ones.

The type of virus that causes polio infection determines the symptoms. The most serious type attacks the nerve cells that control muscle movement, causing severe pain and muscle paralysis. Typically, the muscles of the legs are involved, but the virus can also paralyze the muscles of the arms, the muscles used to breathe, or even the muscles used to eat and swallow.

There is no treatment or medication for polio. Keeping the person comfortable while in bed with the body properly aligned is important. Passive exercise to the affected limb(s) can help maintain muscle strength and joint flexibility while the disease runs its course. Survivors have lasting immunity to the specific polio virus that they were infected with.

Thanks to the polio vaccine, which builds immunity against all three types of polio virus, polio is rare in the United States; however, it is still a major concern in less developed countries. The World Health Organization, an agency of the United Nations that promotes good health for every person in the world regardless of race, nationality, political or religious affiliation, or socioeconomic status, is trying to render the poliomyelitis virus extinct by the turn of the century through worldwide immunization efforts.

RUBELLA

Rubella, also called German measles or three-day measles, is caused by the rubella virus. It is spread by direct contact or by respiratory droplets and is found in the blood, stool, and urine of infected persons. Contact with freshly contaminated objects like a drinking glass or tissue can also cause infection.

Rubella is itself a relatively mild disease with rare complications. It may begin with a mild fever and cold-like symptoms that are soon followed by a rash. The rash is similar to that of measles, except that it lasts only about three days. The greatest concern associated with rubella infection is the devastating effect it can have on an unborn child if a pregnant woman becomes infected with the virus (see page 29). For this reason, immunization of all children is encouraged.

Symptoms of rubella infection can be treated (i.e., acetaminophen for fever) while the disease runs its course. Active rubella infection usually builds lasting immunity, although some people are infected a second time. Immunity can also be achieved with the rubella vaccine.

TETANUS

Although tetanus is not a contagious or infectious disease, because it is not spread from one person to another, it is a significant infection that can be prevented with immunization. Tetanus is caused by the bacteria *Clostridium tetani* which is found in soil and in the intestines of animals and human beings. The tetanus microorganism typically enters the bloodstream through a deep wound or break in the skin; for example, a nail puncture. It can also enter through a gunshot wound, burn, splinter site, or even an insect bite if the wound is contaminated with the tetanus bacteria. The tetanus bacteria does not require oxygen to survive, and once it is deep inside a wound it begins to multiply rapidly.

The tetanus bacteria produces a toxin that attaches to the nerve cells of the central nervous system, causing fever, chills, headache, and muscle stiffness that typically begins with the neck and jaw; this is why tetanus is commonly referred to as "lockjaw." Within hours the muscles of the face, neck, back, abdomen, and extremities become rigid and irritable. Any stimulus, such as a slight draft or the turning on of a light, can initiate severe and painful muscle spasms and convulsion. People keep a clear mind during this time and are aware of the severe spasms and pain.

Tetanus is treated in several ways: with an antitoxin that neutralizes unattached tetanus toxin; a tetanus immune globulin (natural proteins that help fight the tetanus bacteria, if the central nervous system is not yet affected); antibiotics to keep the bacteria from multiplying; and antiseizure and other medications.

Protection against tetanus is achieved with tetanus toxoid (the tetanus vaccine), which helps the body produce protective antitoxin. To ensure long-lasting immunity, a "booster" shot of tetanus toxoid is recommended every 10 years. When a tetanus-prone injury occurs, tetanus toxoid is usually administered if more than five years have elapsed since the person's last tetanus booster, or if his or her immunization history is unknown. Tetanus immune globulin (TIG) may also be given. Everyone should receive a tetanus "booster" shot every 10 years to maintain adequate immunity.

COMMUNICABLE DISEASE NOT PREVENTABLE BY IMMUNIZATION

CHICKENPOX

Chickenpox is caused by a highly contagious virus called varicella-zoster that is spread by respiratory droplet or direct contact with respiratory secretions or fluid from the skin blisters of infected people. Chickenpox can also be spread indirectly by contact with contaminated articles such as clothing or drinking glasses.

Chickenpox infection typically begins with a mild fever and fatigue. Twenty-four hours later a rash begins to appear, first as small red spots on the trunk, then spreading to the arms, legs, and face. Soon the small red spots become raised and filled with a fluid, forming blister-type lesions. This rash is very itchy. The fluid within the blisters is highly contagious because it contains live virus. There may be several "waves" of blisters, but eventually they dry and scab over. Once all the blisters are scabbed over (within 7 to 10 days) and the fever is gone, the person is no longer contagious to others.

Symptoms of chickenpox can be treated (i.e., acetaminophen for fever) while the person is kept comfortable until the disease runs its course; a vaccine will soon be available. Children with depressed immune systems who are unable to fight infection can be given immune globulin (protective protein antibodies) to prevent infection if they have recently been exposed to the chickenpox virus. Chickenpox infection results in long-term immunity. Some people, however, develop a disorder called shingles that is caused by the reactivation of chickenpox virus that has remained dormant within the body.

Chickenpox infection and the use of aspirin and aspirin products to control fever have been linked to the occurrence of Reye syndrome in children (see page 103). When a child has a fever, products containing acetaminophen (such as Tylenol®) should be used instead of aspirin products to treat fever. Aspirin products should not be used (for children) unless specifically prescribed by a physician.

HEPATITIS A

Hepatitis A, also known as epidemic hepatitis or infectious hepatitis, is caused by the hepatitis A virus (HAV). Both hepatitis A and hepatitis B (see page 70) produce similar changes in the liver and have very similar symptoms. Hepatitis A is spread through contaminated food or water and by direct contact with infected body fluids. The major path of transmission is through the fecal/oral route due to poor sanitation practices and poor handwashing techniques. Most outbreaks of hepatitis A infection are seen in children or young adults in day-care centers, schools, and other institutions that house large numbers of people. Illness caused by hepatitis A virus occurs more quickly and appears to be more acute than illness caused by hepatitis B virus.

Hepatitis A infection causes fever, nausea, poor appetite, abdominal pain, muscle aches, headache, extreme fatigue, and jaundice (yellowish skin). Hepatitis A infection is rarely fatal, and recovery usually occurs without long-term complications.

Treatment is mainly supportive, such as acetaminophen for fever and pain, and lots of rest until the disease runs its course. There is no vaccine for hepatitis A, but an injection of immune globulin (protective protein antibodies) is very effective in preventing the disease in people who have recently been exposed to the hepatitis A virus. However, immune globulin does not give lifelong protection. Hepatitis A infection usually builds immunity against future infection.

RHEUMATIC FEVER

See rheumatic heart disease, page 125.

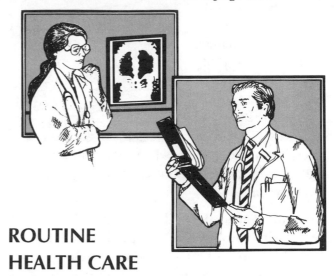

ROUTINE HEALTH CARE

One of the most important measures you can take to maintain an optimal position on the health continuum is to seek regular health care and to follow the instructions and advice of your health-care providers. You should regularly see health-care providers for general medical care, sensory care (sight and hearing), and dental care.

MEDICAL CARE

Specific medical disorders are discussed in depth in Chapters 6 through 18. How often you should seek health care depends on your family history, your age, your degree of exposure to environmental and occupational hazards, and your general health. Although a primary general health-care provider can meet most of your health-care needs, sometimes you need a specialist. If so, make sure that you keep accurate records and copies of important information from each health-care provider and share that information with all providers and family members as needed.

DENTAL CARE

Cavities and periodontal disease are the two most common causes of tooth loss. Cavities are the major culprit in people age 30 or younger, and periodontal disease is the major culprit in people over 40.

CAVITIES

Bacteria within the mouth cause tooth enamel to decay. Bacterial plaque forms along the cracks and crevices of the teeth and builds over time. When it comes in contact with sugars and starches from foods and fluids, an acid is formed that dissolves tooth enamel, creating a cavity. If the cavity is not treated, it continues to grow until it reaches the root of the tooth. The root 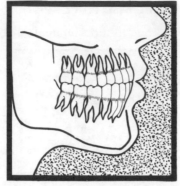 houses the tooth nerve, and when it is reached by decay there is severe pain. Without treatment by a dentist, tooth loss can result.

Cavities can also form along the root of a tooth. As gums recede with age or from periodontal disease, bacterial plaque can attach to the exposed root and cause cavities. The roots are easy targets for decay because they do not have the protective enamel coating that the upper portion of the teeth have. Roots are coated with dentin, a softer material that is easily dissolved by acids. It is estimated that more than 60% of people over age 65 have root decay.

PERIODONTAL DISEASE

Periodontal disease causes inflammation, ulceration, and infection of the gums, ligaments, and bones that support the teeth. By causing these supportive structures to loosen, periodontal disease can lead to tooth loss. There appears to be a genetic connection to periodontal disease in some families. If you have a family history of periodontal disease, you may begin to have symptoms as early as age 25. Several chronic diseases such as diabetes or thyroid disease, certain medications, and tobacco use also increase your risk of periodontal disease.

Periodontal disease can either progress slowly over the years without causing pain or other noticeable symptoms, or occur rather abruptly. You should see your dentist immediately if you notice any of these signs of periodontal disease:

- gums bleed with toothbrushing;
- gums are tender and/or inflamed (red and swollen);
- gums are separating from teeth;
- pus drains from gums;
- teeth have recently shifted or are loosening;

- there is a change in the way your teeth fit together when you chew or bite down;
- mouth has a new, persistent bad taste or smell.

The condition and health of your teeth and gums are determined by several factors, one of which is genetic. The structure and strength of your teeth is genetically influenced, which may explain why some children seem to always have cavities even though they practice good dental hygiene. Periodontal disease is three times more common in women than in men; this may be because of hormonal influences.

The condition and health of teeth and gums also depend on how well you care for them on a daily basis (brush at least twice and floss daily), how often you have regular dental checkups, and how much sugar and starch you eat.

Fluoride has proved to be effective in reducing tooth decay in people of all ages and is often added to local water supplies. Ask your dentist about the use of fluoride supplements or mouthwashes.

OTHER HEALTH HISTORY INFORMATION

ALLERGIES

An allergic reaction is an inappropriate response by the body's immune system (see page 200) to something that should not ordinarily cause a reaction. Things that trigger an allergic reaction are called allergens. An allergic reaction occurs when a person comes in contact with an allergen to which he or she has already developed a hypersensitivity because of previous exposure(s). Common allergens include house dust, molds, pollens, grasses, foods, animal dander, medications, and insect venom. The probability of having allergies increases if there is a family history of allergies because the susceptibility is genetically influenced. Although the tendency to have allergies is inherited, the specific type of allergy is not. For example, a mother and father may both have allergies to pollens, causing their hay fever symptoms, but their child may develop an allergy to animal dander, causing hives.

Allergies can develop at any time. It is possible to become allergic to something that has never before caused an allergic reaction, such as medications or

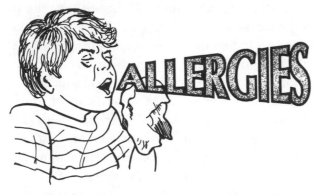

environmental elements that the individual has been exposed to for years. A fairly large percentage of children outgrow their allergies, while others have a change in the type of allergy symptom. For example, a child with allergic asthma may outgrow asthma symptoms only to develop hay fever symptoms as an adult.

Allergies can cause a wide variety of reactions. Symptoms may include itchy skin with the formation of hives, eczema, rhinitis (a runny nose), watery eyes, swelling of body tissues in a local or general area, and allergic asthma, which can cause coughing, wheezing, and difficulty breathing. Some people experience gastrointestinal reactions such as vomiting, abdominal cramping, or severe diarrhea. Allergies are certainly no fun and can leave a person feeling tired and washed out. And although allergy symptoms are frequently "only" irritating, annoying, and/or uncomfortable, some reactions are very serious and can lead to profound shock and death.

Once the specific allergen that triggers an allergy is identified by blood or skin testing, the best treatment is avoidance of the allergen. This, however, is not always possible or realistic. Medications can usually help control and/or relieve allergy symptoms. A series of injections to "desensitize" the immune system to a specific allergen is sometimes given, but results vary.

ANESTHETIC COMPLICATIONS

MALIGNANT HYPERTHERMIA

This genetic disorder occurs in people who are susceptible to certain anesthetic agents. Symptoms include extreme muscle rigidity and high fever, which occur during the surgical or early recovery periods. Malignant hyperthermia is inherited through an autosomal dominant inheritance pattern. It can be life threatening if not recognized and treated immediately.

PSEUDOCHOLINESTERASE DEFICIENCY

Also called serum cholinesterase deficiency.

This genetic disorder involves the absence or deficiency of an enzyme that breaks down certain paralyzing agents used for anesthesia. People with pseudocholinesterase deficiency have trouble "waking up" and resuming breathing on their own after receiving certain anesthetic agents. Difficulty resuming spontaneous breathing also occurs in people who are carriers of the mutant gene which causes this enzyme deficiency.

Tell your health-care provider if you suspect that you are at risk for the occurrence of malignant hyperthermia or pseudocholinesterase deficiency should you ever require anesthetic. Safe anesthetic agents are available that are not associated with these disorders.

LEARNING DISABILITIES

Learning disabilities (LDs) are thought to be caused by abnormalities within the central nervous system that interfere with the individual's ability to store, process, or produce information, thereby interfering with the ability to learn. This creates a gap between the person's potential and his or her actual performance. LDs tend to run in families, which suggests a genetic component may be involved. (Researchers are currently closing in on a gene thought to be responsible for some cases of dyslexia.) LDs affect both children and adults. The National Center for Learning Disabilities states that 10% of the U.S. population has some type of LD, although some experts believe the percentage is even higher.

There are various types of LDs. They can affect visual, auditory, or verbal learning; interfere with motor ability; or interfere with communication or logic abilities. LDs are not the same as learning problems due to mental retardation, autism, deafness, blindness, or behavioral disorders.

Some types of LDs, listed here by permission of the National Center for Learning Disabilities, include:

- **APRAXIA (DYSPRAXIA):** the inability to "motor plan"—to make an appropriate body response.

- **DYSGRAPHIA:** difficulty with the act of writing, both in the technical as well as the expressive sense; also difficulty with spelling.

- **DYSLEXIA:** difficulty with language in its various uses (not always reading).

- **DYSSEMIA:** difficulty with signals, such as social cues.

- **AUDITORY DISCRIMINATION:** perceiving the differences between sounds and the sequence of sounds.

- **VISUAL PERCEPTION:** the ability to understand and put meaning to what one sees.

- **ADD/ADHD (ATTENTION DEFICIT [HYPERACTIVITY] DISORDER):** may be accompanied by learning disabilities (about 20% of children with LDs may have accompanying ADD); characterized by hyperactivity, distractibility, and impulsivity; interferes with the individual's availability for learning.

Symptoms vary greatly depending on the type of learning disability. LDs can affect a person's ability to read, to comprehend what is read, to retain information, to express oneself orally or in writing, or to compute math. Affected children may have trouble listening, paying attention, or concentrating, and they learn less from life experiences. Therefore, they may appear to act without thinking of the consequences of their actions, and they may act impulsively and misperceive situations.

Discovering LDs early is crucial. Children with undiagnosed LDs undoubtedly suffer feelings of frustration, despair, shame, anger, low achievement, and low self-esteem. These children may be labeled lazy, disruptive, or slow, and are all too often held back in school. Being held back a year (retainment) has not been shown to help children with LDs; on the contrary, it delays for another year appropriate diagnosis and needed special education. This can be disastrous for the child academically, socially, and emotionally. Children with undiagnosed LDs have increased risk of school failure and dropout, juvenile delinquency, difficulties in social and interpersonal relationships, drug and alcohol use, and adult illiteracy.

Accurate diagnosis of the exact type of LD is the first step in helping the child. Diagnosis involves a psychoeducational evaluation of the child that assesses his or her intelligence, education/school skills, language, attention, behavior, motivation, and approach to tasks, as well as other nonacademic/social skills. Hearing and vision testing are also included.

Testing identifies the existence of LDs, the type, and the child's areas of strength. Once the LD is identified, an individualized education program (IEP) is constructed for the child, which among other things outlines the particular type of special education and related services to be provided for the child, and who should provide them. Special education methods, including the use of oral testing, calculators, computers, word processors, and one-on-one instruction may be included in the child's IEP. Public law 94-142m and the Individuals with Disabilities Education Act (IDEA) provide every child the right to receive testing for LDs upon request of a parent, or on the suggestion of a teacher, counselor, or other professional, such as the child's doctor, with parental permission. Also ensured is the right to receive free education through the public school system. The importance of parents taking an active advocacy role to ensure that their child is receiving the education guaranteed them by the public school system cannot be overemphasized. Parents too often don't know what their parental rights are, what their child's rights are, or what the public education system is mandated to provide. For a start, parents can contact their state's department of education or write for information from the National Center for Learning Disabilities, 381 Park Avenue South, Suite 1420, New York, NY 10016; 212-545-7510.

Children and adults with LDs have difficulty learning from standard teaching methods despite having average to above-average intelligence. For them, learning is achieved through teaching methods that bypass their problem area and utilize their strong areas. Although there is no cure for LDs, receiving appropriate special education from the early learning years on helps the individual learn how to compensate for his or her LD and thereby overcome it. Children with LDs are bright and imaginative and have a lot to offer themselves, families, and society. Therefore, a great injustice is done to all when a child's LD is not discovered.

SUDDEN INFANT DEATH SYNDROME (SIDS)

Also known as crib death.

In 1990 the National Institute of Child Health and Human Development defined SIDS as "the sudden death of an infant under one year of age that remains unexplained after a complete postmortem investigation that includes an autopsy, examination of the scene of death, and review of the case history."

Source: National Institute of Child Health and Human Development, 1990. Reprinted from *SIDS Alliance Greater Illinois Chapter Newsletter* (1992), Vol. 7, p. 4.

SIDS occurs in all races, ethnic groups, and socio-economic levels, causing 7,000 to 10,000 deaths each year in the United States alone. It is the main cause of death in infants aged one month to one year, with most cases occurring between the ages of two and four months. The cause of SIDS and the exact way the babies die are unknown. Theories as to the cause vary from viral infection to infant apnea (periods of absent breathing). Many experts, however, believe that a combination of factors contribute to SIDS and suspect these infants were born with conditions that made them sensitive or vulnerable to both internal and external stresses. Risk factors associated with the incidence of SIDS can be categorized as prenatal (before birth) or postnatal (after birth).

PRENATAL (BEFORE BIRTH) RISK FACTORS:

- maternal cigarette smoking during pregnancy
- maternal age less than 20 years
- lack of prenatal care
- maternal drug use
- maternal anemia

POSTNATAL (AFTER BIRTH) RISK FACTORS:

- infant of low birth weight
- infant of multiple birth (twin, triplet, etc.)
- infant of premature birth
- infant of male sex
- infant of parents who have had a previous child die from SIDS

These recognized risk factors are often, but not always, associated with SIDS. SIDS has also occurred in infants who had none of these risk factors present. Early and continuous prenatal care and avoidance of cigarette smoking and other drug use during pregnancy may maximize chances of avoiding SIDS.

Recent studies have shown a lower rate of SIDS in infants who are put to bed on their backs instead of on their stomachs. Therefore, this is the current recommendation by the American Academy of Pediatrics.

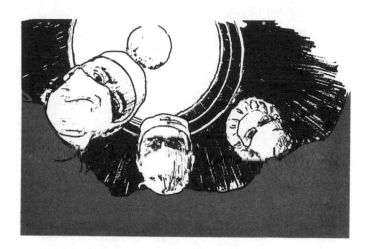

SURGICAL HISTORY

Surgical procedures are performed to treat disease, repair injuries, correct defects (deformities), and relieve pain or other symptoms of disease. Recording an accurate history of the surgical procedures you have had, and why and when they were performed, is an important aspect of your complete medical history. It helps the professionals who provide you with health care reach a more accurate diagnosis, especially if they are unfamiliar with you or your health status.

SECTION 5
GENERAL HEALTH INFORMATION

5.1 Are healthful eating practices in general followed? List any special diets followed for significant periods, such as vegetarianism.

5.2 List the date(s) and results of blood cholesterol screenings.

5.3 Indicate participation in routine exercise.

5.4 If alcohol is or was used, describe its intake as occasional, frequent, daily, etc. Be as specific as possible. List ages when alcohol consumption began and ended, if applicable.

5.5 If tobacco has ever been used, indicate if cigarettes, chewing tobacco, or snuff. If cigarettes, list number of packs per day. List ages when tobacco use began and ended, if applicable.

5.6 If ever exposed to second-hand smoke (e.g., at work or living with someone who smoked), document how many hours a day of exposure and number of years.

5.7 Indicate presence of a chemical dependence. Document the specific substance of abuse; for example, alcohol, cocaine, or other. Record the age at which the abuse and/or dependence began. Document treatment(s) received for the substance abuse, if known. Document the age when chemical use ended, if applicable.

5.8 Document any sleep disorders: insomnia, narcolepsy, sleep apnea syndrome, sleepwalking (as an adult), sleep-eating, other. Record the age at which the disorder began. List treatment(s), if known.

5.9 If an accident occurred resulting in injury or trauma, list the type of accident and age at the time (e.g., boating, hunting, motor vehicle, near drowning, near suffocation, sports injury, electrical shock, lightning strike, or other). List treatment(s) required, if known. Document any permanent mental or physical limitations or impairments related to the accident.

5.10 Document the occurrence of the following diseases or immunizations against them, and age at the time: chickenpox, diphtheria, haemophilus influenza type B, hepatitis A, hepatitis B, measles (rubeola, black measles, seven-day measles), mumps, pertussis (whooping cough), poliomyelitis (polio), rubella (German measles, three-day measles), tetanus, or other. Describe any permanent physical or mental limitations or impairments related to the infection(s). If immunized, document complications, if any.

5.11 Indicate whether medical examinations are routine. List primary care physician, his or her address, and phone number.

5.12 Indicate whether dental care is routinely received. List occurrence of periodontal disease, dentures, partial plates, bridges, or dental implants.

5.13 If allergies are or were present, list them. Include allergies to foods, medications, pollens, grasses, molds, animal dander, insect venom, other.

5.14 If a learning disability is or was present, document the specific type, if known.

5.15 List surgeries, their dates, age at the time, the medical facility, surgeon's name, and the reason for the procedure, if known.

5.16 List any complications that have occurred with general anesthesia. Include disorders such as pseudocholinesterase deficiency and malignant hyperthermia. Describe other abnormal reactions to anesthetic agents.

5.17 If desired, list the medications being taken, including the name of the prescribing physician, why prescribed, age when the medication was begun, and when the medication was discontinued (if applicable). (List only those medications taken on a long-term basis.)

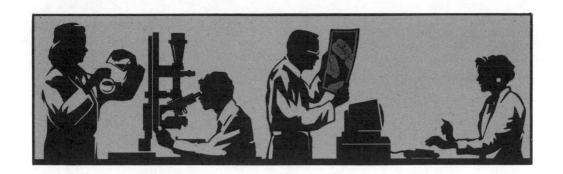

UNIT II
YOUR BODY SYSTEMS

CHAPTERS 6 THROUGH 18

Chapters 6 through 18 discuss the different systems of the body. A body system is a unit of the body that works to perform specific tasks. Each body system is presented for you in "head to toe" order, beginning with **The Eyes and Ears** (Chapter 6) and finishing with **The Integumentary (Skin) System** (Chapter 18).

These chapters present three types of information:

1. **STRUCTURES AND FUNCTIONS.** This type of information is an overview of the structures (anatomy) of the particular system and how it functions (physiology).

   It is important to read this overview. It will help you understand the medical terminology used in many health documents, including the *HEALTH HISTORY FORM.*

2. **STRUCTURAL DEFECTS.** This type of information covers a select group of structural defects present at birth that can occur in the particular body system. These are presented in alphabetical order.

3. **DISEASES AND DISORDERS.** This type of information covers a select list of diseases and disorders, both genetic and infectious, that affect or involve the particular body system. These are also presented in alphabetical order. Body systems and their disorders frequently overlap. For example, a neuromuscular disease involves both the muscles (muscular) and the nervous (neuro-) system. Diseases and disorders that involve more than one body system are cross-referenced in each chapter.

Read the first part of each chapter dealing with structures and functions before completing the corresponding section of your *HEALTH HISTORY FORM.* It is NOT necessary to read about every structural defect or every disease and disorder. If you have a particular disease or disorder, or if you find that a blood relative has it, read the information to learn if there could be a genetic component to the disease.

If you have a disease or disorder that you cannot find described, check the index to see where it is listed. Also check the glossary for information about some diseases and disorders that are not included in this book.

If you still cannot find the disease mentioned, it does NOT mean it is insignificant. On the contrary, it should be documented on your *HEALTH HISTORY FORM* under "Other diseases and disorders."

Later, ask your health-care provider about the significance of that disease to your own health and that of your children.

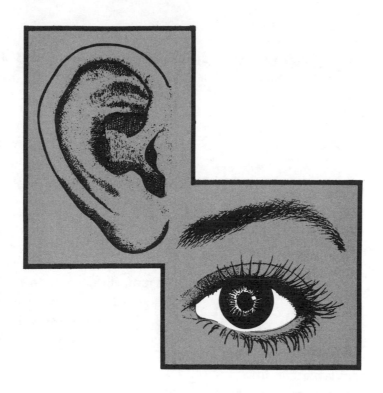

CHAPTER 6
THE EYES AND EARS

T he five major senses are sight, smell, taste, hearing, and touch. Following is a discussion on sight and hearing and some of the health disorders that can affect them.

THE EYES — STRUCTURES AND FUNCTIONS

Sight is made possible by the complex functions of the eyes (see figure 6.1) in conjunction with specialized areas in the brain. The eyes lie within the bony sockets of the skull, and each eyeball is moved by six extraocular muscles attached to its outermost layer.

The eye has three layers. The outer layer, called the sclera, is the tough, white, fibrous layer that surrounds the eye on the back and sides. The forward portion of the sclera is the cornea, which is the clear tissue that bulges slightly from the eye over the iris and pupil.

The middle layer of the eye, called the uvea, is the color layer. It consists of the choroid, which is thick with blood vessels that nourish the retina at the back of the eye, and the iris and ciliary body in the front of the eye. The iris, which is the ring of color visible in the eye, is made of muscle fibers that contract and relax to change the size of the pupil (the opening in the center of the iris) which controls the amount of light that enters the eye. The ciliary body consists of muscle fibers at the outer edge of the iris that produce fluid to maintain pressure within the front of the eye and that change the shape of the lens in order to focus light rays on the retina.

The inner lining of the back of the eye is the retina, which houses nerves and photoreceptors (light

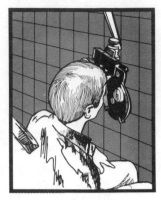

receivers) that catch the light as it enters the eye. The two types of photoreceptors in the retina are cones and rods.

Cones are located most densely within the center of the retina in an area known as the macula. Cones work well in full light and provide clear, sharp central vision (visual acuity) and color discrimination; rods work well in dim light and are most prevalent along the outside of the retina. Rods are used for peripheral and night vision.

Light passes through the cornea, the fluid within the eye, the pupil, and the lens. In the process, light rays are refracted (bent) so that they focus on the back wall of the eye along the retina, stimulating the photoreceptors. These in turn send a message to the optic nerve, which exits through the back of the eye. The optic nerve carries the message to the back of the brain, which sees the message as a visual image. Depth perception is the result of the brain's receiving a message from both eyes.

Vision loss and blindness have many causes. They can be present at birth (congenital) or develop during childhood or adulthood. Vision loss may result from infection, injury, genetic diseases or disorders, or from complications of a health disorder such as diabetes or high blood pressure; or vision loss may be due to age-related deterioration of eye structures. Legal blindness occurs when vision can be corrected to only 20/200 or less. This measurement means that a person must stand 20 feet from an object to see it clearly, whereas a person with normal vision would see that same object clearly from 200 feet.

Loss of vision can be abrupt or slow. Visual disturbances should be checked immediately by an ophthalmologist, a physician who specializes in disorders of the eye. Children should receive routine

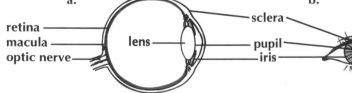

Figure 6.1. Structures of the eye:
a. internal structures   **b. visible structures**

retina — macula — optic nerve — lens — sclera — pupil — iris

vision screenings and be referred for a complete eye examination when abnormalities and/or deficits are noted.

Young adults should have routine eye examinations at least every few years. People aged 35 and older should have yearly examinations with glaucoma screening. People with a family history of glaucoma should be checked every year.

DISEASES AND DISORDERS

CATARACTS

When the lens of the eye becomes cloudy (opaque) a cataract has formed. Some cataracts are congenital (present at birth) as a result of prenatal infection or genetic disease. Cataracts that occur as a result of aging are called senile cataracts and are the most common. Other causes of cataract formation include eye injury, health disorders such as diabetes, long-term use of medications such as steroids, and long-term exposure to sunlight.

SIGNS AND SYMPTOMS. Cataract formation can significantly limit sight. Symptoms include dimming, blurring, and glaring of vision, and a decreased ability to see colors or to see at night. The pupil of the eye may appear white or cloudy in some people.

TREATMENT. A lens that has a cataract can be surgically removed, and vision can be corrected with an implanted artificial lens or with eyeglasses or contact lenses.

CONJUNCTIVITIS

The conjunctiva is the clear membrane that lines the inner eyelids and the front of the eye. Conjunctivitis is an inflammation of the conjunctiva as a result of infection, chemical or environmental irritation, injury, allergic responses, or other health disorders.

SIGNS AND SYMPTOMS. Conjunctivitis causes eye redness, itching and pain, and the production of purulent drainage.

TREATMENT. Conjunctivitis can be treated with ophthalmic (eye) antibiotics or other solutions.

GLAUCOMA

Glaucoma is increased pressure within the eye (intraocular pressure) that can lead to varying degrees of blindness. There are a variety of causes. Although some forms of glaucoma can be caused by other medical disorders, the majority are classified as primary glaucomas that affect both eyes and have a strong genetic influence.

SIGNS AND SYMPTOMS. The most common form of primary glaucoma is open-angle glaucoma, which usually has a very slow onset. Because it often has no noticeable symptoms as it progresses, permanent eye damage may already be extensive by the time symptoms begin. Peripheral vision is usually lost first, resulting in tunnel vision (see figure 6.2) that can continue to progress until complete loss of vision occurs. People with a family history of glaucoma must have yearly checkups to catch it in its early stages if vision loss is to be prevented.

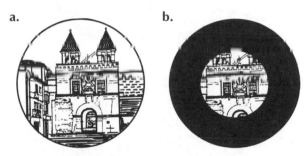

Figure 6.2. Effect on peripheral vision loss:
a. normal vision   b. tunnel vision

Closed-angle or angle-closure glaucoma is a less common form of glaucoma. It usually occurs suddenly and abruptly, causing severe eye pain and swelling, headache, and vision changes (such as blurred vision and "halos" around lights) resulting from a sudden increase in eye pressure. If not treated immediately, vision loss and blindness can occur.

TREATMENT. Regardless of the type of glaucoma, early treatment can reduce and maintain intraocular pressures within normal limits. By doing this, damage to the retina and the optic nerve is spared or minimized. Treatment may include oral medication, eyedrops, laser surgery, and/or conventional surgery.

REFRACTIVE ERRORS

Refractive errors or disorders occur when light rays that pass through the front of the eye (the cornea and lens) are not refracted (bent) sufficiently to focus them on the retina. Some refractive disorders are congenital (present at birth) with a genetic influence, while others are the result of a loss of elasticity and stretch within the lens and other anterior eye structures that normally lengthen and shorten to refract (bend) light rays. Refractive errors may occur singularly or in combination and can be corrected by eyeglasses or contact lenses. Refractive errors include:

- **HYPEROPIA (farsightedness).** With hyperopia the eye is too short from front to back, causing light to be focused behind the retina, making it impossible to focus clearly on close objects without corrective lenses (see figure 6.3).

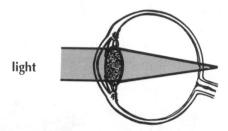

Figure 6.3. Hyperopia: the eye is short from front to back, causing light to focus beyond the retina

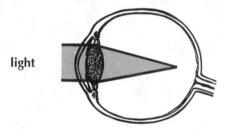

Figure 6.4. Myopia: the eye is long from front to back, causing light to focus in front of the retina

- **MYOPIA (nearsightedness).** With myopia the eye is too long from front to back, causing light to be focused in front of the retina and making it impossible to focus clearly on distant objects without corrective lenses (see figure 6.4).

- **ASTIGMATISM.** The usual cause of astigmatism is an uneven curvature of the cornea that causes light entering the eye from different angles to be focused at different points. This makes sharp vision, both near and far, difficult without corrective lenses.

RETINAL DETACHMENT

If the retina tears away from the vascular choroid, a partial or total loss of vision can result. Causes of retinal detachment include injury, congenital defect, infection, tumor, and degenerative changes within the

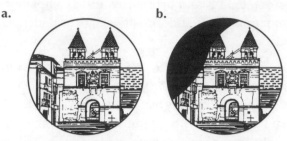

Figure 6.5. Effect of vision loss: a. normal vision b. draping shadow seen with retinal detachment

retina or its supportive tissues. Some health disorders such as high blood pressure and diabetes can increase the risk of retinal detachment. People with a family history of retinal detachment should be examined periodically so that early degenerative changes such as lattice degeneration or retinal holes, which can be identified only by a physician (ophthalmologist), can be treated early. Retinal detachment may be an autosomal dominant disorder in some cases.

SIGNS AND SYMPTOMS. Retinal detachment may cause floaters (specks that seem to float across the field of vision), flashing bursts of light within the eye, and a dark, curtain-like shadow that drapes across the field of vision (see figure 6.5). A loss of central vision can occur if the macular area is detaching.

TREATMENT. Retinal detachment requires immediate attention. Laser surgery and/or conventional surgery can stabilize the retina and prevent further loss of vision.

RETINITIS PIGMENTOSA (RP) AND OTHER RETINAL DEGENERATIVE DISORDERS

Retinitis pigmentosa (RP) is a group of disorders that cause a slow breakdown (degeneration) of the photoreceptor cells within the retina, resulting in loss of sight. Symptoms of RP may begin in childhood and steadily worsen with age. Most cases of RP are thought to be the result of new gene mutations. Once mutation occurs, the disorder can be passed to future generations. All three inheritance patterns are seen in various types of RP (autosomal dominant, autosomal recessive, and X-linked). The specific risk of transmitting the disorder to future generations depends on the specific type of inheritance pattern. For an overview of inherited diseases associated with RP and retinal degeneration, see table 6.1.

TREATMENT. There currently is no effective cure for retinal degenerative diseases. Early diagnosis is imperative to retain optimal vision. Routine eye examination by an ophthalmologist, especially when there is a family history, increases the probability of early diagnosis. Good nutritional practices may help prevent progressive damage. Wearing ultraviolet-blocking sunglasses may greatly reduce the risk of developing some retinal degenerative diseases, such as age-related macular degeneration (see table 6.1).

RETINOBLASTOMA

Retinoblastoma is a congenital or pediatric malignant tumor of the retina that can be either nongenetic or genetic in cause. The genetic form usually affects both eyes and follows an autosomal dominant inheritance pattern.

SIGNS AND SYMPTOMS. The retinal tumor is usually evident at birth or by the age of two years. As the tumor grows, the child's pupil may reflect a white glow as light entering the eye reflects off the tumor.

TREATMENT. Depending on the size of the tumor and how much eye tissue is affected, treatment can include radiation therapy, tumor freezing (cryotherapy), laser therapy, chemotherapy, or removal of the eye (enucleation). Early detection and treatment are important to halt (arrest) tumor growth, prevent its spread (metastasis), and preserve as much sight as possible.

INHERITED DISEASES CHARACTERIZED BY RP AND/OR RETINAL DEGENERATION		
Name	**Inheritance Pattern**	**Description & Symptoms**
Bardet-Biedl syndrome	Autosomal recessive	Multiple physical problems, including RP, extra fingers and/or toes, obesity, mental retardation, and kidney disease. Not all of these occur in every person with this disease.
Bassen-Kornzweig syndrome (Abetalipoproteinemia)	Autosomal recessive	RP, progressive neurologic problems, and oddly shaped red blood cells.
Best disease (vitelliform dystrophy)	Autosomal recessive	Characterized by a lesion in the central retina (the macula) that often leads to impaired central vision in one or both eyes.
Choroideremia	X-linked	Similar to RP, including night blindness followed by loss of peripheral vision, degeneration of the retina and choroid. It affects only males.
Gyrate atrophy	Autosomal recessive	Associated with a deficiency in the enzyme ornithine aminotransferase. Symptoms include myopia (nearsightedness), night blindness, reduction in peripheral vision, and cataracts.
Leber congenital amaurosis	Autosomal recessive	Severe visual impairment from birth or very early childhood.
Age-related macular degeneration	Unknown	The leading cause of central degeneration vision loss in people over the age of 60. The first symptom is usually a blank spot in the center of the visual field or a distortion of normal central vision. It is occasionally found in more than one member of a family.
Refsum syndrome	Autosomal recessive	RP, hearing loss, neurologic problems, and dry and/or flaky skin.
Stargardt disease	Autosomal recessive	A form of macular degeneration that usually appears before the age of 20. Symptoms are reduced central vision with a preservation of peripheral vision.
Usher syndrome	Autosomal recessive	Combination of RP and congenital hearing impairment. Different types occur: Type I: Profound hearing impairment, problems with balance, and early onset of RP. Type II: Moderate hearing impairment, and later onset of RP.

Source: Jill C. Hennessey, M.S., *The Inheritance of RP and Allied Retinal Degenerative Diseases*, RP Foundation Fighting Blindness. Used with permission.

Table 6.1.

STRABISMUS

Strabismus, also known as crossed eyes, is most frequently seen in young children. With strabismus the eyes do not focus on the same object, because one eye deviates from the other (see figure 6.6). The deviation of the affected eye(s) may be toward the nose, the top of the head, the feet, or outward toward the ear. Because the points of focus from each eye are different,

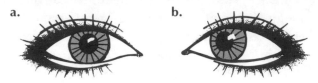

Figure 6.6. Effect of strabismus:
a. normal position of eye
b. eye deviated inward toward nose

sharp vision is difficult. The brain eventually suppresses the message it receives from the deviated eye, and that eye's ability to see weakens. If strabismus is not corrected, the deviated eye will lose all vision from disuse, a disorder known as amblyopia. Some occurrences of strabismus are genetically influenced, while others may be due to injury or disease.

TREATMENT. Strabismus should be corrected in young children as soon as it is detected to prevent permanent vision loss from the development of amblyopia. When excessively long or short extraocular muscles cause strabismus, it can be surgically repaired. Other treatments for strabismus include covering the "good" eye with a patch to force use of the deviated eye, and corrective eyeglasses.

THE EARS — STRUCTURES AND FUNCTIONS

The function of the ear, its structures, and the auditory nerve is to receive and transmit impulses to the brain, which interprets them as sound. The auditory nerve is also called the vestibulocochlear nerve, acoustic nerve, or cranial nerve VIII.

The ear has three sections: the external ear, the middle ear, and the inner ear (see figure 6.7). The parts of the ear that are visible on the sides of the head constitute the external or outer ear. They consist of the pinna (auricle) and the external ear canal, which leads to the eardrum (tympanic membrane). The eardrum separates the external ear from the middle ear.

The middle ear contains three small bones called ossicles that connect to form a continuous chain from

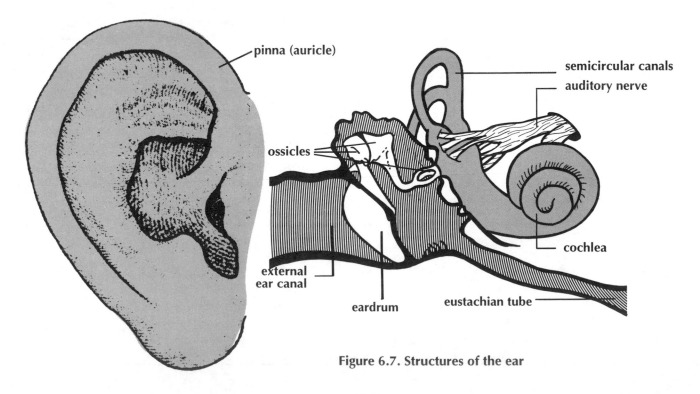

Figure 6.7. Structures of the ear

the eardrum to the inner ear. The eustachian tube is a canal that opens from the middle ear into the area of the throat behind the nose (the nasopharynx). This canal allows air to come and go from the throat to the middle ear to equalize air pressure on both sides of the eardrum. The last ossicle of the middle ear connects with the inner ear.

The inner ear contains two very important fluid-filled structures: the cochlea, which transmits sound; and the semicircular canals, which maintain balance and sense of body position (equilibrium).

As sound waves travel through the air and enter the external ear canal, they cause the eardrum to vibrate. These vibrations are conducted through the ossicles of the middle ear to the fluid-filled cochlea of the inner ear. Within the cochlea, the vibrations are converted into nerve impulses; the auditory nerve transmits these impulses to the hearing (auditory) centers in the brain, which interpret them as sound. Any interruption in this process causes hearing loss.

DISEASES AND DISORDERS
HEARING LOSS

Two major types of hearing loss (deafness) are conductive hearing loss and sensorineural hearing loss. Conductive hearing loss occurs when sound vibrations cannot be transmitted through the external or middle ear canal because of blockage by a foreign object or excessive wax buildup within the ear canal; damage to the eardrum or to the bones of the middle ear; or a congenital deformity or malformation of the ear. Recurrent ear infection (otitis media) can also result in conductive hearing loss because of scarring of the eardrum, which impedes its ability to vibrate.

Sensorineural hearing loss is caused by damage to, or a defect of, the cochlea or the auditory nerve from exposure to infections before birth (prenatal infections), childhood infections, tumor growth, injury, drug toxicity, genetic disease, or aging. Genetic diseases associated with hearing loss include Waardenburg syndrome, Usher syndrome, and many others. Hearing loss present at birth (congenital) can have many causes, but frequently the cause is unknown.

Hearing loss may or may not be treatable. Surgical correction is possible in some types of conductive

hearing loss; hearing aids may be helpful in some types of sensorineural hearing loss.

MENIERE DISEASE

Also known as Meniere syndrome or endolymphatic hydrops.

Meniere disease involves the structures of the inner ear, the cochlea, and the semicircular canals. The symptoms of Meniere disease usually begin between the ages of 30 and 50 and affect more men than women and more Whites than Blacks. Most cases of Meniere disease affect only one ear.

Theories as to the cause of Meniere disease include infection of the inner ear, allergy, chemical disturbance within the body, changes in the blood vessels that serve (supply) the inner ear, psychological factors including stress, and genetic factors. Meniere disease does run in some families, which supports a genetic connection.

SIGNS AND SYMPTOMS. The symptoms of Meniere disease apparently result from the accumulation of too much lymphatic fluid within the inner ear. Three main symptoms must be present for a diagnosis of Meniere disease. The most pronounced symptom is vertigo: an extreme "whirling" dizziness felt whether the eyes are open or closed, causing profound disturbances in balance and difficulty in walking. The remaining symptoms are tinnitus (a continuous buzzing or ringing in the ear), and sensorineural hearing loss. The tinnitus is almost always present, but the vertigo and hearing loss come and go in severe recurring episodes or attacks that literally incapacitate the affected person. Other symptoms associated with these attacks include headache, nausea, vomiting, and jerking eye movements that are most likely related to the vertigo. These attacks may last minutes or hours, but lingering effects can be felt for days. The hearing loss that occurs during attacks is temporary at first; with repeated attacks it can become permanent.

TREATMENT. There is no cure for Meniere disease. Treatment is designed to control the severity of attacks and prevent further hearing loss. A combination of treatments is used. Affected people are encouraged to learn to recognize signs of impending attacks, such as a feeling of fullness in the ear, so that they can avoid activities such as driving and instead find a quiet place where they can remain until the severe symptoms subside. Salt is sometimes restricted, and the use of alcohol, tobacco, and caffeine is discouraged. Medication can be used to relieve and/or control dizziness, nausea and vomiting, and the amount of fluid in the inner ear. Various surgical procedures exist that may help people who are repeatedly incapacitated by Meniere disease and its accompanying tinnitus and vertigo. Unfortunately, these procedures may also result in partial or total hearing loss.

OTITIS MEDIA (OM)

Otitis media is an inflammation of the middle ear. Failure of the eustachian tube to open and allow fluid within the middle ear to drain out can cause OM. OM can also be caused by microorganisms (mainly bacteria) that travel from the throat up the eustachian tube into the middle ear, causing infection. OM is seen most often in infants and children. Children are more prone to OM than adults because their eustachian tubes lie in a horizontal line between the middle ear and that area of the throat located behind the nose (the nasopharynx). As a result, throat secretions and microorganisms have easy access to the middle ear. As children grow, their eustachian tubes become more vertical, making it more difficult for the secretions and microorganisms to get from the throat into the middle ear.

Increased mucus production in children with allergies can increase their risk of developing OM, as do enlarged adenoids (one of the tonsil pairs located behind the nose), which can block the eustachian tubes. Children at risk of upper respiratory infections, for example those who live in households where people smoke, are more likely to have OM.

SIGNS AND SYMPTOMS. With chronic OM, symptoms can include delayed speech development and communication, because the fluid that constantly accumulates in the middle ear causes distorted sound perception or loss of hearing. With acute OM there is sudden and extreme ear pain, irritability, decreased hearing, and difficulty sleeping. Pus-like material usually caused by bacterial infection is often present in the middle ear in cases of acute OM.

TREATMENT. OM is treated with antibiotics. When the course of antibiotics is completed, a follow-up examination confirms whether or not the middle ear is clear of fluid and/or pus. If children have a large amount of pus with OM, the health-care provider may puncture the eardrum and drain the middle ear. Draining the eardrum relieves ear pain and prevents the material from rupturing into the inner ear, which could cause abscess formation, bone infection of the skull, or meningitis.

The eardrum can rupture spontaneously in OM because of the high buildup of pressure within the middle ear. Spontaneous rupture can scar the eardrum; repeated scarring can cause permanent hearing loss. In children who have repeated episodes of OM or who do not respond to medication, the placement of ear tubes and/or the surgical removal of the adenoids may be recommended to prevent potential hearing loss. These treatments should be considered carefully only after seeking a second opinion, preferably from an ear specialist.

OTOSCLEROSIS

Otosclerosis is a disorder that causes conductive hearing loss. It affects women more often than men and usually begins in the teenage or early adult years. Otosclerosis results from the abnormal formation of bone that surrounds the inner ear. The bone blocks the conduction of sound vibrations from the ossicles.

The precise cause of otosclerosis is unknown, but it is thought to follow an autosomal dominant inheritance pattern with reduced penetrance (the mutant gene may be inherited but not always cause otosclerosis). Other suspected causes include ear infections (otitis media) and vitamin deficiencies.

TREATMENT. Hearing can be improved by the use of hearing aids and/or surgery.

SECTION 6
THE EYES AND EARS

Check any of the following diseases and disorders of the eyes that are or were present.

6.1 Cataracts: indicate whether the right, left, or both eyes were affected and at what age(s). List treatment(s), if known. Document if an intraocular lens was surgically implanted into the right, left, or both eyes.

6.2 Conjunctivitis: indicate whether the right, left, or both eyes were affected and at what age(s).

6.3 Glaucoma: document the specific type (open-angle or closed-angle), if known. Indicate whether the right, left, or both eyes were affected and at what age the condition was diagnosed. Document treatment(s), if known.

6.4 Loss of sight (vision): indicate whether the right, left, or both eyes were affected and at what age(s) the loss occurred. Document cause, if known.

6.5 Refractive errors: document as myopia (near-sightedness), hyperopia (farsightedness), and/or astigmatism.

6.6 Retinal detachment: indicate whether it was of the right, left, or both eyes. Indicate at what age(s) the condition occurred and the precipitating event, if known. Document treatment(s), if known.

6.7 Retinal degenerative disorder (see table 6.1, page 85, for a list of retinal degenerative disorders): document the specific disorder, if known, and indicate whether the right, left, or both eyes were affected. Document treatment(s), if known.

6.8 Retinoblastoma: indicate whether the tumor was present in the right, left, or both eyes and at what age the condition was discovered. Document treatment(s), if known.

6.9 Strabismus: indicate whether the right, left, or both eyes were affected and at what age(s). Document treatment(s), if known.

Check any of the following diseases or disorders of the ears that are or were present.

6.10 Hearing loss: indicate whether the right, left, or both ears were affected and at what age(s). Indicate whether deafness was present at birth. Document the type of hearing loss as sensorineural or conductive, if known, and the cause and treatment(s), if known.

6.11 Meniere disease: indicate whether the right, left, or both ears were affected and at what age(s) symptoms began. Document treatment(s), if known.

6.12 Otitis media (OM): indicate whether the right, left, or both ears were affected and at what age(s). Document treatment(s), if known.

6.13 Otosclerosis: indicate whether the right, left, or both ears were affected and at what age(s) the disorder became apparent. Document treatment(s), if known.

6.14 Document any other diseases or disorders of the eyes or ears that are or were present, the age of the individual at onset of the disorder, and treatment(s), if known.

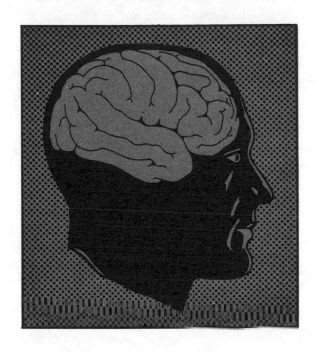

CHAPTER 7

THE NERVOUS SYSTEM

The nervous system is the command center for the entire body. Along with the endocrine system, it regulates and coordinates all body functions by continuously reacting to both internal and external environments, thereby maintaining biologic balances within all body systems.

STRUCTURES AND FUNCTIONS

The structures of the nervous system (NS) are the brain, the spinal cord, and the nerves. These structures are divided into two nervous systems: the central nervous system (CNS), which consists of the brain and the spinal cord, and the peripheral nervous system (PNS), which consists of the nerves. These two systems work together to relay information from body tissues to the brain, process the information, and relay instructions and commands back to the body tissues. This processing and relaying of information is carried out by the neurons, the primary nerve cell of the NS (see figure 7.1). Each neuron consists of a cell body, appendages called dendrites that receive information from a nearby neuron, and other appendages called axons that send the information on to the next neuron. Neurons communicate in this way by releasing chemicals known as neurotransmitters, which in turn stimulate the next neuron, creating a chain reaction that passes on a message to the brain from an area of the body where the message originated. The same process works in reverse to carry a message that originates in the brain to a specific area of the body.

Neurons range in length from less than an inch to several feet. Many of the axon appendages are surrounded by a protecting layer of myelin. Groups of myelinated appendages create the white matter, and groups of nerve cell bodies create the gray matter in nervous system tissue. White and gray matter are found in both the brain and spinal cord.

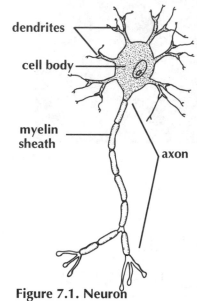

dendrites

cell body

myelin sheath

axon

Figure 7.1. Neuron

THE CENTRAL NERVOUS SYSTEM (CNS)

The CNS consists of the brain and the spinal cord. Because these organs are so vital and sensitive, built-in mechanisms protect them from injury. First, the skull and spine (backbone) surround the brain and spinal cord with rigid bone. Second, the brain and spinal cord have a tough outer covering composed of three membrane layers called the meninges. The meninges protect and help nourish the nerve tissues (neurons) of the brain and spinal cord. Third, a clear fluid called cerebrospinal fluid (CSF) circulates around and through the brain and spinal cord, providing a fluid cushion that helps to support the organs and reduce shock from jarring movement.

CSF is produced in fluid-filled spaces within the brain called ventricles. The ventricles are lined with blood vessels; fluid and other elements in the bloodstream filter from these vessels into the ventricles to create CSF. Once formed in the ventricles, CSF circulates through and around the brain and spinal cord and is eventually reabsorbed into the bloodstream.

Four major arteries in the neck ascend to "feed" the nerve cells of the brain by joining to form a ring or circle at the base of the brain. Blood entering this circle is distributed to various portions of the brain through small arteries that branch off from the circle. This circular configuration, known as the circle of Willis, is yet another protective mechanism: in the event that one of the four major vessels becomes blocked, some distribution of blood into the branching arteries can continue, thereby reducing the number of neurons that are damaged and destroyed.

The linings of all the blood vessels that traverse through the brain are able to keep most harmful agents, such as bacteria or chemical toxins, from entering into the CSF or into brain tissue itself. This special ability is known as the blood-brain barrier; its function is vital to the well-being of the central nervous system.

The brain itself is a collection of regions, each of which is responsible for very specific functions. The three basic parts of the brain are the cerebrum, the cerebellum, and the brain stem (see figure 7.2).

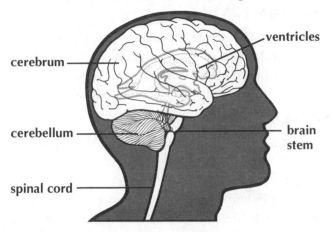

Figure 7.2. Structures of the central nervous system

THE CEREBRUM

The cerebrum is the largest portion of the brain and is divided into right and left sides, or hemispheres. The outer portion of the cerebrum is a lumpy, gray mass of neurons called the cerebral cortex, which is responsible for complex functions such as memory, consciousness, intellect, thought processing, and sensory perception. Each cerebral hemisphere is divided into four regions or lobes: the frontal, parietal, temporal, and occipital lobes, each responsible for specific functions (see figure 7.3).

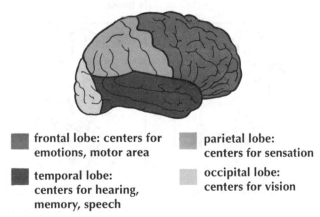

■ frontal lobe: centers for emotions, motor area

■ temporal lobe: centers for hearing, memory, speech

■ parietal lobe: centers for sensation

■ occipital lobe: centers for vision

Figure 7.3. Lobes of the cerebrum and some of their functions

THE CEREBELLUM

The cerebellum lies below the cerebrum in the back portion of the brain; it also has right and left hemispheres. The cerebellum coordinates muscle movement and balance and receives sensory input for hearing, vision, and touch.

THE BRAIN STEM

The brain stem connects the brain to the spinal cord. The cranial nerves that relay sensory and motor (muscle) messages to and from the head and neck region start in the brain stem. Other structures considered to be part of the brain stem include the thalamus, the hypothalamus, the pons, and the medulla oblongata. These structures regulate many automatic body functions, including heart and breathing rates, body temperature, blood pressure, basic reflexes, some sensory and emotional responses, and the release of hormones from glands throughout the body.

THE SPINAL CORD

The spinal cord has its own mass of nerve cells (neurons) that transmit sensory and motor (muscle) nervous system messages. It has tracts or pathways of myelinated nerve axons that relay messages back and forth between body tissues and the brain.

THE PERIPHERAL NERVOUS SYSTEM (PNS)

The PNS consists of 12 pairs of cranial nerves that enter and leave the brain stem and connect with areas of the head, face, and neck—and 31 pairs of spinal nerves that exit and enter the spinal cord through openings between the vertebrae (bones) of the spine. These nerves carry sensory and motor (muscle) messages to and from the brain from all tissues and organs.

The PNS has voluntary divisions, which can be consciously controlled, and autonomic or automatic divisions, which

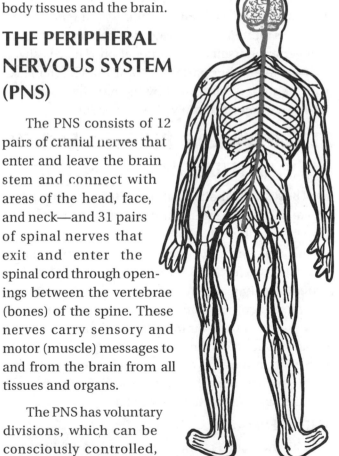

Figure 7.4. The peripheral nervous system

cannot be consciously controlled. The voluntary division allows the brain to sense, for example, a leg itch by means of the sensory message that travels from the leg to the spinal cord to the brain, where the message is analyzed and recognized as an itch. The brain then sends a message through the spinal cord to the muscles of the arm and hand, stimulating them to scratch.

The autonomic nervous system, on the other hand, regulates unconscious activities such as changes in heart rate, breathing rate, gland stimulation, and sweating. Autonomic messages are processed mainly in the brain stem, without conscious thought. For example, the information that the body is overheating is sent up the spinal cord to the brain stem, which tells the sweat glands to release sweat to cool the body.

It is still not understood how the nervous system manages to direct all body reactions and responses within fractions of a second or how it provides for thought, reasoning, and the formation of opinions and emotions. However, although this complex system is apparently powerful enough to do more as a whole than just the sum of its parts, it is very fragile. Once a neuron is injured or destroyed, it usually cannot repair or regenerate itself. Sometimes if an injury is slight, neurons in another part of the brain can learn to take over the task(s) controlled by the damaged neurons, but most often the damage is permanent.

STRUCTURAL BIRTH DEFECTS
NEURAL TUBE DEFECTS (NTDS)

These major malformations of the nervous system are caused by the failure of the skull or spine to form properly during early embryonic development. They include anencephaly, encephalocele, and spina bifida. Neural tube defects (NTDs) sometimes run in families, indicating that a genetic factor may be involved. Among the contributing factors are environmental influences, as for example the mother's nutritional intake of folic acid during the prenatal period. Because both genetic and environmental influences contribute to the occurrence of neural tube defects, they are classified as multifactorial disorders.

ANENCEPHALY

The incidence is approximately 1 in 1,000 births. In anencephaly, most of the skull is absent. The underlying brain tissue may be incompletely or abnormally formed. Spontaneous abortion (miscarriage) or stillbirth occurs in a large number of cases. There is no treatment for anencephaly. Survival for more than one day is rare.

ENCEPHALOCELE

An encephalocele is the herniation of brain tissue through a hole in the skull, usually at the base. The defect can be repaired surgically in some cases, but the amount of damage to the nervous system varies.

SPINA BIFIDA

Incidence is approximately 1 in 500 to 1,000 live births; it is most often seen in females. Prevalence is more common in certain geographic locations, including Ireland. Infants of women whose diets did not contain sufficient folic acid during pregnancy have been found to be at higher risk of spina bifida and other neural tube defects.

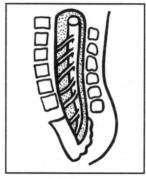

a. normal spine: spinal cord is enclosed within the vertebrae

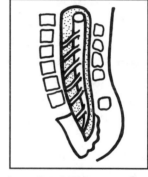

b. spina bifida occulta: back portion of a vertebra is missing

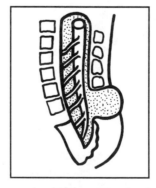

c. spina bifida cystica: back portion of a vertebra is missing, and the meninges, filled with cerebral spinal fluid, protrude from the spine in a sac-like structure called a meningocele

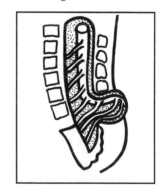

d. spina bifida cystica: meningocele is present as in figure 7.5c, but in this defect the sac-like structure also contains the spinal cord; this defect is called a myelomeningocele

Figure 7.5. Spina bifida

SIGNS AND SYMPTOMS. There are different types of spina bifida. In spina bifida occulta, the back side of one or more vertebrae of the spine fail to form completely, leaving a small opening in the spine; however, the spinal cord itself is not involved (see figure 7.5b). There may be a tuft of hair, a mole, or dimpling in the lower back area, but usually that is all that is apparent. A surprising number of people have spina bifida occulta but are never diagnosed. Some people may develop symptoms later in life, such as leg weakness, gait disturbances, or decreased bladder control. They may be at increased risk to have children with more severe forms of spina bifida.

In the more severe type of spina bifida, spina bifida cystica, there is a sac-like protrusion from the spinal defect. This defect is classified into two types according to which tissues are involved. With a meningocele, the thin membranes surrounding the spinal cord (the meninges) and spinal fluid protrude through the defect in the spine; however, the spinal cord (nerve) does not (see figure 7.5c). There is usually only minimal neuromuscular impairment in this type, if any.

A myelomeningocele (or meningomyelocele) is the most severe type of spina bifida cystica. It is diagnosed when the sac-like protrusion includes the spinal cord, the meninges, and spinal fluid (see figure 7.5d). This defect results in paralysis below the level of the defect.

TREATMENT. Meningoceles are surgically correctable. With myelomeningoceles, surgical closure corrects the defect in the spine, but does not repair the spinal cord or reverse the paralysis.

DISEASES AND DISORDERS
ALZHEIMER DISEASE (AD)

AD is a progressive degenerative disorder resulting in continual mental deterioration that cannot be stopped or reversed. It causes more than 50% of the cases of senile dementia seen in the elderly. It may begin as early as age 25 or as late as age 80. People whose symptoms start at age 58 or earlier are more likely to have familial AD, which is transmitted genetically through an autosomal dominant inheritance pattern. Those whose symptoms start after age 58 may have an autosomal dominant form of the disease, or they may have inherited a susceptibility to AD when exposed to certain environmental factors (a multifactorial form of the disease).

It is unknown whether a single gene or a group of genes causes familial AD; gene mutation on chromosomes 14, 19, and 21 have been associated with its occurrence. People with Down syndrome have three chromosomes 21, and a majority have Alzheimer-type brain deterioration in early adulthood. This finding helped researchers track one of the familial AD genes to chromosome 21, and perhaps partially explains why the risk of having AD is somewhat increased in people with a family history of Down syndrome. Studies also indicate a much higher incidence of AD in people with a history of head injury.

In AD, neurons within the cerebral cortex are destroyed and protein plaques accumulate within the destroyed areas. These changes occur to a lesser degree in people without AD as part of the normal aging process, but are much more pronounced in people with AD.

SIGNS AND SYMPTOMS. Memory loss (especially short-term memory), forgetfulness, personality changes, impaired ability to concentrate, and decreasing ability to perform daily self-care and hygiene activities are signs of AD. Eventually confusion, speech difficulty, loss of muscle control, and emotional outbursts necessitate continuous supervision.

TREATMENT. There is no treatment or cure for AD. In fact, the only way to confirm the diagnosis is by brain biopsy, or by autopsy after death. Most cases are diagnosed by symptoms alone after other causes of dementia have been ruled out following a thorough neurological examination. The accurate diagnosis of AD is extremely important because of the potential genetic connection for other family members.

AMYOTROPHIC LATERAL SCLEROSIS (ALS)

Also known as Lou Gehrig's disease, and motor neuron disease.

ALS is an irreversible, progressive (gradually worsening) disease that results in continuous destruction of muscle neurons within the spinal cord and the lower brain stem. About 10% of ALS cases are familial, and the gene responsible for this type of ALS was only recently identified. The cause of the remaining cases of ALS, called sporadic ALS, is still unknown.

SIGNS AND SYMPTOMS. Muscle weakness and cramping in the arms and legs frequently appear first, usually in people between 40 and 70 years of age. As increasing numbers of neurons are destroyed, a total loss of muscle control occurs and muscles begin to waste away (atrophy) from nonuse. Even the muscles used for breathing, swallowing, and speaking are affected. It is important to note that the mental capacity and function of people with ALS is not affected by the disease.

TREATMENT. There is no cure for ALS. Treatment focuses on maintenance of muscle function and independence and on preventing associated complications for as long as possible. Survival after symptoms appear is usually no longer than 10 years.

CEREBRAL PALSY (CP)

CP is a nonprogressive disorder that primarily affects muscle movement and posture, although there may also be sensory and/or mental impairment.

CP is caused by brain damage that occurs during the prenatal, labor and delivery, or infancy periods. The major cause is lack of oxygen or injury to brain tissue. Lack of oxygen may result from poor placental function, prenatal infection, Rh hemolytic disease, placental bleeding complications, maternal drug and/or alcohol use, or a long and difficult labor and delivery. Injury to the brain can result from infection (meningitis or encephalitis), hemorrhage into brain tissue, head injury, or chemical or metabolic disorders. Children at highest risk for CP are those born premature or with low birth weights.

SIGNS AND SYMPTOMS. Because CP primarily involves muscle function, a delay in accomplishing motor (muscle) tasks is common, including poor sucking and feeding abilities in newborns. CP is often classified according to the type of muscle dysfunction present. In spastic CP, increased muscle tension and deep tendon reflexes affect posture and voluntary muscle movements. Athetoid or dyskinetic CP is manifested by muscle movements that vary from jerking to writhing. People with ataxic CP have difficulty with coordination, balance, and walking. Although many people with CP have normal or even superior intelligence, a significant number have some degree of mental impairment, hyperactivity, or attention deficit disorder. Seizures can occur in severe cases. Vision and hearing problems may also be present.

TREATMENT. There is no treatment or cure for CP. Early identification of affected children allows early initiation of therapy and support to help them develop as fully as possible. Competent prenatal, labor, and delivery health care and the prevention of accidents and injury during the first year of life can significantly reduce the incidence of CP.

CEREBRAL VASCULAR ACCIDENT (CVA)

Also known as stroke. See page 120.

ENCEPHALITIS

Some forms are referred to as sleeping sickness.

This inflammatory disorder of the brain tissue can be caused by bacterial, viral, fungal, or parasitic microorganisms. The most common types of encephalitis are caused by viruses. Encephalitis can occur as a complication of childhood communicable diseases such as mumps, measles, or chickenpox. Some encephalitis-causing microorganisms can be transmitted from animals or insects, including horses, mosquitoes, and ticks, and some can be transmitted from person to person.

SIGNS AND SYMPTOMS. Symptoms can vary from mild to severe and include fever; lethargy with excessive sleeping; alterations in consciousness or behavior; irritability; headache; muscle stiffness; pain involving the neck, back, and extremities; balance problems; dizziness; changes in vision; and nausea and vomiting. Severe symptoms include seizures, paralysis, and even coma. Encephalitis can result in complete recovery, permanent nerve damage, or death.

TREATMENT. Bacterial encephalitis is treated with antibiotics. Viral encephalitis is not usually treatable with antibiotics; antifever and antiseizure medications are given to control symptoms while the body fights the virus. The best treatment for encephalitis is prevention when possible, such as by immunizing children against childhood communicable diseases.

EPILEPSY

Also called seizure disorder or convulsive disorder.

Epilepsy is the occurrence of repeated seizures brought on by a sudden burst of neuron excitation and stimulation that may spread to neurons throughout the brain or stay within a localized area. Some types of seizure involve a total loss of consciousness, with stiff, jerking movements of the arms and legs (called a generalized tonic-clonic or grand mal seizure); other types of seizure involve only a specific function or region of the body (called partial or focal seizures). Epilepsy can result from damage to nerve cells (neurons) of the brain caused by physical trauma or injury, infections such as meningitis or encephalitis, a lack of oxygen due to stroke (CVA) or rupture of an aneurysm, or a brain tumor. Epilepsy is seen in some genetic disorders such as tuberous sclerosis and in some metabolic disorders.

Often the cause of epilepsy cannot be identified. Genetic influences play a larger role in some types of epilepsy than in others. Petit mal seizures have a strong genetic connection, are seen most often among children and adolescents, and are considered to be generalized seizures because of a brief change in or loss of consciousness. They do not involve muscle tensing or jerking. Instead, people having a petit mal seizure are very still and appear to gaze straight ahead as if daydreaming or dazed. Occasionally the eyelids twitch or the eyes move in an unusual way. Petit mal seizures do not last long, but if not correctly diagnosed they can create problems for the individual both at home and at school. Safety is a major concern for people who have epilepsy because of the potential for injury to themselves and others when they suddenly lose consciousness. Some health-care providers classify epilepsy in general as a multifactorial disorder because of the role that both genetic and environmental factors have in its occurrence.

SIGNS AND SYMPTOMS. Symptoms of epilepsy vary and depend on the type of seizures. Loss of consciousness with visible jerking, attention span interruption, loss of muscle tone, and memory loss can all be symptoms. Unusual movement in only one body area, such as smacking of the mouth or tremors of the arms or legs can be signs of seizure activity. Seizure activity in people with epilepsy may be triggered by stimuli such as flashing lights, low blood sugar levels, or excessively low blood sodium levels.

TREATMENT. In some cases epilepsy can be cured by correcting the underlying cause; for example, surgically removing a brain tumor or treating a metabolic disease with medication. If the cause is unknown or cannot be corrected, seizure activity is controlled with medication that raises the person's seizure threshold (decreasing the likelihood of seizure) given for a pro-

longed period of time. After the person is seizure free for a significant period of time (for example, two years), the health-care provider may decrease the dosage of medication and eventually discontinue it altogether. Some children outgrow epilepsy; those who do not require continued medication and regularly scheduled evaluation.

FAMILIAL DYSAUTONOMIA

Also called Riley-Day syndrome.

The incidence is approximately 1 in 10,000 to 20,000 live births. It is an autosomal recessive disease that occurs primarily in Ashkenazic Jewish families (Jews of central and eastern European descent), affecting males and females equally. Sources estimate 1 in 30 to 50 Ashkenazic Jews are carriers of the mutant gene (meaning they have one normal gene and one dysautonomia gene).

Familial dysautonomia is associated with abnormal sensory and autonomic nervous system development. The autonomic nervous system is responsible for many functions, including body temperature regulation, normal blood pressure maintenance, and other involuntary body functions. As a result, symptoms are widespread and involve many body systems.

SIGNS AND SYMPTOMS. Affected people may exhibit a lack of or indifference to the sensation of pain; altered taste and heat perception; difficulty with speech and swallowing; problems with balance and coordination; poor regulation of body temperature and blood pressure; stunted growth; abnormal curvature of the spine (scoliosis); episodes of vomiting and excessive sweating; and low tear production that puts them at risk of eye injury and corneal ulcers. Intelligence is not usually affected by the disorder.

TREATMENT. There is no cure. Care involves supportive measures of specific symptoms, which can vary considerably from person to person.

FEBRILE SEIZURES

To be febrile means to have a fever. Febrile seizures are usually seen with sudden and rapidly rising fevers, usually 102° to 104°F. Febrile seizures are seen most often in children aged five years and younger and occur more frequently in boys. There is usually a family history of febrile seizures, suggesting an inherited susceptibility in its occurrence. Most children who have febrile seizures outgrow them, but children who have them at very young ages may have repeated episodes. Febrile seizures are not usually associated with any permanent neuron damage.

SIGNS AND SYMPTOMS. Febrile seizures are characteristically tonic-clonic seizures—generalized, stiff, jerking movements with a temporary loss of consciousness.

TREATMENT. The health-care provider may prescribe antiseizure medication(s) after a complete evaluation to rule out other possible causes of the seizure. Parents may also be instructed to treat any future fevers aggressively to prevent seizure recurrence.

GALACTOSEMIA

The incidence of this autosomal recessive disorder is approximately 1 in 50,000 to 70,000 live births. Since many states began requiring newborn screening for galactosemia, it has been found to occur more frequently than previously thought.

Galactosemia is an enzyme deficiency that results in an inability to break down the simple sugar galactose or the milk sugar lactose into glucose, the blood sugar the body uses for energy. Types of galactosemia differ depending on the specific enzyme deficiency; two types are harmful.

SIGNS AND SYMPTOMS. In the less frequent form of galactosemia, a deficiency of the enzyme galactokinase causes premature cataract formation, which may be the first noticeable symptom of the disorder. It usually appears within the first year of life.

A deficiency of the enzyme galactose-1-phosphate uridyl transferase, considered the classic form of galactosemia, results in damage to the brain, liver, kidney, and intestines. Symptoms become apparent soon after birth with the start of milk feedings, including breast milk. Irritability, lethargy, feeding problems, and seizures reflect the brain damage caused by the enzyme deficiency. Mental retardation ensues. Other symptoms include liver enlargement and jaundice (yellow discoloration of skin), vomiting, diarrhea, and growth retardation. Cataract formation in both eyes at one to two months of age is typical.

TREATMENT. A milk-free diet is immediately started. Eliminating milk and other lactose-containing foods from the diet may prevent the damage associated with galactosemia. Infants are given soy-based formulas as soon as possible; untreated infants may die within days after birth, which is why immediate diagnosis is so important. The galactose-free diet must be continued for life. Some health-care providers may allow a slight modification in the diet after eight years of age. People with galactosemia must read all food labels closely for the presence of milk and lactose, and for milk-product additives such as casein and whey. Lactose is used as a filler in some medicines, spices, and chewing gum, making them sources of accidental lactose ingestion. A registered nutritionist can help affected individuals with dietary education and planning.

Women with galactosemia have an additional concern related to childbearing because they have a high risk of infertility. They should seek counseling before attempting to conceive. Should pregnancy occur, if the fetus inherits galactosemia and the woman is not on a strict galactose-free diet, the fetus will suffer irreversible damage before birth. Maintaining a strict diet throughout pregnancy may prevent this.

GUILLAIN-BARRÉ SYNDROME (GBS)

Also known as acute idiopathic polyneuritis, post-infectious polyneuritis, Landry's paralysis, and acute polyradiculoneuropathy.

GBS primarily affects the spinal and cranial nerves and areas of the spinal cord. The cause is unknown, but because a significant number of people develop GBS after having a respiratory or gastrointestinal illness, a viral and/or autoimmune cause is suspected.

In GBS the protective layer of myelin that covers the neurons deteriorates, causing the nerves to become inflamed and swollen, thereby disrupting the conduction of nervous system messages to the muscles.

SIGNS AND SYMPTOMS. Muscle weakness results and progresses until muscle paralysis occurs, usually beginning in the legs and moving upward, sometimes even affecting the muscles used to talk, swallow, and breathe. Symptoms may worsen for several days or weeks and reach a plateau for additional days or weeks. Eventually the inflammation dissipates and the myelin is repaired. Muscles usually regain movement in the opposite order that the paralysis occurred.

TREATMENT. Maintaining vital body functions, such as breathing, and preventing complications are all that can be done while GBS runs its course. Mechanical breathing assistance (ventilation) and intensive care may be required during the peak of the illness. Most people fully recover from GBS, but a few have some permanent nerve damage.

HUNTINGTON DISEASE (HD)

Sometimes referred to as Huntington chorea.

Incidence is 1 in 10,000 to 25,000 live births, with a lower incidence among Blacks and Asians than among Whites. It is transmitted through an autosomal dominant inheritance pattern. Huntington disease is characterized by the progressive destruction of nerve cells within certain areas of the brain.

SIGNS AND SYMPTOMS. This is a late-onset disease, and symptoms typically do not appear until age 35 to 45. The destruction of nerve cells within the brain causes involuntary muscle movements of the face, arms, and legs, and eventually interferes with balance and the ability to walk. Speech, swallowing, and breathing are eventually affected. Mental changes such as memory loss, decreased attention span, and emotional and personality changes are seen. Death usually occurs within 10 to 20 years after the onset of symptoms.

TREATMENT. There is no cure. Researchers have recently identified the responsible mutant gene. The finding has led to a presymptomatic test which is available to identify carriers of the Huntington disease gene prior to the onset of symptoms. Comprehensive counseling is recommended, however, for at-risk individuals prior to their actual testing.

HYDROCEPHALUS

Also known as "water on the brain."

Hydrocephalus occurs when too much cerebral spinal fluid (CSF) accumulates in the ventricles of the brain, which can be caused by excessive production of CSF, slowed reabsorption of CSF, or an obstruction of CSF flow through the ventricles. Any of these situations can result from a congenital defect, tumor, infection (such as meningitis or encephalitis), bleeding within the brain, or head injury.

The accumulation of fluid within the ventricles causes the ventricles to enlarge (dilate), compressing surrounding brain tissue against the skull and slowing the flow of blood through the brain. Hydrocephalus may be a chronic condition present at birth or may occur with other disorders later in life. Permanent brain damage and death can result.

SIGNS AND SYMPTOMS. Signs of mental deterioration can occur as pressure within the skull increases and the brain becomes compressed and damaged. Symptoms vary in severity and can include headache, nausea and vomiting, seizure, coma, and death. In infants, skull bones that have not yet fused together separate in response to the increased pressure, resulting in head enlargement.

TREATMENT. If possible, the cause is corrected. In some cases, a surgically placed shunt device drains excess CSF from the ventricles into either the abdominal cavity or the right atrium of the heart. The shunt may need to be surgically replaced or adjusted as the child grows.

INFANTILE AUTISM

Also called pervasive developmental disorder; formerly called infantile or autistic psychosis.

Infantile autism is a rare developmental disorder in which a child does not develop the ability to communicate and interact with his or her environmental surroundings and other people. The child has deficits in mental and thought processing, language and speech development, and social interaction skills. Symptoms usually appear before the age of 2½ years. Sometimes a child appears to develop normally in infancy and then begins to regress. Autism occurs three to four times more often in males than in females; in general, however, affected females have more severe symptoms.

The cause of autism is unknown, although evidence supporting a genetic cause is increasing. Other biological risk factors suspected to cause autism include infections such as meningitis or encephalitis; prenatal (before birth) rubella infection; oxygen deprivation or other brain injury occurring before, during, or after birth; seizure disorders such as epilepsy; chemical imbalances within the brain; and abnormal structural development of the brain itself.

SIGNS AND SYMPTOMS. Autistic children are self-absorbed and withdrawn and usually do not exhibit interest in other people. They may avoid eye contact with others and may appear to be repulsed or bothered by physical contact, such as being held or cuddled. They may form attachments to inanimate objects such as balls or rubber bands, and be fascinated with objects that spin, such as tops or spinning plates. In addition, they might not speak; seem to have a private language that others cannot understand; mimic or repeat words they hear; exhibit rocking, twirling, head banging, or other repetitive movements; exhibit self-mutilation behavior; have a very high or very low perception of pain; and appear to be deaf and unresponsive to verbal communication yet be very sensitive to sound. Mental retardation may be present in varying degrees, yet some autistic children demonstrate a superior mental talent in a particular area or skill, such as memory recall, mathematical calculation, music, or art.

TREATMENT. Treatment usually focuses on helping the child achieve the highest functional level possible; that level is determined on the basis of the type and severity of the symptoms. The majority of children with autism require some degree of lifelong supervision. A variety of treatments are often tried, but unfortunately many are ineffective. Behavior modification is one of the more successful treatments. Family support is very important; national and local support groups such as the Autism Society of America (ASA) and Siblings Helping Persons with Autism through Resources and Energy (SHARE) are often beneficial to family members.

MENINGITIS

Also known as spinal meningitis.

Meningitis is the inflammation of the meninges that cover the brain and spinal cord. It can be caused by infectious agents, including bacterial, viral, or fungal microorganisms; chemical toxins such as lead or arsenic; or any other substances that somehow get into the cerebrospinal fluid and trigger an inflammatory response. Microorganisms in the blood from another site of infection such as the sinuses, nose, throat, or ears can enter the cerebrospinal fluid by crossing the blood-brain barrier, or they may enter directly through an open area in the skull or spine caused by injury or surgery. Some toxic chemical agents taken by mouth can enter through the blood-brain barrier once they are absorbed into the bloodstream.

SIGNS AND SYMPTOMS. The inflammation and swelling within the meninges can cause headache, nausea and vomiting, fever, and soreness and stiffness in the neck, back, and extremities, as well as irritability, lethargy, change in level of consciousness, visual and balance disturbances, seizure, and/or coma.

TREATMENT. Bacterial meningitis can be contagious and is a very serious infection. It can be treated successfully with antibiotics, but early diagnosis is critical because even with early treatment, bacterial meningitis can result in permanent brain damage and death. A vaccine against a major meningitis-causing bacteria, *Haemophilus influenzae* type B, is part of the current recommended immunization schedule for children (another reason immunizations are so very important).

Aseptic meningitis, caused by viral infection, is treatable with antibiotics only when the herpes simplex virus (HSV) is the cause. Fortunately, most forms of aseptic meningitis run their course with no permanent damage to the nervous system.

Treatment of meningitis caused by chemical toxins depends on the specific toxin involved.

MENKES SYNDROME

Also called kinky hair syndrome and Menkes steely-hair syndrome.

The incidence is approximately 1 in 35,000 live male births. It is transmitted through an X-linked inheritance pattern. In Menkes syndrome the body is unable to absorb copper from the diet, resulting in severe copper deficiency.

SIGNS AND SYMPTOMS. Infants have symptoms of central nervous system impairment, including seizures and poor control of body temperature shortly after birth. Their hair is typically twisted and of steel-wool consistency. Bone and artery formation is often abnormal. Central nervous system impairment, including mental retardation, progresses with age, and death often occurs by age three.

TREATMENT. There is no cure. The administration of copper has not been successful in humans; treatment is primarily supportive.

MIGRAINE HEADACHES

Migraine headaches are thought to be caused by alternating periods of narrowing (constriction) and widening (dilation) of cerebral arteries, which result in tissue swelling and changes in certain chemical levels. The exact cause of migraines is unknown, but they do run in families and occur more frequently in women. Some people can identify factors such as certain foods, stress, or medications that almost always cause or trigger their migraines.

SIGNS AND SYMPTOMS. Severe pain that is often limited to one side of the head can occur with a migraine headache, as can nausea, vomiting, and visual disturbances, such as seeing rings around lights or seeing in zig-zag patterns. Symptoms often begin in adolescence and decline during the middle adult years. Anyone with any type of severe headache should be thoroughly examined to rule out other possible causes of head pain, such as brain tumor.

TREATMENT. Migraine headaches can be treated with medication. In some instances dietary changes, stress reduction, and an increase in the amount of sleep/rest received may help reduce the frequency and/or severity of migraine headaches.

MULTIPLE SCLEROSIS (MS)

MS is a degenerative disease that affects the brain and spinal cord and interferes with muscle strength and movement. In MS the protective myelin sheath that surrounds many nerve axons is destroyed, greatly slowing the transmission of messages from neuron to neuron. Eventually, plaques form along the axons where myelin has been destroyed, causing irreversible damage along the nerve pathway and preventing the conduction of messages to body muscles. The exact cause is unknown, but MS does occur more often in some families than in the general population, and occurs most often in females. MS is thought to be related to both genetic and environmental factors. For example, one theory proposes that an inherited defect in the body's immune system does not become apparent until triggered by a specific virus.

SIGNS AND SYMPTOMS. Symptoms of MS, which usually begin between the ages of 20 and 40, initially come and go in episodes of relapses and remissions. Symptoms include muscle weakness, lack of coordination, tingling or burning sensations, and sometimes muscle pain. In time, as the nerve damage becomes irreversible, muscle movement in the arms and legs is lost, and muscle weakness affects even speech and vision.

TREATMENT. MS cannot be cured or prevented at this time. People with MS need proper rest and nutrition. Emotional stress, excessive physical exertion, and infection can cause a relapse or worsening of symptoms and should be avoided.

MYASTHENIA GRAVIS (MG)

In MG, physical exertion causes progressive muscle weakness that is relieved by rest. Some people with MG have weakness only in the eye muscles, while others have weakness in muscles throughout the body. The exact cause is unknown, but MG is suspected to be an autoimmune disorder; that is, a disorder in which the body has produced antibodies that attack its own tissue.

The muscle weakness in MG is thought to result from interference in the transmission of nervous system messages to the muscles. Although the muscles look normal on examination, they gradually lose their strength when they are used. Intellect and sense of touch are not affected.

Myasthenia crisis is a life-threatening complication of MG. Severe muscle weakness, usually brought on by emotional stress, infection, surgery, or injury, is so severe that intensive care and mechanical breathing assistance (ventilation) are required until the crisis runs its course.

SIGNS AND SYMPTOMS. Drooping eyelids; double vision; difficulty swallowing, speaking, and breathing; and arms and legs that weaken upon exertion, such as walking stairs or lifting—all are symptoms and can begin at any time from ages 20 to 50.

TREATMENT. MG can be treated with medication and, in some cases, surgery.

NEUROFIBROMATOSIS (NF1)

Also called von Recklinghausen disease and mistakenly called the "elephant man" disease.

Incidence is approximately 1 in 3,000 to 4,000 live births. NF1 is transmitted through an autosomal dominant inheritance pattern. It affects both males and females and occurs in all races and ethnic groups worldwide. Approximately 50% of cases are the result of a new gene mutation in the egg or sperm. Nerve tissue overgrowth forms multiple tumors called neurofibromas.

SIGNS AND SYMPTOMS. NF1 can be associated with a wide variety of symptoms. The first evidence of the disease is usually the presence of six or more skin lesions called café au lait spots. Many times these lesions are present at birth. Small lumps (neuro-fibromas) form beneath the skin or deeper along nerve pathways, causing complications that may include skeletal deformities and blindness. A small percentage of people may develop brain tumors that can cause seizures and/or intellectual handicap, but most people with NF1 have normal intelligence, although a significant number (40%) have learning disabilities. (Seizures can also occur in people without brain tumors.) Unfortunately, there is no way to predict how severe the disease will become in an individual. Some people with NF1 have increased symptoms during adolescence and/or pregnancy; others experience a continual progression (worsening) of symptoms as they age.

TREATMENT. NF1 has no cure. Surgical removal of the tumorous growths may be necessary if the eyes or ears are involved. Growths are sometimes removed for cosmetic reasons; however, many times the growths return. Body braces for bone deformities are sometimes needed. Children with NF1 need medical evaluation every 6 to 12 months so that complications can be diagnosed and treated early. Physical examinations and hearing and vision screenings should be done regularly. Adults need medical evaluation at least once a year. In 1990, scientists discovered a similarity between the protein formed by the NF gene and a protein associated with cancer. It is now known that the NF1 gene, when normal, is a recessive cancer repressor gene.

PARKINSON DISEASE

Also known as paralysis agitans.

Although the exact cause of Parkinson disease is unknown, it is thought to be caused by the destruction of the neurons deep in the center of the brain that produce a chemical called dopamine, which helps maintain normal conduction of nerve messages from the brain. In Parkinson disease, communication between the brain and muscles weakens (perhaps because of decreased amounts of dopamine). Mainly, Parkinson disease affects people aged 50 and older, but it is also seen in younger people. Some families have a higher incidence of Parkinson disease; a genetic susceptibility is suspected but has not yet been proved. A multifactorial cause, in which heredity is combined with an environmental cause such as a virus, may be responsible. Parkinson disease can also develop after a brain injury such as infection or trauma and can be induced by certain antipsychotic drugs.

SIGNS AND SYMPTOMS. People with Parkinson disease have hand and foot tremors (especially while at rest), difficulty in getting the body to move, a shuffling, stiff-legged walk, forward slumping of the posture, rigid muscle tone, and an expressionless, mask-like facial appearance. Usually, mental capacity is affected only in severe cases, but depression is not uncommon.

TREATMENT. The symptoms of Parkinson disease can be markedly reduced with medication to replace the chemical dopamine, although this treatment does not stop the disease from progressing. Physical therapy and social and psychological support are important elements of treatment as well.

PHENYLKETONURIA (PKU)

The incidence of PKU is highest among whites in the United States and northern Europe. Although it occurs in all races, it is rarest among African, Japanese, and Jewish populations. Reported incidence in the United States is 1 in 5,000 to 6,000 live births. In northern Ireland the incidence is reported to be as high as 1 in 4,500. PKU is an autosomal recessive disease.

The liver enzyme phenylalanine hydroxylase, which breaks down (metabolizes) the amino acid phenylalanine into another amino acid called tyrosine, is absent in people with PKU. Tyrosine is necessary for the production of certain body regulators (including some thyroid hormones) and melanin. Although the body needs phenylalanine for normal growth and cell repair, the excessive amount that accumulates in the bloodstream in PKU is toxic to brain tissue and causes permanent brain damage. Children with undiagnosed and/or untreated PKU have poor muscle coordination, growth delay, and mental retardation, and may have tremors and seizures. Because early detection and treatment are necessary, U.S. law requires all newborns to be screened for PKU soon after birth. The test is often repeated at around two weeks of age.

SIGNS AND SYMPTOMS. Children with PKU tend to have lighter coloring (pigmentation) than other members of their families because of decreased melanin production. In light-skinned populations children typically have fair skin, blond hair, and blue eyes. These children are also prone to eczema or other skin irritations related to their lack of melanin.

TREATMENT. A child diagnosed with PKU is immediately placed on a low-phenylalanine diet which, if initiated within the first few days or weeks after birth, prevents mental retardation and allows the child to lead a normal, healthy life. Low-phenylalanine formula is available for infants with PKU, but as children become older the diet becomes more difficult to follow because phenylalanine is present in many protein foods, including meat, eggs, milk, cake, pudding, and even soda. Parents should get help with meal planning and nutritional assessments from a registered nutritionist. Blood phenylalanine levels are evaluated frequently to assess the adequacy of dietary control.

How long a child with PKU should remain on the low-phenylalanine diet is somewhat questionable, but most experts suggest a strict diet at least until the child is eight years of age. At that time some health-care providers allow a slightly higher amount of phenylalanine to be consumed. Studies indicate that children who no longer adhere to a phenylalanine-restricted diet can have disturbances in behavior and decreasing intelligence quotients. These findings support the continuation of a controlled phenylalanine diet throughout life. Once brain destruction has occurred, diet cannot repair it.

Women with PKU have an additional concern during pregnancy. If the woman does not adhere to a strict low-phenylalanine diet during pregnancy, her elevated phenylalanine levels will cross the placental membrane and cause irreversible brain damage in the fetus. It is therefore recommended that women with PKU who have been off the PKU diet get back on it at least three months before they conceive. It is imperative that these women get preconceptional and genetic counseling and be closely monitored throughout pregnancy.

RABIES

Rabies is a fatal infection that attacks the central nervous system. It is caused by the rabies virus, which is most often transmitted to human beings through the saliva of an infected animal, usually with a bite. Warm-blooded wild animals and unvaccinated domestic pets can be infected with the rabies virus.

SIGNS AND SYMPTOMS. In human beings with untreated rabies infection, symptoms develop anywhere from days to months after exposure. Lethargy, fever, and a sore throat may appear first, but the infected person quickly enters an excitement phase and exhibits maniacal behavior, seizures, severe spasms, and paralysis of muscles, including those used for breathing and swallowing. Death occurs within days of the onset of symptoms.

TREATMENT. Prevention of the infection after exposure involves a series of vaccinations given over a period of time. If treatment is not given before symptoms appear, death will occur.

The best treatment for rabies is prevention of the disease in animals. All pet owners should have their pets vaccinated against rabies on a regular basis as recommended by their veterinarian. People should be wary of overly friendly wild animals, because many infected animals go through a "friendly" stage before entering the "rage" stage in which they bite everything. An unprovoked bite is a more likely sign than a provoked bite that an animal has rabies.

Any animal bite should be cleaned immediately and checked by a health-care provider. If the animal can be caught, it can be observed for signs of rabies infection. If the animal cannot be found, rabies treatment must be started. If the animal is destroyed or found dead, it should immediately be sent for testing, because examination of brain tissue will quickly show whether it had rabies.

RETINOBLASTOMA

See page 85.

REYE SYNDROME (RS)

RS involves swelling and increased pressure within the brain. The function of other body organs, especially the liver, is also affected. The exact cause of RS is unknown, but RS usually affects children 18 years of age and younger. The children are usually recovering from a recent viral illness, most commonly influenza or chickenpox. The relationship between RS and these viral infections is unknown, but aspirin-containing medication used to treat symptoms of these viral illnesses has also been linked with RS. Therefore, children should be given nonaspirin products such as acetaminophen (Tylenol®/Tempra®) instead of aspirin products during influenza, chickenpox, or any other illness with fever, unless instructed otherwise by a health-care provider. Some over-the-counter medications such as Pepto Bismol® contain aspirin (which may be listed as ASA or acetylsalicylic acid), and should also be avoided. Children should never be given any medication without direction from a health-care provider.

SIGNS AND SYMPTOMS. Lethargy, repeated vomiting, irritability, disorientation, slurred speech, and a staggering walk are symptoms of RS and lead to coma, during which time the child may require mechanical breathing assistance (ventilation).

TREATMENT. Early diagnosis is essential because the child must be closely observed in a hospital intensive care unit. Although there is no cure, medications, intravenous fluids, and mechanical breathing assistance (ventilation) can help counteract the damage from RS while it runs its course. With early treatment, the child usually recovers without permanent damage. Without early treatment the rate of death from RS is very high. Fortunately, there has been a significant drop in RS cases in recent years.

TAY-SACHS DISEASE

Also called GM2 gangliosidosis.

This is the most well known of the Jewish genetic diseases and is an autosomal recessive disorder. The incidence among the Ashkenazic Jewish population (Jews of central and eastern European descent) is approximately 1 in 3,600 live births; the estimated carrier rate is 1 in 30. The incidence is also as high in French Canadians from eastern Quebec. The incidence among the non-Jewish populations and non-French Canadians is approximately 1 in 90,000 to 360,000 live births; the estimated carrier rate is 1 in 150 to 300. Tay-Sachs disease is caused by a deficiency of the enzyme hexosaminidase A, which makes the body unable to break down (metabolize) fats in the brain. Without adequate amounts of this enzyme, harmful fatty substances build within brain and nerve cells and destroy them.

SIGNS AND SYMPTOMS. Infants typically begin to show symptoms at 4 to 6 months of age. A previously healthy, normal child begins to lose muscle coordination and by one year is unable to perform even simple tasks. The child begins to have muscle spasms and seizures and eventually becomes paralyzed. Progressive mental deterioration, blindness, and deafness also occur, with death occurring by age five.

TREATMENT. There is no treatment for this disease. Providing as much comfort and support as possible to the child and family is important. Testing to identify people who carry the mutant gene is available.

TOURETTE SYNDROME (TS)

Generally classified as a tic disorder, Tourette syndrome is thought to be transmitted through an autosomal dominant inheritance pattern with varying degrees of expression. Recent studies indicate it to be fairly common and perhaps associated with attention deficit hyperactivity disorder, obsessive-compulsive disorder, and some anxiety and depressive disorders. The syndrome is seen more often in males than in females, with symptoms first beginning between two and 15 years of age.

SIGNS AND SYMPTOMS. Symptoms include uncontrolled, recurrent twitching of the face, head, and shoulders, with shouting episodes (sometimes of obscenities), other verbal noises (including snorting sounds), and obsessive-compulsive behavior. Symptoms vary greatly from person to person.

TREATMENT. Medication has had varying degrees of success. Most cases of Tourette syndrome are mild and do not require medication. Behavioral therapy may be helpful.

TUBEROUS SCLEROSIS (TS)

The incidence is approximately 1 in 10,000 to 50,000 live births, with perhaps greater than 50% of cases being the result of new mutation in the egg or sperm. It is transmitted through an autosomal dominant inheritance pattern. Tuberous sclerosis causes a wide range of symptoms among affected people. It causes abnormal tissue growths or tumors on the skin and in internal organs. A small percentage of people develop cancerous tumors.

SIGNS AND SYMPTOMS. Tuberous sclerosis occurs in varying degrees and can cause a variety of benign skin tumors and/or lesions, including a red rash on the face, white birthmark lesions, or tumors around the nails or in patches along the skin. The lesions can also occur in the brain, eyes, and heart. Mental retardation, mental deterioration, and seizures may accompany brain involvement.

TREATMENT. There is no cure for tuberous sclerosis; support for the individual and the family is important.

TUMORS OF THE NERVOUS SYSTEM

Tumors can arise anywhere in the nervous system (NS). NS tumors can be primary tumors, meaning they started within the NS, or secondary tumors, meaning they started somewhere else in the body and spread (metastasized) to the NS. NS tumors can be cancerous (malignant) or noncancerous (benign). Brain tumor is the most common type of solid tumor occurring in children and is second only to leukemia as the most common type of childhood cancer. Although most types of NS tumors are not genetic, a few are. NS tumors are usually named after the type of NS tissue they involve.

SIGNS AND SYMPTOMS. Specific symptoms depend on the areas of brain/nervous system involved. Brain tumor growth usually obstructs the flow of cerebrospinal fluid through the ventricles, resulting in increased pressure in the brain (intracranial pressure). Although NS tumors cause a variety of symptoms, headaches and unexplained vomiting are practically universal. Other symptoms include vision or hearing disturbances, loss of coordination and/or balance, numbness, and muscle weakness or paralysis. Any persistent or unexplained symptoms like these should be checked immediately by a health-care provider.

TREATMENT. If possible, the NS tumor is surgically removed; radiation and chemotherapy may also be used. Nonmalignant tumors are usually easier to surgically remove than malignant tumors unless they are in a difficult-to-reach area. The rate of successful removal of NS tumors has improved due to recent advancements in surgical methods and techniques. Untreated tumors, malignant and nonmalignant, can result in death. Relatives of children with brain tumors should receive regular health evaluations because their risk of developing brain tumors is higher than the general population's.

SECTION 7
THE NERVOUS SYSTEM

Check any of the following structural defects of the nervous system that were present at birth.

7.1   Encephalocele: document how it was treated, if known. Document any permanent mental or physical limitations or impairments resulting from the encephalocele.

7.2   Spina bifida occulta or spina bifida cystica: if cystica, indicate if the spinal cord and nerves were involved (meningomyelocele or myelo-meningocele). Document treatment, if known, and any associated permanent mental or physical limitations or impairments (such as long-term hydrocephalus, paralysis, etc.).

7.3   Document any other structural defects of the nervous system, if present, and treatment, if known.

Check any of the following diseases and disorders of the nervous system that are or were present.

7.4   Alzheimer disease (AD): indicate at what age symptoms began. Document treatment, if known.

7.5   Amyotrophic lateral sclerosis (ALS, also known as Lou Gehrig's disease): indicate at what age symptoms began. Document treatment, if known.

7.6   Cerebral palsy (CP): document the type of CP as spastic, athetoid (dyskinetic), ataxic, or other, if known. Document the cause of cerebral palsy, if known.

7.7   Encephalitis: indicate at what age(s) and the type or cause (viral, bacterial, fungal, or parasitic) of encephalitis for each occurrence, if known. Document any mental or physical limitations or impairments resulting from the encephalitis.

7.8   Epilepsy: indicate at what age epilepsy began. Indicate the type of epilepsy, type of seizure activity, and any triggering events, if known. Document treatment, if known.

7.9   Familial dysautonomia (Riley-Day syndrome).

7.10   Febrile seizures as an infant or young child: document ages when febrile seizures occurred.

7.11   Galactosemia.

7.12   Guillain-Barré syndrome (GBS): indicate at what age symptoms began. Indicate treatment, if known.

7.13   Huntington disease (HD): indicate at what age symptoms began.

7.14   Hydrocephalus: indicate if present at birth (congenital) or, if developed later, indicate at what age. Document the cause of the hydro-cephalus and treatments, if known.

7.15   Infantile autism: indicate the age symptoms began. Document treatments, if known.

7.16   Meningitis: indicate at what age(s) and the type or cause (viral, bacterial, chemical, etc.) of meningitis, if known. Document any mental or physical limitations or impairments resulting from the encephalitis.

7.17　Menkes syndrome.

7.18　Migraine headaches.

7.19　Multiple sclerosis (MS): indicate at what age symptoms began.

7.20　Myasthenia gravis (MG): indicate at what age symptoms began.

7.21　Neurofibromatosis (NF1): if another type of neurofibromatosis, indicate which type. List the age it was diagnosed.

7.22　Parkinson disease: indicate at what age symptoms began. Indicate treatment, if known.

7.23　Phenylketonuria (PKU).

7.24　Rabies: indicate if the rabies was treated.

7.25　Reye syndrome (RS): indicate at what age.

7.26　Tay-Sachs disease.

7.27　Tourette syndrome (TS): indicate at what age symptoms began. Document specific behaviors, if known.

7.28　Tuberous sclerosis (TS).

7.29　Tumors of the brain or spinal cord: indicate at what age(s) these were diagnosed and whether malignant (cancerous) or benign (noncancerous). If malignant, document whether the cancer was primary (began in the brain or spinal cord) or secondary (spread from a cancer site elsewhere in the body), if known. Indicate the specific type of tumor, if known, and how treated. If the tumor was a primary cancer, document any areas/organs of the body to which the cancer spread (metastasized), if known.

7.30　Document any other diseases or disorders of the nervous system that are or were present, the age of onset, and treatment(s) received, if known.

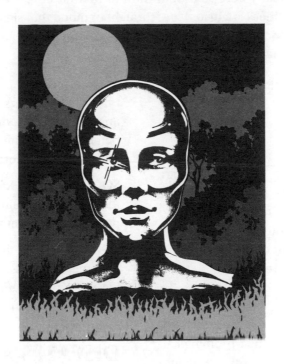

CHAPTER 8
MENTAL ILLNESS

STRUCTURES AND FUNCTIONS
CAUSES OF MENTAL ILLNESS
DISEASES AND DISORDERS

o universally accepted definition of mental illness exists. In general,
mental illness is a disorder of thought or mood that significantly impairs
judgment, behavior, the capacity to recognize reality, or the ability to cope with
the ordinary demands of living.

STRUCTURES AND FUNCTIONS

There are no clear-cut structures or functions of the psychological part of a human being as there are with the physical systems of the body. Rather, the psychiatric or mental aspect of an individual seems to involve an integration of physiological well-being, personality development, intellect, emotion, self-concept, spirituality, and social interaction.

CAUSES OF MENTAL ILLNESS

Experts do not always agree on the exact cause of mental illness. Current theories focus on biological, psychological, behavioral, and social-interpersonal factors. Some mental illnesses occur at much higher rates of incidence within some families than in the general population. Whether this occurs because of genetic transmission of a mental illness or because certain behaviors are learned from family members and close friends who have mental disorders is controversial. As more is learned about human genes and the traits and characteristics they control, the causes of many mental illnesses may be discovered.

BIOLOGICAL THEORISTS propose that physical factors cause mental illness. Possible physical causes include the inheritance of gene mutations that can be passed from one generation to the next, the presence of chemical imbalances in the brain, physical diseases, physical injuries, or a combination of these.

PSYCHOLOGICAL THEORISTS propose that faulty development of the mind and personality are the cause of mental illness. They suggest that early childhood experiences mold the mind and personality for life. Thus, responses to situations as an adult are based on early childhood experiences. The belief, then, is that negative or harmful experiences can cause inadequate psychiatric development and contribute to the onset of mental illness at any time during the lifespan.

BEHAVIORAL THEORISTS propose that behavior is learned. Reinforcing some behaviors and not rein-

forcing others causes certain behaviors to be learned and others to be dropped. The belief, then, is that behaviors associated with mental illness are somehow reinforced and therefore learned.

SOCIAL-INTERPERSONAL THEORISTS propose that mental illness results from the interactions between people and their environment.

It is possible that no single theory fully explains any mental illness. There are probably many factors, both genetic and environmental, that can increase or decrease a person's risk of developing mental illness at any time.

DISEASES AND DISORDERS

ANXIETY DISORDERS

Anxiety describes apprehension, uneasiness, uncertainty, or dread that results from feeling threatened or stressed.

Anxiety disorders, in general, seem to occur more often in females than males. Suspected risk factors include family history, certain medical conditions such as thyroid gland abnormalities and adrenal gland abnormalities, chemical substance intoxication or withdrawal, exposure to physical or psychological danger or threats, long-term exposure to criticism or disapproval, and the holding of unrealistic goals or beliefs. Anxiety in normal levels is essential for human survival. Normal anxiety is the force that makes people do things like study for a test, stop at red lights, and pay bills. However, anxiety can reach harmful levels. The higher the level of anxiety, the more likely the person will have trouble concentrating, learning, solving problems, and thinking logically. In addition, as anxiety levels increase, the person may talk louder and faster, feel restless, have body tremors, be disorganized and irritable, and engage in seemingly purposeless repetitive behaviors (e.g., hand wringing or pacing).

SIGNS AND SYMPTOMS. Many people occasionally exhibit symptoms of anxiety disorder without actually having an anxiety disorder. The frequency and severity of symptoms and the impact those symptoms have on interpersonal relationships and job, school, and home responsibilities determine whether there is a serious problem. Anxiety disorders include obsessive-compulsive, panic, phobic, and post-traumatic stress disorders.

OBSESSIVE–COMPULSIVE DISORDER (OCD)

Obsessions are thoughts, urges, or emotions that a person cannot stop thinking about. Compulsion is the uncontrollable performance of seemingly senseless, repetitive acts (rituals) that a person carries out in an attempt to prevent something bad from happening. Trying to resist the compulsion only increases anxiety. Common ritualistic behaviors seen in people with OCD include washing and cleaning excessively, checking and rechecking, or behaving according to very rigid guidelines (for example, putting on and removing socks exactly 11 times before putting on shoes). OCD usually first appears during adolescence or young adulthood.

PANIC DISORDER

Panic disorder is characterized by recurrent and usually unpredictable episodes of anxiety that reach a level of panic or terror and last from minutes to hours. Panic disorder usually first appears in late adolescence to early adulthood.

PHOBIC DISORDER

The primary feature of phobic disorders is an irrational fear of an object, activity, or situation that precipitates extreme anxiety, causing a person to go to great lengths to avoid it. Experts believe that the phobic person is not really afraid of the trigger itself, but is unconsciously displacing the real source of anxiety (such as guilt or a fear of losing a personal relationship) to an external source (such as a fear of social situations, enclosed spaces, animals, etc.). Phobic disorders can appear at any time from childhood through late adulthood.

POST-TRAUMATIC STRESS DISORDER (PTSD)

PTSD is characterized by anxiety symptoms that occur after a traumatic experience, such as being raped, being held prisoner of war, or having a home devastated. The person with PTSD may relive the traumatic event in nightmares and daydreams, avoid people and situations associated with the incident, have insomnia, be irritable, and suppress emotions. PTSD can occur at any time, even years, after the traumatic event.

TREATMENT. Depending on the specific anxiety disorder, treatment may include individual, group, and/or family therapy, relaxation techniques, behavior modification, and use of antianxiety or antidepressant medication. Hospitalization may be required.

EATING DISORDERS

People with eating disorders are preoccupied with food and their own physical appearance. Suspected risk factors include family history (with mounting evidence supporting a genetic predisposition), chemical imbalances in the brain, history of depression, low self-esteem, feelings of powerlessness, high expectations from family members, perfectionistic behaviors, and life in a society that worships thinness. Two eating disorders are anorexia nervosa and bulimia nervosa.

ANOREXIA NERVOSA

Anorexia nervosa is a potentially fatal self-imposed starvation that maintains an inappropriately low body weight for a person's age and height and is based on an unrealistic fear of becoming or being fat. Although anorexia nervosa is seen in both sexes, it most frequently occurs in adolescent girls and in women.

SIGNS AND SYMPTOMS. People with anorexia nervosa continue to diet even after reaching a weight below that appropriate for their height and age; they "feel fat" despite extreme weight loss and an emaciated appearance; and they become obsessed with thinness and counting calories. Some people become engrossed with nutrition and food preparation, and may in fact become expert gourmet or health food cooks, although they do not themselves eat the food they prepare. People often hoard and hide food without eating it, exercise excessively, have low self-esteem, lack assertiveness, and are confused and anxious about their sexuality and about taking on adult roles. Some people with anorexia nervosa have episodes of eating a large quantity of food in a short period of time (a food binge) followed by self-induced vomiting and/or the overuse of laxatives or diuretics (a purge)—behavior that is commonly seen in people with bulimia nervosa (see page 112). Anorexia nervosa eventually causes physical symptoms and body changes. These include the cessation of menstruation, changes in the distribution of body hair, muscle weakness, dehydration, anemia, low blood pressure and slowed heart rate, constipation, mouth sores and tooth decay, a decrease in the rate of body metabolism, and a drop in body temperature. Longstanding anorexia can affect the function of the heart, liver, and bone marrow and cause a loss of calcium from bones (osteoporosis).

TREATMENT. Treatment usually includes diet therapy to attain sufficient nutrition to promote a gradual weight gain; individual, group, and/or family therapy; and medication to treat anxiety and depression. Hospitalization may be required for treatment because weight loss can be so severe it is life threatening.

BULIMIA NERVOSA

Bulimia nervosa involves repeated episodes of binging (eating a tremendous quantity of food in a short period of time) with little self-control. The binging episode usually stops when abdominal pain, interruption, or physical exhaustion occurs. Foods most commonly eaten during binging are high calorie carbohydrates such as sweets, pastries, and other deserts. Bulimia nervosa is also frequently associated with purging (self-induced vomiting and/or overuse of laxatives and diuretics) to rid the body of food eaten during a binge period so as to prevent weight gain, and in a sense to regain self-control. Unlike people with anorexia nervosa who weigh much less than they should, people with bulimia nervosa often have an average weight for their age and height. Although binging and purging behavior is sometimes seen in people with anorexia nervosa, the two eating disorders are recognized as separate entities. Bulimia nervosa usually occurs in adolescent and young adult women, although it is being diagnosed in men and in older women more now than in the past.

SIGNS AND SYMPTOMS. People with bulimia nervosa have binging and purging episodes, sometimes more than 10 a week. They often participate in strict dieting between binges, feel guilty and depressed because they realize that their eating pattern is abnormal and they cannot control it, are dissatisfied with their body weight but do not have the distorted body image common in people with anorexia nervosa, have low self-esteem, and feel powerless. Physical symptoms include weakness, dehydration, low blood pressure and irregular heart rate, numbness and tingling of the hands and feet, tooth decay and discoloration (due to continued exposure of the teeth to stomach acids during self-induced vomiting), and abrasions on the knuckles (from scraping against the front teeth as the fingers are put down the throat to induce vomiting). Bulimia nervosa can become life threatening.

TREATMENT. Treatment usually involves assisting the person to gain control over eating habits; individual, group, and/or family therapy; and antidepressant medication. Hospitalization may be required.

MOOD DISORDERS

These disturbances of emotions, mood, and behavior can range from extreme elation and euphoria to extreme depression. Suspected risk factors include family history, chemical imbalances in the brain, neurological disorders such as brain tumors and Alzheimer disease, and loss or change in lifestyle such as death of a loved one, divorce, loss of job, or illness. Mood disorders are sometimes the side effects of physical illness and of certain medications such as hormones, sedatives, and anticancer agents. Two mood disorders are unipolar and bipolar depression.

UNIPOLAR DEPRESSION

Also known as major depression.

Unipolar depression can appear in children and adults, both male and female. Women, however, are more likely to seek treatment for depression than men.

SIGNS AND SYMPTOMS. Depression causes feelings of extreme sadness, helplessness, a sense of loss of control, hopelessness, low self-esteem, worthlessness, and decreased interest in routine activities such as practicing personal hygiene, eating, meeting job and school requirements, and socializing. Thoughts of and attempts to commit suicide may be signs of depression. Children with depression may be withdrawn, aggressive, or problematic in school, or have frequent unwarranted physical complaints. No matter at what age depression occurs, symptoms can range from mild to severe and last from weeks to years.

TREATMENT. Depending on the type or severity of symptoms, hospitalization may be necessary. Treatment may involve antidepressant medication and individual, group, and/or family counseling. Electroconvulsive (shock) therapy may be indicated for some individuals.

BIPOLAR DISORDER

Formerly called manic depression.

Bipolar disorder is characterized by mood swings from mania (episodes of euphoria and excitability) to severe depression. It occurs in both women and men, usually first appearing after age 30. For bipolar disorder to be diagnosed, at least one episode of manic symptoms must have occurred, although current and predominant symptoms may be those of depression.

SIGNS AND SYMPTOMS. During the manic phase, the person may have elated moods, hyperactivity, hallucinations (hearing, seeing, or smelling things that others do not hear, see, or smell), delusions (beliefs that do not agree with reality), poor judgment, rapid speech, irritability, racing thoughts, feelings of extreme importance, decreased sleeping and eating, impulsiveness, and aggressive behavior. Job, school, and social skills may be impaired. The severity of manic symptoms range from mild to severe.

Manic behavior in children and adolescents may also include hyperactivity, temper outbursts, short attention span, trouble with the law, disturbances in school performance, and problems in interpersonal relationships.

During the depressive phase, the person exhibits symptoms of unipolar depression (see page 112).

TREATMENT. Treatment for bipolar disorder varies with the type and severity of symptoms and may involve antimanic and antidepressant medication, and individual, group, and/or family therapy. Hospitalization may be necessary.

PSYCHOTIC DISORDERS

SCHIZOPHRENIA

Schizophrenia is a collective diagnosis for a group of chronic disorders characterized by intermittent episodes of disturbance in thoughts, beliefs, emotions, behaviors, and interpersonal relationships. Schizophrenia is classified as disorganized, catatonic, paranoid, undifferentiated, or residual. Schizophrenia is equally common in men and women; it usually appears in late adolescence or early adulthood, but it can occur earlier or later in life.

Suspected risk factors include family history (many experts believe schizophrenia is a genetic disorder); chemical imbalances in the brain; physical conditions such as head injury, brain tumor, or stroke; feelings of loss of love and nurturing early in life; and stressful events such as a loss, change in health or lifestyle, or physical or sexual assault.

SIGNS AND SYMPTOMS. Depending on the specific type of schizophrenia, symptoms commonly include delusions (beliefs that do not agree with reality), hallucinations (hearing, seeing, or smelling things that others do not hear, see, or smell), confused thinking, withdrawal into self, staying in one position for long periods of time or moving about almost constantly, disturbances in speech, and paranoia.

Schizophrenia does not involve multiple personalities and should not be confused with multiple personality disorder.

TREATMENT. Depending on the type and severity of symptoms, treatment can include antipsychotic medication; individual, group, and/or family therapy; social skills training; and hospitalization.

INSTRUCTIONS: To be sure your health-care provider has all the information needed to plan and individualize your health care, answer the following questions after you read Chapter 8, Mental Illness. Write your answers in Section 8 of the *GENETIC CONNECTIONS*™ *HEALTH HISTORY FORM,* which you will find at the back of this book. Use a separate *HEALTH HISTORY FORM* for each family member.

NOTE: Check any of the following mental illnesses that are or were present.

SECTION 8
MENTAL ILLNESS

8.1 Anxiety disorder: indicate the type as obsessive-compulsive disorder, panic disorder, phobic disorder, or post-traumatic stress disorder; or specify others, if known. Indicate at what age symptoms began. Document any treatment(s) received, if known.

8.2 Eating disorder: indicate the type as anorexia nervosa or bulimia nervosa; or specify other, if known. Indicate at what age symptoms began. Document treatment(s), if known.

8.3 Mood disorder: indicate the type as unipolar depression (major depression) or bipolar depression (manic depression), if known. Indicate at what age symptoms began. Document any treatment(s), if known.

8.4 Schizophrenia: indicate the type of schizophrenia as disorganized, catatonic, paranoid, undifferentiated, or residual, if known. Indicate at what age symptoms began. Document treatment(s), if known.

8.5 Document any other mental illnesses that are or were present, the age of the individual at the onset of the disorder, and treatment(s) received, if known.

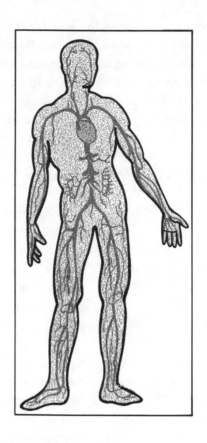

CHAPTER 9

THE CARDIOVASCULAR SYSTEM

STRUCTURES AND FUNCTIONS
COMMON RISK FACTORS
STRUCTURAL BIRTH DEFECTS
DISEASES AND DISORDERS

The cardiovascular or circulatory system consists of the heart and all the blood vessels, including the arteries and veins. The cardiovascular system circulates blood throughout the body, delivering oxygen and nutrients to and transporting waste away from each cell. Arteries are the vessels that lead away from the heart and distribute oxygen and nutrients throughout the body's tissues; veins are the vessels that collect blood returning from the body's tissues and carry it back into the heart. The heart itself is the pump that keeps the blood flowing through the vessels. As long as the heart pumps effectively and the vessels of the body remain intact and open, the circulatory system can function.

STRUCTURES AND FUNCTIONS

The heart lies within the chest (thoracic) cavity between the lungs and behind the breastbone (sternum), extending more into the left side of the chest than the right. The heart is surrounded by a sac-like membrane called the pericardium. Between the pericardium and the slick surface of the heart is a small amount of fluid (pericardial fluid) that both lubricates and reduces friction between the two surfaces, allowing the heart to beat freely. The pericardium also helps to keep the heart in place.

The heart is made of muscle and is about the size of a fist. Blood flows through four hollow spaces in the heart called chambers: the right atrium and the left atrium, which collect blood returning to the heart; and the right ventricle and the left ventricle, which fill with blood from the atria and pump it into arteries for circulation. Valves within the heart act like one-way swinging doors, which open and close as the heart contracts and relaxes, to keep blood moving through the heart in one direction. There are four heart valves: one between each atrium and ventricle and one between each ventricle and the large vessels that exit them (see figure 9.3).

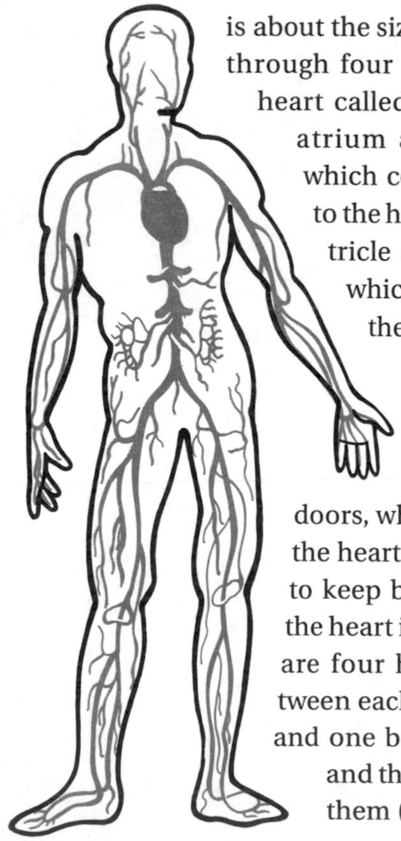

Figure 9.1. Arteries of the body

Heart muscle is made of specialized cells that make it unlike any other organ, allowing it to rhythmically and continuously contract and relax as one unit. The heart beats as the result of stimulation from specialized pacemaker cells located within the heart muscle itself. These pacemaker cells connect with one another and spread throughout the heart, forming a type of electrical conduction system (see figure 9.4). This conduction system allows the pacemaker's stimulation to travel throughout the entire heart muscle, causing the heart to beat again and again in coordinated movement. In adults, the heart's primary pacemaker cells stimulate the heart approximately 60 to 100 times per minute.

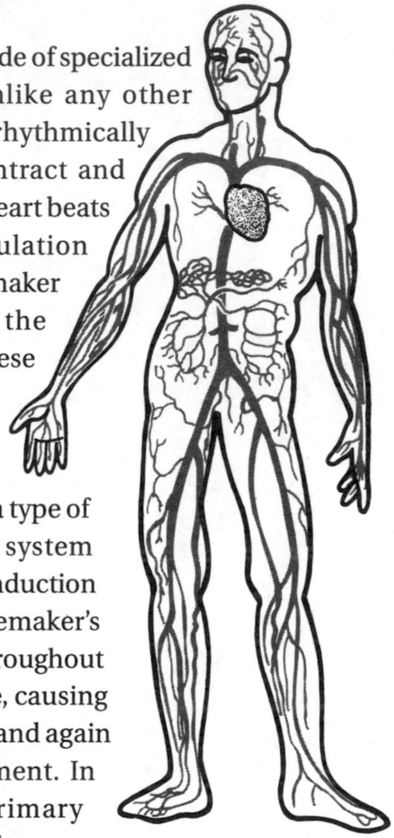

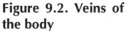

Figure 9.2. Veins of the body

Although the heart functions as one unit, it has right and left sides. These sides are separated within the heart by a muscular wall called the septum, so that blood flowing through one side does not cross over within the heart into the other side.

The right side of the heart consists of the right atrium and the right ventricle, which is the right heart's main pumping chamber. The right ventricle receives blood returning from the body through the veins and pumps it to circulate around the lungs. As this blood travels around the lungs it releases the carbon dioxide it has carried from the body's tissues, and then it loads up with oxygen.

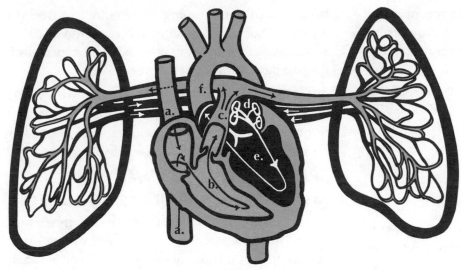

a. blood returning from the body enters the right atrium

b. it flows through the right atrio-ventricular valve into the right ventricle

c. the blood is then pumped through the pulmonic valve into the pulmonary artery to circulate around the lungs, where it releases carbon dioxide waste and picks up oxygen

d. the oxygenated blood flows to the left atrium

e. it then flows through the left atrio-ventricular valve into the left ventricle, which pumps the blood through the aortic valve

f. blood flows into the aorta to circulate throughout the body

Figure 9.3. Structures of the heart and the circulation of blood

The left side of the heart consists of the left atrium and the left ventricle, which is the left heart's main pumping chamber. The left ventricle receives the oxygen-rich blood from the lungs and pumps it throughout the body's arteries, supplying all body tissues with oxygen and other nutrients (see figure 9.3). The heart muscle itself expends a great deal of energy because of its continuous workload, and therefore it requires a great deal of oxygen and nutrients. The blood flowing through the coronary arteries supplies the heart with oxygen and nutrients.

Cardiovascular diseases affect the heart (cardio) and/or the body's arteries and veins (vascular). These cardiovascular diseases include atherosclerosis, coronary artery disease, hypertension, cerebral vascular accident (stroke), and peripheral vascular diseases. Often these disorders are interrelated and share common risk factors, and often one disorder contributes to the occurrence of another. The number of deaths attributed to cardiovascular disease has decreased steadily in recent years, in part due to public awareness of risk factors and healthier lifestyles. Despite these decreases, however, cardiovascular disease remains the number one killer of both men and women in the United States.

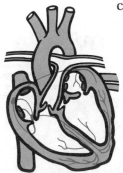

Figure 9.4. Electrical conduction system of the heart

COMMON RISK FACTORS OF HEART DISEASE

One very important risk factor associated with cardiovascular disease is family history. The incidence of heart disease within families strongly suggests that heredity directly contributes to its occurrence. People with a family history of cardiovascular disease, especially in family members aged 55 years or younger, should tell their health-care provider so they can receive appropriate annual screenings and testings.

Risk factors for cardiovascular disease can be divided into two groups: modifiable, meaning they can be changed or controlled, and nonmodifiable, meaning they cannot be changed or controlled.

MODIFIABLE RISK FACTORS

These include:

- high-fat/high-cholesterol diet
- high blood pressure
- cigarette or other tobacco use
- obesity
- lack of exercise
- diabetes
- oral contraceptives—which have been shown to cause high blood pressure, high cholesterol and blood sugar levels, and increased risk for blood clot formation in some women. Combined with cigarette smoking, oral contraceptives increase the risk for the development of cardiovascular disease, including stroke. New studies are examining the use

of new "low-dose combination" oral contraceptives that seem to minimize the cardiovascular risks and may prove to actually reduce or slow the process of atherosclerosis. Women should discuss their family history and other cardiovascular risk factors with their health-care provider before choosing a method of birth control.

NONMODIFIABLE RISK FACTORS

These include:

- family history
- increasing age
- gender: men with cardiovascular disease still outnumber women, but the gap is rapidly closing; after menopause the incidence of cardiovascular disease for women is almost equal to that for men
- race: the incidence for Blacks is higher than for Whites, especially in combination with high blood pressure, which itself contributes to other forms of cardiovascular disease including atherosclerosis and stroke.

STRUCTURAL BIRTH DEFECTS
CONGENITAL HEART DEFECTS (CHD)

Also called congenital heart disease.

The incidence is approximately 1 in 200 live births, male or female. CHDs are abnormalities in the structures of the heart or of the two large vessels leaving the heart: the pulmonary artery and the aorta. More than one CHD may be present. The heart is one of the first organs formed in embryonic development. By week 4 of pregnancy the heart is already beating, and by week 7 all four chambers and valves of the heart are formed. A disruption in fetal development during these early, critical weeks can result in CHDs. Factors associated with their occurrence include family history, maternal rubella infection during pregnancy, maternal diabetes during pregnancy, and prenatal exposure to alcohol or cocaine. CHDs occur at higher rates with some chromosome disorders (e.g., Down syndrome).

SIGNS AND SYMPTOMS. CHDs vary in severity. Symptoms depend on the location, size, and type of defect, how it interferes with blood flow through the heart and body, and whether delivery of oxygen to body tissues is impaired. When present, general symptoms of CHD include fatigue, intolerance of exercise, susceptibility to respiratory infections, shortness of breath, and sometimes a blue color to the skin (cyanosis) because of a lack of oxygen. Although CHDs are present at birth, they may not become evident until the first days or weeks of life, or even later.

TREATMENT. Not so long ago children with CHDs rarely survived, but thanks to advances in medical technology and surgical techniques, a great number of children survive to live long and healthy lives.

SPECIFIC TYPES OF CHD
ATRIAL AND VENTRICULAR SEPTAL DEFECTS

These defects are characterized by the presence of "holes" in the heart where there should be none. Atrial septal defects (ASD) are openings in the wall between the two upper chambers of the heart (the atria); ventricular septal defects (VSD) are openings in the wall between the two lower chambers of the heart (the ventricles) (see figure 9.5). Because the pressure in the left side of the heart is greater than the pressure in the right side, blood is shunted across these openings from left to right. ASD and VSD do not cause cyanosis, because the blood shunting across the defect already contains oxygen; however, the excess blood entering the right side of the heart causes an increase in blood sent to the lungs. This can damage the lungs or cause congestive heart failure if the defect is large. Many septal defects close spontaneously by the age of five or six years; some require surgical closure.

PATENT DUCTUS ARTERIOSUS (PDA)

PDA occurs when a blood flow channel that was necessary during fetal life, but not needed after birth, fails to close. When it stays open (patent), normal blood circulation is impaired. Some PDAs eventually close spontaneously, some respond to medication, and some require surgical closure (see figure 9.5).

STENOSIS

Some defects involve a narrowing (stenosis) of the structures of the

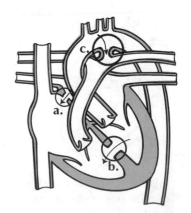

Figure 9.5.
Congenital heart defects:
a. atrial septal defect
b. ventricular septal defect
c. patent ductus arteriosus
Source: D.L.Wong, *Whaley & Wong's Essentials of Pediatric Nursing*, 4th ed. (1993). Used by permission. Modified.

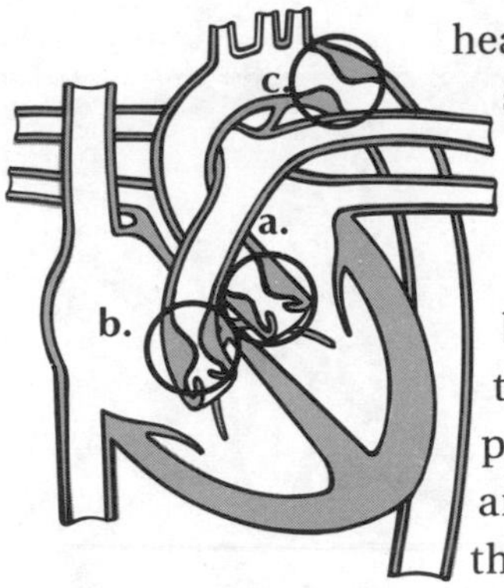

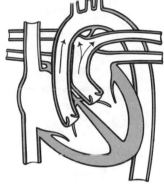

Figure 9.6. Stenosis:
a. aortic stenois
b. pulmonary stenosis
c. coarctation of the aorta
Source: D.L.Wong, *Whaley & Wong's Essentials of Pediatric Nursing*, 4th ed. (1993). Used by permission. Modified.

heart or the great vessels, obstructing the normal flow of blood through and/or out of the heart. Stenosis can occur at the valve areas, below the valves, or above the valves. Aortic stenosis, pulmonary stenosis, and coarctation (constriction) of the aorta are examples of obstructive defects (see figure 9.6). Except in severe cases they do not cause cyanosis; instead, they usually lead to pressure buildup in front of (before) the stenosis and decreased pressure beyond (after) the stenosis. Stenosis significantly increases the workload of the heart. Surgical correction is usually required.

TRANSPOSITION

Some CHDs involve malformations of heart structures. Transposition of the great vessels is a CHD in which the aorta arises from the right side of the heart and the pulmonary artery from the left side—the exact opposite of their normal positions—resulting in two totally non-communicating systems, with oxygenated blood going right back to the lungs over and over, and unoxygenated blood recirculating throughout the body again and again (see figure 9.7). If extra channels between the left and right heart are not present, such as an ASD, VSD, or PDA, death occurs. Surgical correction is indicated and a series of operations may be needed.

HYPOPLASTIC LEFT HEART SYNDROME

In this malformation, structures of the left side of the heart are underdeveloped. The major structure involved is the left ventricle, the major pump muscle of the heart. This defect is fatal without intervention, but

Figure 9.7.
Transposition of the great vessels: aorta and pulmonary artery
Source: D.L.Wong, *Whaley & Wong's Essentials of Pediatric Nursing*, 4th ed. (1993). Used by permission. Modified.

intervention is not always possible. Surgical correction or heart transplantation may be attempted.

TETRALOGY OF FALLOT

Tetralogy of Fallot involves four different defects: VSD, hypertrophy (enlargement) of the right ventricle, pulmonary artery stenosis (narrowing), and an enlargement of the aorta that is shifted toward the heart's right side. Commonly associated with cyanosis, tetralogy of Fallot usually requires surgical repair.

DISEASES AND DISORDERS

ANEURYSM

An aneurysm is a weakened or damaged area in the blood vessel wall that pouches or balloons out under the pressure within the vessel. Aneurysms occur primarily in arteries, but can also occur within the heart muscle itself. If arterial aneurysms rupture, they can result in severe hemorrhage (bleeding) and death. The weakened area in the vessel wall can be a congenital defect (present at birth) or can be associated with a genetic disorder such as Marfan syndrome. Because aneurysms can be caused by atherosclerosis, people with heart disease are at higher risk of aneurysm development.

SIGNS AND SYMPTOMS. An aneurysm frequently causes no symptoms. On physical examination the health-care provider may note pulsations or feel enlarged areas of the aorta within the abdomen, may hear whistling noises over some aneurysms with use of a stethoscope, or may note a decrease in blood pressure in arteries distant from the location of the aneurysm.

TREATMENT. Aneurysm may be treatable with surgical repair depending on its location. Surgical repairs made before rupture are usually highly successful. If an aneurysm ruptures, however, death may result rapidly unless repaired immediately. Some aneurysms are not treated immediately; before surgical repair is recommended, the aneurysm is reevaluated frequently to see whether it is enlarging.

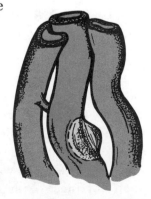

Figure 9.8. Aneurysm

ATHEROSCLEROSIS

Also known as hardening of the arteries.

Atherosclerosis is a process of plaque formation, which is made of fat and cholesterol. With atherosclerosis, plaque builds up inside the arteries, making the inside of the artery narrower and the artery itself stiff and hard (see figure 9.9). As the inside of the artery gets narrower, less blood can travel through the vessel and less oxygen and nutrients are delivered to the body tissues served by that vessel. Atherosclerosis causes many other cardiovascular disorders including coronary artery disease, myocardial infarction, high blood pressure, stroke, and peripheral vascular disease. It progresses slowly over many years and often begins during childhood.

SIGNS AND SYMPTOMS. See other cardiovascular disorders that follow.

TREATMENT. See the specific cardiovascular disorder.

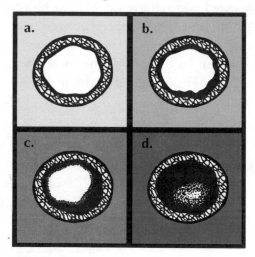

Figure 9.9. Progression of atherosclerosis:
a. normal artery b. atherosclerosis beginning
c. atherosclerosis progressing d. artery totally blocked

CEREBRAL VASCULAR ACCIDENT (CVA)

Also known as stroke.

CVA occurs when blood flow through an artery within the brain is interrupted (blocked), depriving the brain cells fed by that artery of the oxygen and nutrients they need to function and survive. Interruption may be the result of atherosclerosis that has narrowed the artery to the point of complete blockage; a blood clot that has formed within the artery; a circulating blood clot, piece of plaque, or any other debris in the blood that has traveled through the bloodstream from another part of the body; or the rupture or tear of an artery within the brain. The rupture of an artery in the brain can be caused by high blood pressure, especially if the vessel is hardened by atherosclerosis, or from injury (trauma) to the head. Regardless of the cause, a

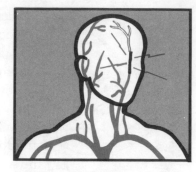

Figure 9.10. CVA (stroke): the result of an interruption in the blood supply to the brain

stroke can be fatal or result in permanent disability.

SIGNS AND SYMPTOMS. The effects of a stroke depend on the area of the brain involved and the functions controlled by that area; therefore, symptoms vary a great deal from one individual to another. There may be a loss of balance or muscle control of a specific body area or profound weakness and paralysis to an entire side of the body. Speech or the ability to comprehend another's speech may be impaired. People having a CVA may be disoriented, confused, emotionally erratic, or unresponsive. Regardless of the symptoms, immediate medical attention is necessary.

TREATMENT. The best treatment for stroke is prevention by minimizing the risk of atherosclerosis and other cardiovascular diseases; for example, controlling high blood pressure and diabetes. With treatment and rehabilitation some of the effects of stroke can be minimized; some resolve completely. Many people, however, have some remaining physical and/or neurological impairment.

CONGESTIVE HEART FAILURE (CHF)

In CHF, the heart fails to pump effectively. The general circulation of oxygen and nutrients is impaired and blood flow through the heart backs up, causing congestion. Many disorders can lead to congestive heart failure, including coronary artery disease, myocardial infarction (heart attack), hypertension (high blood pressure), rheumatic heart disease, and congenital heart defects.

SIGNS AND SYMPTOMS. CHF may cause mild to severe symptoms and can result in death. The symptoms depend on whether the right, left, or both sides of the heart are failing. If the left side fails, blood congests around the lungs. This causes difficulty in breathing, because fluid is forced from the congested blood vessels into the lungs themselves (see figure 9.11). Rapid breathing, cough, rapid heart rate, bluish or pale skin, and eventual mental confusion can result. If the right side fails, which can occur by left heart failure (and vice versa), blood congests in the peripheral veins, causing fluid to leak from the veins into the tissues of the lower legs and feet and into the abdominal organs, including the liver (see figure 9.11). This results in swelling (edema) of the legs, feet, and other dependent areas, and in abdominal discomfort.

As the heart muscle weakens, it enlarges and becomes less efficient. To compensate, the rate at which the heart beats increases. This actually works for a while, but in the long run the increased heart rate adds to the work of the heart and worsens the failure.

TREATMENT. CHF can be treated by first correcting underlying causes when possible, initiating lifestyle and dietary modifications as needed, and using medications. Lifelong medical management is generally required.

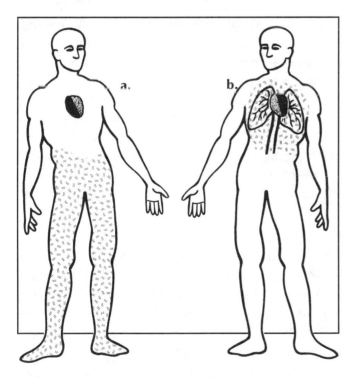

Figure 9.11. Congestive heart failure:

a. **congestive failure of the heart's right side—fluid accumulates in lower extremities and abdominal organs**

b. **congestive failure of the left side of the heart—fluid accumulates in and around the lungs**

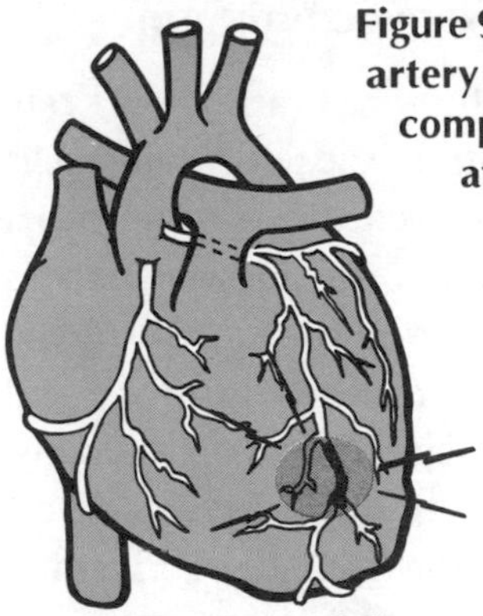

Figure 9.12. Narrowing of a coronary artery because of atherosclerosis: complete blockage causes heart attack (myocardial infarction)

CORONARY ARTERY DISEASE (CAD)

Also called coronary atherosclerotic heart disease (CAHD).

CAD occurs when atherosclerosis narrows the coronary arteries that supply the heart (see figure 9.12). As the *insides* of these arteries narrow, less oxygen and nutrients pass through to the heart muscle. This may not cause problems at rest, but when the heart has to work harder due to physical activity or emotional stress, its oxygen demands increase significantly.

SIGNS AND SYMPTOMS. When the extra oxygen cannot be supplied because of the narrowed coronary arteries, the heart muscle begins to ache and hurt. This type of chest pain is called angina pectoris, which literally means a choking, suffocating pain. Anginal pain may cause discomfort in the chest that radiates to the neck, jaw, or arms (usually the left arm); it may mimic indigestion.

TREATMENT. Rest alone may relieve angina, but to manage and/or prevent its recurrence, medications and lifestyle modifications are used. Anyone whose angina is not relieved by rest and/or medication within 5 to 10 minutes should be taken for immediate examination and evaluation, because unrelieved angina is a symptom of heart attack (myocardial infarction).

ELECTRICAL CONDUCTION DISORDERS
Also called dysrhythmia and arrhythmia.

Disturbances of the heart's rate or rhythm can be caused by abnormalities in the heart's electrical conduction system. The stimulus to beat (contract) travels along the conduction system and causes the heart muscle to beat in a top-to-bottom coordinated movement. The heart beats approximately 60 to 100 times per minute in most healthy adults. If the stimulus to beat (contract) comes from a different area than normal, if there is more than one stimulus, or if the stimulus repeats too rapidly or too slowly, an abnormal heart rate or rhythm results. These abnormal rates and rhythms are called dysrhythmias. Examples of dysrhythmia include: atrial flutter, a rapid heart rate in which the stimulus comes from the pacemaker cells of the atrium; ventricular tachycardia, a rapid heart rate in which the stimulus comes from pacemaker cells within the ventricles; atrial fibrillation, in which the atria do not contract in coordinated motion; and ventricular fibrillation, in which the ventricles do not contract in coordinated motion. Abnormal electrical conduction pathways may be the result of a congenital defect (present at birth) or damage or injury to the heart.

SIGNS AND SYMPTOMS. Some dysrhythmias are harmless and cause no symptoms, while others cause irregular heart rates that create the sensation of skipped beats or a racing, pounding heart, lightheadedness, and/or chest pain. Ventricular tachycardia and ventricular fibrillation are serious dysrhythmias that can cause sudden death.

TREATMENT. Many dysrhythmias are treatable with medication; others may require surgical or catheter intervention such as the insertion of an electrical pacemaker or an implantable cardioverter-defibrillator (ICD), which shocks the heart automatically should a life-threatening dysrhythmia occur; or eliminating (ablating) the pacemaker site that is causing the abnormal rhythm.

ENDOCARDITIS

Infection causes this inflammation of the inner lining of the heart and the heart valves. People with rheumatic heart disease and congenital heart defects are susceptible to it. Endocarditis can also occur after invasive heart procedures (for example, open heart surgery or catheter procedures) or after minor surgical procedures that sometimes introduce bacteria or other microorganisms into the bloodstream, such as dental, gastrointestinal, or gynecological procedures.

SIGNS AND SYMPTOMS. Signs of general illness, including fever, fatigue, cough, and signs of congestive heart failure or the presence of a heart murmur can occur with endocarditis.

TREATMENT. Endocarditis requires hospitalization and can have serious complications, including congestive heart failure and stroke. Antimicrobial medication for the specific microorganism causing the infection is given in treatment. Endocarditis can result in permanent damage to the heart valves and can recur.

FAMILIAL HYPERCHOLESTEROLEMIA
Also called type II hyperlipoproteinemia.

The incidence is variable, from 1 in 200 to 500 live births, with the disorder being transmitted through an autosomal dominant inheritance pattern. This is the most common hereditary disorder related to elevated blood fats. It results in elevated blood levels of fats (lipids), including triglycerides, cholesterol, and low-density lipoprotein (LDL, the "bad" cholesterol). It is sometimes categorized as type A, which is associated with increased cholesterol, and type B, which is associated with increased cholesterol and triglycerides. Both types A and B of familial hypercholesterolemia are associated with premature atherosclerosis, the underlying disorder of many cardiovascular diseases, including angina, heart attack, and stroke. This association is one reason heart disease runs in families and a good reason for people with a family history of hypercholesterolemia to seek early, regular health evaluations, especially if family members have been affected by cardiovascular disease before age 55.

SIGNS AND SYMPTOMS. Many people with familial hypercholesterolemia have yellowish fat nodules or plaques, called xanthomas, on the skin or eyes from the deposit of excess blood fats. Xanthomas can also be located internally within bones or organs, including the heart. If there is a history of familial hypercholesterolemia, children should be screened beginning at age three. Earlier screening is not recommended because infants and young toddlers need to maintain adequate amounts of fat in their diets for normal development of the central nervous system (brain).

TREATMENT. Diet modifications to limit the intake of fats and cholesterol are recommended, although low-fat diets generally fail to lower blood fat levels very much. Medication can also help reduce blood cholesterol levels.

HYPERTENSION (HTN)
Also known as high blood pressure.

Blood pressure is the force at which blood is circulated (pushed) within the arteries. Arteries contain oxygen-rich blood from the left side of the heart, which pumps at a much higher pressure than

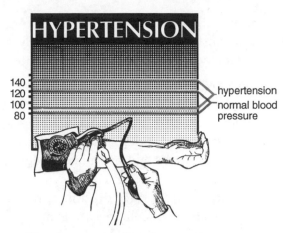

Figure 9.13. A blood pressure of 140/90 mmHg or greater indicates hypertension, commonly known as high blood pressure

the right side. As the heart muscle beats (contracts), blood is ejected with great force from the left ventricle into the arterial vessels. The pressure at this point is the maximum pressure the arteries are subjected to. This maximum pressure is represented by the top number of a blood pressure reading and is called the systolic pressure. As the heart relaxes between beats, the pressure within the arteries drops to a much lower pressure. This residual pressure is represented by the bottom number of a blood pressure reading and is called the diastolic pressure. This is the lowest pressure the arteries are subjected to. The normal average pressure for adults is 120/80 millimeters of mercury (mm Hg); however, deviations are normal, depending on a person's age and sex. Hypertension is defined as a consistent blood pressure of 140/90 or greater.

If untreated, the high force of blood flow begins to wear and tear on the arteries and other body organs, particularly the heart, brain, kidneys, and eyes. The constant high pressure exerted against the walls of the arteries causes damaged areas that are prone to plaque formation; in fact, hypertension causes atherosclerosis to progress more quickly and makes people with hypertension more likely to have heart attacks, strokes, and kidney disease, which often contribute to or cause death. Extreme hypertension can result in sudden, unexpected death from heart failure or hemorrhage (bleeding) from a ruptured artery within the brain.

Hypertension can be caused by other medical conditions, such as an obstruction in the artery that leads to the kidney, kidney disease, or some types of tumor. However, 90% to 95% of the time the exact cause is unknown; it is most likely caused by genetic or environmental factors, or the interaction of the two. Hypertension with unknown cause is called essential hypertension.

SIGNS AND SYMPTOMS. Some people experience headaches, dizziness, flushed skin, or nosebleeds. Usually there are no symptoms; thus, hypertension is known as the silent killer. In fact, it has been estimated that more than half the people who have high blood pressure do not know they have it. Children are not immune to high blood pressure: the American Heart Association estimates that more than two million children in the United States between the ages of 6 and 17 have hypertension. Children, regardless of their age, should have their blood pressure checked during their yearly physical exam, especially if there is a family history of hypertension.

TREATMENT. Hypertension can be controlled by losing weight, changing lifestyle and diet, quitting the use of tobacco, exercising regularly, reducing stress, and reducing the use of salt, alcohol, and/or medication. If medication is prescribed, it is important to continue taking it even though symptoms may subside.

MARFAN SYNDROME

The incidence worldwide is approximately 1 in 10,000 live births. Marfan syndrome is seen in both sexes and in all races and ethnic groups, and it is transmitted through an autosomal dominant inheritance pattern. As many as 25% of cases may be the result of a new mutation that occurred in the egg or sperm. The severity of Marfan syndrome varies greatly among affected people; this may be the result of a variety of different gene mutations that cause the disorder.

A protein called fibrillin, which normally makes the connective tissues within the body strong and elastic, is produced in a weak form in people with Marfan syndrome. The body tissues affected include the heart, blood vessels, bones, ligaments, and eyes.

Many people with Marfan syndrome are not diagnosed until adolescence or young adulthood; unfortunately, some are not diagnosed until tragedy has struck from deadly complications. For example, U.S. Olympic volleyball star Flo Hyman and University of Maryland basketball player Chris Patton both died suddenly as a result of Marfan syndrome, both from ruptures of weakened aortas. Thus, it is very important for people with a family history of Marfan syndrome to be tested (DNA testing is available to identify people who carry the Marfan gene). In women who have undiagnosed Marfan syndrome, death in late pregnancy or childbirth from aortic rupture is also a frequent event.

SIGNS AND SYMPTOMS. People with Marfan syndrome are usually tall and slim with unusually long and thin arms, legs, fingers, and toes. Muscle development is sometimes decreased, and people are typically loose jointed. Complications of Marfan syndrome include weak or prolapsed heart valves, weakness and aneurysm formation in the walls of the aorta and other major arteries (including arteries that feed the heart), scoliosis, and vision problems such as nearsightedness, with or without dislocation of the optic lens.

TREATMENT. People with Marfan syndrome can live long and productive lives, but they must be continually monitored so that heart, bone, and eye complications can be diagnosed and treated early. Cardiologists closely monitor the heart valves and the aorta (the large artery that exits the left side of the heart) for signs of weakness and aneurysm formation. Weakened areas can be surgically repaired to prevent sudden rupture. In some instances, medication is prescribed to decrease blood pressure and lessen the work of the heart to reduce the risk of vessel rupture. Braces or other support devices for Marfan-related scoliosis are sometimes recommended. An eye specialist should monitor eye involvement and prescribe necessary treatment. Corrective lenses for associated nearsightedness are almost always needed.

MYOCARDIAL INFARCTION (MI)

Also known as heart attack.

MI occurs when a coronary artery or one of its branches becomes totally blocked (occluded) (see figure 9.12). Complete occlusion of the artery may be the result of atherosclerosis, a blood clot, or a piece of plaque that has broken off and wedged into a narrower part of the artery. Whatever the cause, the results are the same. With the artery closed, the portion of heart muscle it served is deprived of oxygen and nutrients and begins to deteriorate and die, a process known as infarction. In most cases this causes extreme angina

(chest pain); however, some people have small infarctions and do not realize it or simply ignore their symptoms and avoid seeking medical attention.

SIGNS AND SYMPTOMS. Angina that occurs with MI typically begins suddenly, is not relieved by rest or medications, and progressively worsens. It is not always associated with physical exertion or stress like "typical" angina is, but often occurs during times of rest, even during sleep. Other symptoms include difficulty in breathing, dizziness, nausea and/or vomiting, and pale, cool, sweaty skin.

TREATMENT. MI is a medical emergency. If medical care is not received within the first few hours after the onset of symptoms, permanent damage to the heart muscle will result. If treatment is begun soon enough it can prevent or minimize the extent of permanent damage to the heart. Treatments, including the administration of medication that can dissolve the blood clot, or the use of a small balloon inserted and inflated in the area of blockage in the coronary artery (a method known as PTCA, percutaneous transluminal coronary angioplasty), can sometimes open the blocked coronary artery and restore blood supply to the infarcted area. Regardless of the situation and treatment regimen, the first hours and days after an MI are critical and require intensive care. If the MI is massive, death may occur regardless of treatment.

MYOCARDITIS

This inflammation of the heart muscle can be caused by infection, a reaction to medication, the progression of endocarditis or pericarditis, or unknown causes.

SIGNS AND SYMPTOMS. With myocarditis there may be no symptoms, or mild symptoms, including fatigue and fever, or serious symptoms, including congestive heart failure.

TREATMENT. People with myocarditis are treated according to the specific cause and usually require hospitalization.

PERICARDITIS

This inflammation of the membranous sac surrounding the heart (the pericardium) can be caused by infection, health disorders such as systemic lupus erythematosus or rheumatoid arthritis, or injury to the chest.

SIGNS AND SYMPTOMS. Pain in the chest that grows worse with breathing or twisting of the body may occur, or difficulty in breathing.

TREATMENT. People who develop pericarditis are treated according to the specific cause and generally need to be hospitalized.

PERIPHERAL VASCULAR DISEASE (PVD)

PVD involves the vessels along the outer parts (periphery) of the body. More specifically, PVD involves vessels beyond the heart such as those in the arms and legs. PVD can occur in arteries and veins (see figure 9.14).

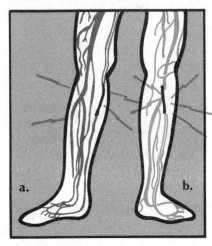

Figure 9.14.
Peripheral vascular disease:
a. in a leg vein   b. in an artery

PVD in arteries is frequently caused by atherosclerosis, although other things, such as injury to the arteries, can be responsible as well. In veins, blood clots (thrombosis or thrombophlebitis) or injury are frequent causes.

SIGNS AND SYMPTOMS. Blocked or impaired arterial blood flow causes pain, tissue death beyond the obstruction, and the formation of ulcers that often become infected with gangrene. If normal circulation is not restored, amputation may be required to halt gangrene infection. Blocked or impaired flow through the veins prevents blood from freely returning to the heart, causing local tissue swelling (edema) and the formation of varicose veins. Broken areas in the skin called stasis ulcers often develop because of the swelling and congestion of blood; they heal very slowly unless normal circulation is restored.

TREATMENT. The type of treatment for PVD depends on whether the arteries or veins are affected. People with PVD are taught to do exercises and to position their legs (which are most affected by PVD) in ways that improve blood circulation. Medications that improve blood flow, control pain, prevent blood clot formation, or treat infection may be a part of therapy. Surgery may

be required to improve blood flow or remove stasis ulcers or gangrenous tissue. Catheter procedures can be used to restore blood flow in some instances.

RHEUMATIC HEART DISEASE

In rheumatic heart disease one or more valves of the heart have been permanently damaged by rheumatic fever. Rheumatic fever can occur after an untreated strep throat infection and can affect the skin, joints, brain, and heart. When rheumatic fever affects the heart, minute pearl-like growths called vegetations or Aschoff's bodies occur along the heart valves and eventually form scar tissue. This scarring interferes with a valve's ability to function. In time the scar tissue begins to pull and draw tight, deforming the valve. With this distortion, the valve stops opening or closing completely, and either the heart muscle has to contract more forcefully to squeeze the normal amount of blood through the smaller opening, or blood continually leaks (regurgitates) back through the valve. A tendency to develop rheumatic fever has been noted to run in families, indicating a possible genetic predisposition.

SIGNS AND SYMPTOMS. Rheumatic heart disease usually causes no symptoms initially, but years down the road a new heart murmur caused by the disturbance in blood flow through the valve develops. Enlargement (hypertrophy) of the heart and heart failure can eventually result because of the increased work caused by leaking (incompetent) valve(s).

TREATMENT. Heart surgery to replace the damaged heart valve(s) is sometimes indicated; but the best treatment for rheumatic heart disease is to prevent rheumatic fever by recognizing and effectively treating strep throat infections. Since the discovery of antibiotics used to treat strep throat, the incidence of both rheumatic fever and rheumatic heart disease has dropped dramatically in developed countries, but worldwide it remains a major health threat.

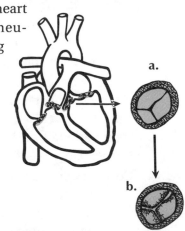

Figure 9.15.
Rheumatic heart disease:
a. normal heart valve
b. rheumatic heart valve

INSTRUCTIONS: To be sure your health-care provider has all the information needed to plan and individualize your health care, answer the following questions after you read Chapter 9, The Cardiovascular System. Write your answers in Section 9 of the *GENETIC CONNECTIONS™ HEALTH HISTORY FORM,* which you will find at the back of this book. Use a separate *HEALTH HISTORY FORM* for each family member.

SECTION 9
THE CARDIOVASCULAR SYSTEM

Check any of the following structural defects of the cardiovascular system that were present at birth.

9.1 Congenital heart defects, also known as congenital heart disease: document the specific type(s) as atrial septal defect, ventricular septal defect, coarctation of the aorta, aortic stenosis, pulmonary stenosis, transposition of the great vessels, tetralogy of Fallot, hypoplastic left heart syndrome, or others. Document treatments, if known.

9.2 Document any other structural defects of the heart or blood vessels, if present, and treatment(s), if known.

Check any of the following diseases and disorders of the cardiovascular system that are or were present.

9.3 Aneurysm: document the location of the aneurysm, if known, and how it was treated. Document any complications resulting from the aneurysm, if known.

9.4 Atherosclerosis (also known as hardening of the arteries).

9.5 Cerebral vascular accident (stroke, CVA): indicate at what age(s) and the area of the brain in which the stroke occurred, if known. Document any residual mental and/or physical limitations or impairments resulting from the stroke.

9.6 Congestive heart failure (CHF): indicate at what age it first occurred. Document whether it was right heart failure, left heart failure, or both, if known. Document treatments, if known.

9.7 Coronary artery disease (CAD), also known as atherosclerotic heart disease (ASHD): indicate at what age symptoms began. Document treatment, if known.

9.8 Abnormal heart rate or rhythm known as a dysrhythmia: indicate at what age it was first diagnosed (some are present at birth while others develop later). Document how it was treated.

9.9 Endocarditis (infection of the inside lining of the heart): indicate at what age(s), and how it was treated, if known.

9.10 Familial hypercholesterolemia: document type A or B, and treatment, if known.

9.11 High blood pressure (hypertension, HTN): indicate at what age it was diagnosed and how it was treated, if known.

9.12 Marfan syndrome: document treatments, if known.

9.13 Heart attack (myocardial infarction, MI): indicate at what age(s), and how it was treated, if known.

9.14 Myocarditis (infection of the muscle layer of the heart): indicate at what age(s), and how it was treated, if known.

9.15 Pericarditis (infection of the outer lining of the heart and the surrounding sac): indicate at what age(s), and how it was treated, if known.

9.16 Impaired circulation to the extremities (arms, legs, hands, feet) known as peripheral vascular disease (PVD): indicate at what age symptoms began, and whether it involved arteries (arterial PVD) or veins (venous PVD), if known.

9.17 Rheumatic heart disease: indicate at what age it was diagnosed and how it was treated.

9.18 Other heart valve disorders, such as mitral valve prolapse (MVP): document other specific heart valve abnormalities, if known, and how they were treated.

9.19 Document any other diseases or disorders of the cardiovascular system that are or were present, the age of onset, and treatment(s) that were received, if known.

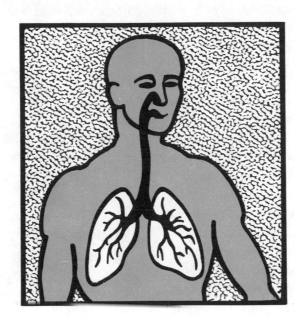

CHAPTER 10
THE RESPIRATORY SYSTEM

STRUCTURES AND FUNCTIONS
STRUCTURAL BIRTH DEFECTS
DISEASES AND DISORDERS

The respiratory system consists of the airway passages and structures from the nose to the lungs. The main job of the respiratory system is to get oxygen into and carbon dioxide out of the blood; this gas exchange is called respiration.

STRUCTURES AND FUNCTIONS

Breathing is an automatic task; it is performed without conscious thought or effort. It is controlled by the respiratory center located in the part of the brain stem called the medulla. The rate or depth of breathing can be controlled consciously, but the respiratory center is the main regulator responsible for continuous breathing. Because the respiratory system has direct contact with the outside environment, it has built-in protective structures. For example, the respiratory tracts (air passages) are lined with a moist, mucus-producing membrane that traps germs and other debris as they are breathed into the body. This lining has tiny hairs called cilia that flap in a wave-like motion to move the mucus and trapped particles toward the throat (see figure 10.1), where they are coughed out, sneezed out, or swallowed. Some special cells along the respiratory tract can actually surround and engulf invading germs, a process known as phagocytosis.

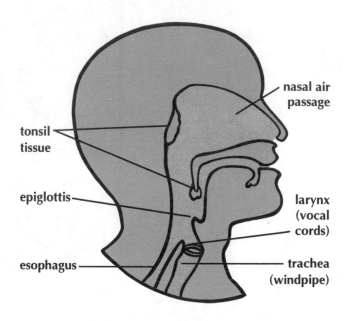

Figure 10.2. Structures of the upper respiratory tract

in the area called the laryngopharynx, the tract divides into two passages: the esophagus, which goes to the stomach, and the larynx, which houses the vocal cords and is the opening to the trachea (windpipe) (see figure 10.2).

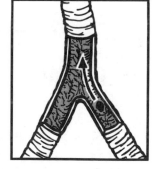

Figure 10.1. Cilia "sweeping" a foreign particle up and out of the lungs

Other protective mechanisms are performed by: the tonsils and adenoids, which help filter germs that enter the nose and mouth; nasal hairs, which filter dust and debris; inner body heat, which warms and moistens air as it passes through the nose, throat, and lungs to prevent the air passages and their linings from drying; and protective automatic reflexes like gagging and coughing, which help keep food and other objects from entering the lungs. These protective mechanisms help keep the airways of the respiratory system open and free from infection.

The respiratory system is often classified as having two sections, the upper and lower tracts. The upper respiratory tract includes the nose, sinuses, tonsils, adenoids, and throat (pharynx). Deeper in the throat,

Once air passes through the larynx, it enters the lower respiratory tract, which consists of the trachea and the lungs (see figure 10.3). From the larynx, the air flows through the trachea into the right and left bronchi, which branch into smaller and smaller passages after they enter the lungs.

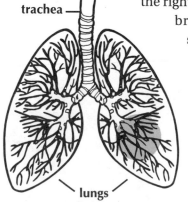
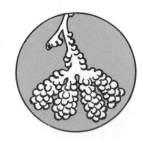

Figure 10.3. Structures of the lower respiratory tract and an enlargement showing clusters of alveoli

Bronchi eventually narrow into small passages called bronchioles, which branch repeatedly into even smaller passages and lead to the alveoli. The alveoli are small, sac-like structures in which the process of respiration (gas exchange) actually occurs. An adult has approximately 300 million alveoli. These alveoli, along with the air passages and the mass of blood vessels that surround the alveoli, make up the lungs.

The lungs lie within the chest cavity; each lung, as well as the chest wall, is lined with a layer of slick membrane called the pleura. A small amount of fluid present between these membranes makes it possible for the lungs to inflate and deflate freely without creating friction between the lung and the tissues of the chest wall.

STRUCTURAL BIRTH DEFECTS

CHOANAL ATRESIA

Choanal atresia is a birth defect in which the nasal passages are blocked at the back of the nose by either a tissue membrane or bone. This defect, which may occur in one or both nasal passages, makes it difficult for infants to breathe, because they breathe primarily through the nose.

SIGNS AND SYMPTOMS. Most noticeably, infants with choanal atresia have difficulty eating because they have trouble breathing and swallowing at the same time.

TREATMENT. Surgery to open the membrane or remove the obstructing bone can correct the defect.

TRACHEOESOPHAGEAL FISTULA

See page 141.

DISEASES AND DISORDERS

ACUTE BRONCHITIS

Sometimes called tracheobronchitis.

Acute bronchitis is the inflammation of the large air passages, including the trachea (windpipe) and bronchi. Acute bronchitis is most commonly seen in young children and elderly people. It is a short-term, reversible disorder, unlike the chronic form of bronchitis which causes long-term, permanent damage. Acute bronchitis is often associated with upper respiratory infections caused by viruses but can also be caused by bacterial infection, allergic reaction, or irritation of the airways when certain gasses or chemicals are inhaled into the lungs. Tissues along the large air passages swell and mucus production increases.

SIGNS AND SYMPTOMS. A dry, hacking cough that worsens at night is characteristic of acute bronchitis. The cough usually becomes wet (produces mucus) within a few days.

TREATMENT. Acute bronchitis is usually self-limiting and requires no treatment. If bacterial infection is the cause, antibiotics are prescribed. Adequate intake of fluids and rest are important. Medications can be used to treat associated fever or pain.

ASTHMA

Asthma is a periodic narrowing of the airways that obstructs the passage of air through the lungs. Asthma attacks vary in severity, from mild coughing and wheezing to severe life-threatening airway obstruction. There are different types or classifications of asthma. Extrinsic asthma, also called allergic, atopic, or immunologic asthma, is thought to be caused by an allergic-type response to certain things that always cause or trigger an attack in the person, such as animal dander, dust, molds, pollens, or foods. This type of asthma is usually seen in children and young adults who often have other symptoms of allergy, including eczema or an inflamed, itchy, runny nose (rhinitis). Most people with extrinsic asthma have a family history of asthma, usually have positive results from allergy skin testing, and have increased levels of a specific antibody in their blood.

The second type of asthma is intrinsic asthma, also called nonallergic or nonimmunologic asthma. The cause of this type of asthma is not clearly understood, although symptoms are the same as those seen in extrinsic asthma. With intrinsic asthma, something that triggers one attack will not necessarily trigger another. Triggers that sometimes cause intrinsic attacks are inhalation of cold air; a reaction to infection, exercise, or stress; and changes in weather, humidity or temperature. Intrinsic asthma commonly begins in late adolescence or adulthood. People with intrinsic asthma may not have a family history of asthma, usually have negative results on allergy skin testing, and show no increase in the specific blood antibody that is usually elevated in people with extrinsic asthma. Attacks can become more severe with time and can contribute to irreversible lung tissue damage and chronic lung disease.

SIGNS AND SYMPTOMS. When an asthma attack is triggered, the bronchi and bronchioles (and sometimes the trachea) narrow, causing tightness in the chest and difficulty breathing. The lining of the airways becomes swollen, worsening the narrowing and preventing the cilia from moving. The mucus-producing cells in the airway lining begin producing more and thicker mucus, which clogs small air passages and traps air within the lungs. Breathing becomes difficult and labored; even exhalation, which is normally a passive act, requires great effort and the use of accessory chest muscles to force air out of the lungs. Sneezing, coughing, wheezing, air hunger (gasping for air), bluish discoloration of the skin (cyanosis) due to low blood oxygen, apprehension, and confusion are all symptoms that can occur with an asthma attack.

TREATMENT. There is no cure for asthma, but it can be managed by avoiding known triggers when possible and by taking medication. Medication used in the management and treatment of asthma is often inhaled so that it can act directly to reduce swelling and open up the air passage to ease breathing. Most episodes or attacks of asthma can be managed at home; however, serious attacks require hospitalization for treatment and observation.

BRONCHIOLITIS

Bronchiolitis is the inflammation of bronchiolar air passages, characterized by tissue swelling and increased mucus production that block the flow of air through the lungs. Bronchiolitis is usually caused by viral infection and primarily affects children 18 months of age or younger.

SIGNS AND SYMPTOMS. Bronchiolitis may develop a few days after the onset of an upper respiratory infection, causing increasing breathing difficulty. As the infant breathes, nostrils (nares) may flare and the chest may heave. Fever may or may not be present and episodes of severe coughing come and go. Heart and breathing rates increase. Young infants may develop apnea (episodes of nonbreathing), have trouble eating, and be irritable.

TREATMENT. Because bronchiolitis is usually caused by a virus, treatment is primarily aimed at the relief of symptoms. Humidifying the air, using nonaspirin products to control fever, and ensuring the intake of adequate fluid and rest are important measures. Some children develop extreme respiratory distress and require hospitalization and oxygen therapy. An antiviral medication may be used if bronchiolitis is caused by infection from the respiratory syncytial virus (RSV) and if the infant has lung or heart disease, a compromised immune system, or severe illness.

CANCER OF THE LARYNX
Also called laryngeal cancer or throat cancer.

Cancer of the larynx (voice box and vocal cords) occurs more frequently in men than in women. A major risk factor for cancer of the larynx is tobacco use, especially when combined with long-term exposure to other inhaled pollutants. Other suspected risk factors include long-term alcohol use, persistent and chronic laryngitis, and long-term straining of the vocal cords. Cancer of the larynx may involve only the vocal cords or all surrounding tissues as well.

SIGNS AND SYMPTOMS. Progressive (worsening) or persistent hoarseness is an early sign of laryngeal cancer. Other symptoms include constantly feeling as if there were a lump in the throat, and pain or burning in the throat after drinking citrus juices or hot liquid. Difficulty swallowing or persistent bad breath may be late symptoms.

TREATMENT. Cancer of the larynx may be curable depending on the exact location of the tumor, the amount of tissue involved, and whether metastasis (spread of the cancer to other tissue) has occurred. Treatment can involve radiation therapy and/or surgical removal of affected tissues, including all or part of the larynx itself.

CANCER OF THE LUNG
Also called lung cancer.

Lung cancer occurs more often in males than in females, but its incidence in females is increasing. Lung cancer is the number one cause of death from cancer in both men and women. It seems to run in some families, which suggests a possible genetic influence. The ability to recognize genetic predisposition to such cancers is just opening up. A major risk factor in the development of lung cancer is smoking, with risk increasing the longer and more heavily a person smokes. Other risk factors include exposure to second-hand smoke and occupational, environmental, and industrial air pollutants. Cancer tumors can develop within the air passages, along the chest wall, or within the membranous sac (pleura) surrounding the lungs. Cancerous tumors can be classified as primary tumors, meaning those cancers that originated in the lungs, or as secondary tumors, meaning those cancers that have spread (metastasized) to the lungs from another cancer site in the body. Lung cancers are usually seen in people aged 50 years or older.

SIGNS AND SYMPTOMS. Unfortunately, because symptoms do not appear until late in the disease, the majority of lung cancers are not found until the cancer is advanced. The first symptoms usually include a persistent cough and the presence of bloody mucus (sputum) coughed up from the lungs. More symptoms appear as the cancer worsens and spreads (metastasizes) into surrounding body structures and/or distant organs. The majority of people do not survive more than five years after being diagnosed.

TREATMENT. The specific type of cancer and the degree to which it has advanced determine the treatment for lung cancer. If detected in its earliest stages (often from chest x-rays performed as part of a routine annual physical examination or screening), surgical removal of part or all of the lung may totally remove the cancer. Unfortunately, many people do not have annual physical examinations and therefore miss the opportunity for early diagnosis. Other treatments include chemotherapy and/or radiation therapy.

CHRONIC BRONCHITIS

In chronic bronchitis, the mucus-producing cells that line the bronchial air passages within the lungs enlarge and start producing too much mucus. The linings of these airways swell and are permanently damaged. The swelling narrows the passages, making it difficult to get air into and out of the deep sections of the lungs (alveoli) where oxygen and carbon dioxide gasses are exchanged. To make things worse, the swelling of the air passages prevents the cilia along these passages from working properly, which means that neither the extra mucus nor the airborne germs entering the lungs can be swept up and out of the

airways. As a result, respiratory infections (including acute bronchitis infections and pneumonia) are common complications that further compromise respiratory function.

SIGNS AND SYMPTOMS. The first symptom associated with chronic bronchitis is a persistent cough which brings up mucus (a "productive" cough), especially on rising in the morning. As the disease progresses, breathing difficulty increases, especially with physical activity. Late in the disease the skin may take on a bluish color (cyanosis) from low blood-oxygen levels. Body swelling and bloating sometimes occur. Both congestive heart failure and acute respiratory arrest can be fatal complications of chronic bronchitis.

TREATMENT. People with chronic bronchitis should avoid cigarette smoke (both first-hand and second-hand), other airborne pollutants, and respiratory infections. Practicing good nutritional habits and drinking plenty of fluids are also important. Medications that open the air passages and reduce inflammation help the lungs achieve the best gas exchange possible. Extra (supplemental) oxygen is sometimes required on a continuous or as-needed basis. People with lung disease can learn special exercises and new breathing techniques to enhance relaxation, strengthen breathing muscles, and achieve maximum lung function. The lung tissue damage associated with COPD (see below) and its associated diseases (including chronic bronchitis) cannot be cured, but can be managed so the individual achieves the highest level of activity, independence, and freedom for as long as possible.

CHRONIC OBSTRUCTIVE PULMONARY DISEASE (COPD)

COPD is a lung condition caused by other lung disorders, including asthma, chronic bronchitis, and emphysema. Although each of these is a separate disease, they all block (obstruct) air flow in and out of the lungs and interfere with oxygen and carbon dioxide gas exchange. Asthma is a reversible obstructive disorder, but on a long-term basis it can cause permanent damage to the air-passage linings and contribute to the development of COPD. And while some people with COPD may have symptoms of only one of the associated diseases, many have symptoms of all three. Cigarette smoking is a major risk factor for

COPD; however, some sources classify COPD as a multifactorial disorder, meaning that it is caused by a combination of environmental factors (including behaviors such as cigarette smoking) and genetic factors. The number of deaths from COPD has increased in recent years, and although more men are affected than women, more and more women develop COPD each year. Read the discussion on each of the separate lung disorders that can cause COPD:

- **ASTHMA** See page 129.

- **CHRONIC BRONCHITIS** See page 131.

- **EMPHYSEMA** See page 133.

CROUP

Also called laryngotracheobronchitis (LTB) and viral croup.

Croup is an inflammation and swelling of the larynx (vocal cords), trachea (windpipe), and the large bronchi, and is usually caused by a viral infection, although some cases are caused by bacterial infection. The inflammation causes swelling and narrowing of the airways, hindering the movement of air both in and out of the lungs and making breathing difficult. Swelling in the vocal cords themselves causes the brassy, seal-like barking cough associated with croup. Croup is seen more frequently in boys and usually occurs in children between the ages of three months and five years. Contributing factors may include genetic predisposition and allergic reaction.

SIGNS AND SYMPTOMS. Symptoms of croup can appear suddenly, frequently at night. They may improve during the day only to reappear the next night. A characteristic brassy cough, described as sounding like the bark of a seal, develops. Hoarseness, noisy breathing (which produces a crowing sound), and anxiety occur. Crying worsens symptoms. A low-grade fever may be present. Symptoms generally last from three to six days.

TREATMENT. Cool or warm mist vaporizors may help relieve the swelling and improve breathing. If there is any indication of respiratory inadequacy or distress, such as labored breathing, bluish discoloration of the skin (e.g., around the mouth), a change in the level of consciousness, or high fever, the child should be seen immediately by a physician. Hospitalization may be required. A croup tent, medication to decrease airway swelling, and oxygen therapy may be used.

CYSTIC FIBROSIS (CF)

The incidence is approximately 1 in 2,000 live births in Whites and about 1 in 16,000 live births in African Americans; it is rarely seen among Asians. CF is an autosomal recessive disease that causes the mucus produced by the body to be exceptionally thick. The thickened mucus causes blockages in ducts through which mucus normally flows freely. The organs affected most are the pancreas and the lungs.

Within the pancreas, the mucus-clogged ducts prevent digestive enzymes from flowing from the pancreas into the small intestine. These enzymes are needed for the breakdown (digestion) and absorption of proteins, fats, and carbohydrates; their absence leads to malnutrition, vitamin deficiencies, and delayed growth. Thick mucus produced within the lungs pools and obstructs the small airways, impairing the movement of air both in and out of the lungs.

SIGNS AND SYMPTOMS. Because the mucus is so thick, people with cystic fibrosis have great difficulty coughing and clearing the mucus from their lungs. Pulmonary (lung) disease resulting from chronic infection is the major complication. The sweat of people with cystic fibrosis has an extremely high chloride content that gives their skin a "salty" taste.

TREATMENT. There is no cure for cystic fibrosis, but it can be managed. Enzymes that help digest food are taken with all meals and snacks to prevent malnutrition. A diet of foods that are high in protein, calories, and salt is recommended, and vitamin supplements help correct vitamin deficiencies. Aggressive lung treatments that loosen and clear lung secretions include medicated aerosol breathing treatments and drainage of the chest three or more times every day. Chest drainage involves pounding, clapping, or vibrating areas of the chest and back while the person is positioned so that gravity helps the loosened secretions flow out of the lungs (percussion and postural drainage). Antibiotics may be given on an everyday basis to prevent or reduce the risk of infection. Clinical trials with gene therapy are under way and may one day provide a cure to people with cystic fibrosis. DNA testing can identify people who have the CF gene.

EMPHYSEMA

Also called pulmonary emphysema.

The lung damage of emphysema occurs deeper within the lung passages than the lung damage of chronic bronchitis. Emphysema causes narrowing and blockage in the deepest sections of the lungs, permanently damaging the lining and walls of the alveoli and/or the small air passages that enter the alveoli. Exhaling, normally a passive act, requires great effort with emphysema. Air that reaches the alveoli is trapped because it cannot passively flow back through the narrowed, tiny passages. Exhaling requires the use of additional muscles and energy to force the trapped air out of the lungs. The exchange of oxygen and carbon dioxide gasses within the alveoli is compromised because of the tissue damage and obstruction.

One type of emphysema, alpha-1 antitrypsin deficiency (AATD) emphysema, is a genetic disorder thought to be transmitted through an autosomal recessive inheritance pattern. People with this disorder produce low (deficient) amounts of a protective protein called alpha-1 antitrypsin. The purpose of this protein is to protect healthy lung tissue from enzymes that the lungs produce to destroy inhaled germs and other debris. Without adequate amounts of alpha-1 antitrypsin, the enzymes also destroy healthy lung tissue. This process causes permanent lung damage and emphysema. People with this inherited form of emphysema usually develop severe emphysema earlier than normal; even sooner if they smoke.

Some studies show that cigarette smoke increases the production of destructive enzymes within the lungs, which may explain why emphysema develops even in smokers who have normal amounts of the alpha-1 antitrypsin protein and why smoking is a big factor in nongenetic occurrences of emphysema.

SIGNS AND SYMPTOMS. Usually not seen until after significant lung damage has occurred, symptoms include shortness of breath and difficulty breathing, at first with exertion but eventually even at rest. People with emphysema may be thin, with a barrel-shaped chest and reddish-colored (ruddy) skin, and exhale through pursed lips as if blowing out a candle.

TREATMENT. The treatment for emphysema is similar to that for chronic bronchitis; it varies depending on the extent of disease, as noted above. People with alpha-1 antitrypsin deficiency emphysema can be treated with medication that replaces the missing protein to prevent further lung tissue damage.

EPIGLOTTITIS

Bacterial infection causes this inflammation and swelling of the epiglottis, which lies just above the larynx (vocal cords). The symptoms of epiglottitis are similar to those of croup (laryngotracheobronchitis), but epiglottitis can be life threatening. It is a medical emergency because the epiglottis can become so red, swollen, and sensitive that it completely closes off the airway above the vocal cords (the larynx). Epiglottitis is usually seen in infants and young children and is sometimes preceded a day or two by a cold, sore throat, or sinus infection.

SIGNS AND SYMPTOMS. Epiglottitis causes a croupy cough (a brassy, seal-like barking noise), difficulty breathing, and sore throat. Children with epiglottitis often sit up, lean forward, and thrust their chins forward in order to get air past the swollen epiglottis. Drooling may occur because swallowing is painful and difficult. Respiratory distress may become severe.

TREATMENT. Epiglottitis requires hospitalization, but it responds very well to treatment with intravenous antibiotics. A temporary artificial airway to the lungs may be required until epiglottal swelling diminishes.

PHARYNGITIS

Also known as sore throat; some cases are strep throat.

This mild or severe inflammation and swelling of the throat (pharynx) can be caused by viral or bacterial agents. Bacterial infections sometimes appear to be more severe than viral infections. Streptococcal pharyngitis is a throat infection known as "strep throat." Complications of an untreated strep throat infection can include rheumatic fever or poststreptococcal glomerulonephritis.

SIGNS AND SYMPTOMS. Sore throat with pain on swallowing, fever, chills, headache, and cough may be present. Strep throat infection may also be accompanied by abdominal pain.

TREATMENT. Bacterial pharyngitis, such as strep throat, is treated with antibiotics. Otherwise, treatments to relieve symptoms include medications that reduce fever and pain, adequate intake of fluids, and rest.

PLEURISY

Also called pleuritis.

Pleurisy is an inflammation and swelling of the outer membrane (the pleura) covering the lungs and the chest cavity. Pleurisy can be caused by infection, tumor growth, or traumatic injury to the chest.

SIGNS AND SYMPTOMS. Inflammation of the pleura creates pain when a deep breath is taken and when body movement causes the chest to be turned from side to side.

TREATMENT. The specific cause determines the treatment and may include antimicrobial and/or anti-inflammatory medications.

PNEUMOCONIOSIS

Pneumoconioses are lung disorders caused by long-term exposure to air that contains damaging dust pollutants. Pneumoconioses are considered occupational diseases because most pollutants are associated with industrial and/or occupational exposure. These diseases develop when long-term exposure to damaging pollutants results in irreversible lung-tissue damage, causing "stiff lungs" and a decreased ability to exchange oxygen and carbon dioxide.

Lung cancers are seen more often in people with some types of pneumoconiosis, especially if they are cigarette smokers. Silicosis, asbestosis, and coal worker's pneumoconiosis are some of the types.

SILICOSIS

Silicosis is seen in foundry workers and miners (including sand-blasting and rock-cutting workers) who are exposed to silica dust.

ASBESTOSIS

Asbestosis is seen in asbestos miners and people who process or use products made with asbestos fibers, such as roofers and demolition workers. People who work with asbestos and who smoke cigarettes are 90 times more likely to develop lung cancer than smokers who have never worked with asbestos.

COAL MINER'S PNEUMOCONIOSIS

Also known as black lung disease, this disorder is seen in coal workers and miners who are exposed to coal dust, silica, and other dust pollutants associated with coal mining.

SIGNS AND SYMPTOMS. Symptoms of pneumoconiosis vary greatly and develop gradually over the years. Included are recurrent respiratory infections, shortness of breath that increases with exertion, chronic cough, and decreased lung capacity. Lung damage is usually evident on chest x-rays; respiratory failure may develop in severe cases.

TREATMENT. There is no cure for the lung damage caused by pneumoconiosis. The best treatment is prevention: wearing protective clothing, breathing masks, and other safety devices recommended by occupational safety standards designed to protect the lungs. State health departments and the Occupational Safety and Health Administration (OSHA) have information on specific occupational hazards and on recommended and required safety precautions.

PNEUMONIA

Pneumonia is an inflammatory disorder of the lungs that may involve one area of one lung or all lung tissue. Fluid and other mucus debris collect within the alveoli and air passages of the lungs, creating congestion and consolidation that interfere with the exchange of oxygen and carbon dioxide. Pneumonia can be caused by infectious agents, including bacterial, viral, fungal, and protozoal organisms, or by irritating chemical agents that are inhaled into the lungs. Pneumonia can also be caused by another disease or can be a complication of injury (trauma) or prolonged bed rest.

SIGNS AND SYMPTOMS. Pneumonia is characterized by fever and chills, coughing, difficulty breathing, and anxiety, which may begin slowly or suddenly. Fatigue, sore throat, and pleuritic-type chest pain may also occur. Pneumonia still causes many deaths each year, especially among infants and elderly persons.

TREATMENT. Bacterial pneumonia can be treated with antibiotics. Supportive measures include adequate intake of fluids, rest, and medication to reduce fever and associated pain. Hospitalization may be required, especially in young children and elderly adults. Oxygen therapy may be indicated in some cases. Gentle rhythmic thumping of the chest (chest percussion) is sometimes done to dislodge the accumulated mucus and debris within the lungs so these obstructions may be expelled by coughing.

TONSILLITIS

Tonsillitis is the infection and swelling of the tonsils. The palatine tonsils, visible in the back of the throat, are most often involved. Inflammation of the adenoid tonsils is called adenitis. The tonsils are thought to help clear the body of germs that enter by mouth and nose. Tonsillitis is usually seen in children.

SIGNS AND SYMPTOMS. Symptoms of tonsillitis include sore, swollen tonsils that can make breathing difficult and swallowing painful. Children may also develop a middle ear infection (otitis media) caused by swelling and enlargement of the adenoid tonsils.

TREATMENT. Bacterial tonsillitis is treated with antibiotics. Tonsils are not surgically removed unless tonsillitis occurs repeatedly.

TUBERCULOSIS (TB)

The bacteria *Mycobacterium tuberculosis* causes TB infection, which mainly affects the lungs. In the early 1900s, TB was a leading cause of death in older Americans. With the discovery of antituberculin medications, the incidence dropped dramatically. Alarmingly, since the late 1980s the incidence of TB has steadily increased, and today TB is seen most commonly in people aged 25 to 45 years. Some modern TB strains are immune to standard medical treatment; this has made the treatment and containment of TB difficult and has once again rendered the disease a major public health concern.

TB is spread by droplets of mucus from the respiratory tract of an infectious person. Some strains of TB can be contracted by drinking milk from infected cows, although this rarely happens in the United States or other countries where the process of pasteurization kills the TB bacteria. The severity of the initial (primary) infection depends on the overall health of the exposed person and the amount and strength of the specific strain of TB bacteria.

SIGNS AND SYMPTOMS. Primary TB (the initial infection) frequently has no symptoms, and the infected person does not appear to be ill. In the meantime, the body's immune system develops antibodies that attack the TB bacteria, and defense mechanisms within the lungs surround and "wall off" the bacteria into cyst-like lesions. The TB bacteria may die or lie dormant within these "cysts." If the bacteria lie dormant, they can break free from these cysts at a later time and multiply rapidly, causing TB pneumonia and/or the spread of bacteria throughout the body to other organs, including the central nervous system. Stress that weakens the body's immune response, such as another illness or malnutrition, can cause repeated reactivation of the TB infection. This chronic, active TB infection causes serious damage to the lungs; it can also spread to and damage other organs, and it can be fatal. Chronic, active TB can be prevented by treating the initial (primary) infection with antituberculin drugs, which are prescribed for 6 to 12 months.

TREATMENT. A skin test can identify people who have been exposed to TB. The most common TB screening method used today is the Mantoux skin test (also referred to as the PPD). Dead tuberculin bacteria are injected under the skin of the inside forearm. If a raised area at least 10 mm in diameter appears at the injection site within 48 to 72 hours, the test result is considered positive and indicates exposure to TB.

After a positive test result, the case is evaluated. Treatment is begun to kill all TB bacteria within the body, prevent the development of chronic active TB disease, and reduce the spread of the disease. With the recent increase in cases of TB in the United States, it may become prudent for everyone to receive annual PPD skin testing so that treatment can be started before damaging disease occurs. Not everyone who has an initial (primary) TB infection develops chronic active TB, but for those who do, TB can be debilitating and fatal, and a significant health risk to others.

SECTION 10

THE RESPIRATORY SYSTEM

Check any of the following structural defects of the respiratory system that were present at birth.

10.1 Obstruction (choanal atresia) of one or both nostrils (nares): indicate how it was treated.

10.2 Document any other structural defects of the respiratory system, if present, and treatment(s), if known.

Check any of the following diseases and disorders of the respiratory system that are or were present.

10.3 Acute bronchitis (sometimes called tracheo-bronchitis): document dates, if known.

10.4 Asthma: document age at which symptoms began and any items known to trigger the asthma. If the symptoms disappeared or changed later in life, document in what way and at what age, if known.

10.5 Bronchiolitis: document dates, if known.

10.6 Cancer of the throat and/or vocal cords (known as cancer of the larynx): list the age at which the cancer occurred and treatment. Document whether the cancer was primary (began in the throat and/or vocal cords) or secondary (spread from a cancer site elsewhere in the body), if known. If it was a primary cancer of the throat and/or vocal cords, document any areas and organs of the body to which the cancer spread (metastasized), if known.

10.7 Cancer of the lungs: document which lung was involved, at what age the cancer occurred, and treatment. Document whether the cancer was primary (began in the lungs) or secondary (spread from a cancer site elsewhere in the body), if known. If it was a primary cancer, document any areas and organs of the body to which the cancer spread (metastasized), if known.

10.8 Chronic lung disease (COPD, chronic obstructive pulmonary disease): list which of the following diseases contributed to the chronic lung condition: asthma, chronic bronchitis, and/or emphysema. Indicate at what age the chronic lung disease (COPD) developed and how it was treated.

10.9 Croup (also called laryngotracheobronchitis, LTB): indicate at what age or ages it developed and how it was treated.

10.10 Cystic fibrosis (CF).

10.11 Emphysema (document your response above at 10.8).

10.12 Epiglottitis: indicate at what age it developed and how it was treated.

10.13 Pharyngitis: document dates, if known.

10.14 Pleurisy (also known as pleuritis): document dates, if known, and how it was treated.

10.15 Lung disease classified as pneumoconiosis (caused primarily by long-term exposure to occupational or industrial air irritants and pollutants): document the specific type, such as silicosis, asbestosis, coal miner's pneumoconiosis, etc., if known. Indicate at what age the symptoms developed and how the disease was treated.

10.16 Pneumonia: document the dates, if known, and how it was treated.

10.17 Tonsillitis: document the dates, if known, and how it was treated.

10.18 Tuberculosis (TB): list the dates of TB skin testing and test results. If TB was present, document at what age it was diagnosed and how it was treated.

10.19 Document any other diseases or disorders of the respiratory system that are or were present, the age of onset, and treatment(s), if known.

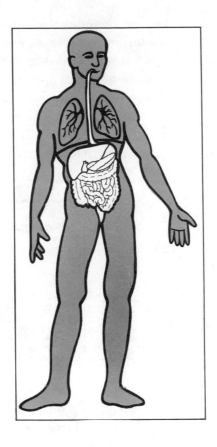

CHAPTER 11
THE GASTROINTESTINAL SYSTEM

The gastrointestinal (GI) system includes the mouth, throat (pharynx), esophagus, stomach, small intestine (small bowel), large intestine (colon or large bowel), and anus. These structures are linked together to form a continuous hollow tube with an opening at each end; these openings are called the mouth and the anus. The liver, pancreas, and gall bladder are also included in the GI system because they have important GI functions. The main job of the GI system is to break down, digest, and absorb food nutrients for distribution to all body cells, and to eliminate the waste products of digestion from the body.

STRUCTURES AND FUNCTIONS

The hollow tube that makes up the GI system runs from the mouth to the anus. Called the GI or digestive tract, this tube is lined with a special layer of tissue called the mucosa, which contains two major kinds of cells: cells that produce the mucus that forms a protective barrier along the GI tract, and cells that produce the enzymes and acids that break down and digest food. The outer layer of the GI tract is made of muscles that contract in wave-like motion (peristalsis) to move food down the tract. The muscular contractions are controlled by the autonomic nervous system and are involuntary, meaning they happen automatically. The only muscles of the GI system that can be voluntarily controlled are those of the mouth, pharynx, and the anal opening (anal sphincter). The production and release of acids, enzymes, and other fluids from the mucosal cells, pancreas, and gall bladder are also controlled by the autonomic nervous system and by hormones within the GI tract.

MOUTH

Digestion begins in the mouth as food is ground into small particles by the teeth and mixed with saliva during chewing. Saliva lubricates the food, making it easier to swallow, and contains enzymes that begin breaking down starches. Chewing allows better digestion of nutrients because digestive enzymes work only on the food surfaces they come in contact with. The more the food is chewed, the more surfaces it has and the better it is digested.

ESOPHAGUS

Once chewed, the food ball (bolus) is pushed to the back of the throat (pharynx) by the tongue and is

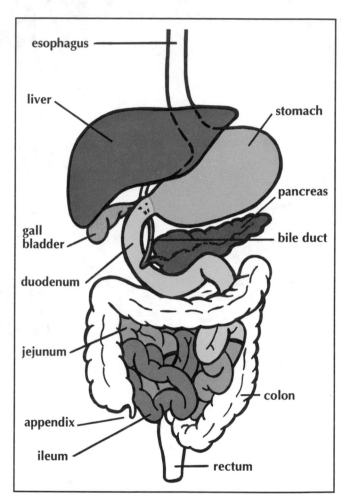

Figure 11.1. Structures of the gastrointestinal system

automatically swallowed. A flap of tissue called the epiglottis, which lies above the vocal cords in the throat, covers the vocal cords during swallowing to prevent food from entering the windpipe (trachea). The section of the GI tract that leads from the throat to the stomach is called the esophagus. It passes through the hiatus, a ring-like opening in the diaphragm (the large muscle that separates the chest and abdominal cavities). Swallowing causes the food bolus to enter the esophagus and be propelled toward the stomach.

STOMACH

As the food bolus reaches the stomach (10 seconds or less after swallowing), it passes through the cardiac sphincter (also called the gastroesophageal sphincter), a muscular ring that momentarily opens to allow the food bolus to pass into the stomach. The presence of food within the stomach stimulates gastric (stomach) cells to release hydrochloric acid and enzymes, which break down the food particles into smaller units. Although the inside of the stomach is very acidic because of the hydrochloric acid, the mucus barrier produced by the mucous glands of the mucosa protects the stomach tissue from the acid. As stomach muscles contract, the food is churned into liquid and propelled toward the lower muscular sphincter, the pylorus. The pyloric sphincter is a small opening through which the liquid passes into the small intestine (small bowel). Large food particles that cannot pass through the pylorus remain in the stomach until they are broken down more.

SMALL INTESTINE

The small intestine is divided into three segments: the duodenum, jejunum, and ileum. Within the small intestine, the final breakdown (digestion) of food particles occurs and most nutrients (including carbohydrates, protein, fats, vitamins, and minerals) are absorbed through the intestinal wall into the bloodstream. When the stomach contents empty into the duodenum (the first segment of the small intestine), the presence of food particles and stomach acid stimulates the release of digestive fluids from the pancreas, gall bladder, and mucosa of the duodenum. Digestive enzymes and acid-neutralizing fluids from the pancreas enter the duodenum via the pancreatic duct. Bile, produced by the liver and stored in the gall bladder, is released into the duodenum via the common bile duct to help dissolve fats, enabling them to be broken down (digested) and absorbed. Bile also aids the absorption of the fat-soluble vitamins A, D, E, and K.

As food is propelled through the small intestine, nutrients, water, and other substances are absorbed through the intestinal wall into the surrounding blood vessels. This nutrient-rich blood is transported to and filtered through the liver. The filtered, nutrient-rich blood is transported to the heart, which circulates it throughout the body to distribute the nutrients to all body tissue.

COLON

Any food contents remaining in the small intestines continue moving toward the colon (large intestine or large bowel). The food residue passes into the colon through the ileocecal valve (another muscular sphincter), which opens momentarily as the food residue approaches. In the colon, water and elements such as sodium and potassium continue to be absorbed into the bloodstream. The remaining waste (feces or stool) within the colon completes its journey through the colon to the rectum, where it is stored until it is eliminated from the body during a bowel movement.

The GI system is not sterile. Foods and liquids contain microorganisms and other impurities. The acidity within the stomach is enough to kill most of these potentially infectious agents. The colon, however, normally contains a large number of bacteria (called normal flora) that play an important role in the breakdown of waste products within the colon and in the transformation of vitamin K into a form the liver can use to produce several blood-clotting factors. This normal bacterial flora within the colon actually helps maintain balance within the GI system and the body as a whole.

LIVER

The liver is considered to be an organ of the GI system, although it performs many regulatory functions for the body. It is located beneath the diaphragm in the upper right side of the abdomen and extends to the upper left side.

The liver cleanses and purifies blood from the GI system by removing bacteria and other harmful agents. The liver changes and/or removes drugs, alcohol, and other toxins found in the blood, including harmful waste products that result from normal metabolism (cell function). Nutrients entering the liver from the GI system are either stored within the liver or changed into other substances that are usable by the body. The liver can store and release large amounts of glucose (the body's main source of energy) and fats. If necessary, the liver can actually make new glucose from either fat or protein. Many vitamins and minerals (including iron) are stored within the liver.

The liver can also act as a holding tank for extra blood if the vascular system becomes congested or overloaded. The liver synthesizes (forms) most blood proteins (important for maintaining water balance within blood vessels), lipoproteins, triglycerides, and several blood-clotting factors (important for controlling and preventing bleeding). All are needed by the body.

The liver also produces bile, which digests fats. Bile contains excess cholesterol, bilirubin, and other waste elements. Bile is carried to the gall bladder, where it is concentrated and stored until the presence of food in the duodenum causes it to be emptied into the duodenum via the common bile duct. Bile is then eliminated from the body with feces.

STRUCTURAL BIRTH DEFECTS

CLEFT LIP AND CLEFT PALATE

The incidence of some degree of clefting is approximately 1 in 700 to 1,000 live births and varies among ethnic groups. Incidence among Japanese is 1.7 in 1,000; 1 in 1,000 in Whites; 0.4 in 1,000 in African Americans. Cleft lip with or without cleft palate tends to occur more frequently in males, while cleft palate alone occurs more frequently in females; both occur more frequently in Asian populations and less frequently in Black populations. Cleft lip and cleft palate are two distinct yet related defects that may or may not occur together. Cleft lip results when the lip and nose structures do not fuse properly (see figure 11.2). Normal fusion occurs around week 5 to 8 of embryonic development. Cleft lip and cleft palate are associated with some chromosomal defects, but also occur independently. The risk of recurrence in subsequent offspring of the same parents increases with severity of the defect. Cleft lip and cleft palate are considered multifactorial defects.

SIGNS AND SYMPTOMS. Cleft lip occurs in varying degrees, ranging from a slight notch in the upper lip to a complete separation (cleft) in the lip that extends upward into the floor of the nose and backward into the upper gum. It can occur on one side (unilateral) or both sides (bilateral) of the upper lip.

Cleft palate also occurs in varying degrees. There may be a separation (cleft) in the soft palate (the soft roof of the mouth farthest back in the throat), in part or all of the hard palate (the hard roof of the mouth), or in both. Cleft palate occurs more often in combination with cleft lip than it does alone.

TREATMENT. Cleft lip and cleft palate each can be surgically repaired with excellent results soon after birth or within the first 18 months of life.

DIAPHRAGMATIC HERNIA

In this defect, the fetus's diaphragm muscle, which separates the chest and abdominal cavities, does not join or fuse completely during embryonic or fetal development. This leaves an opening in the diaphragm that lets the abdominal contents, usually the intestines and/or stomach, enter the chest cavity, crowding the heart and lungs and resulting in immature, arrested development of the lungs (see figure 11.3). The incidence is approximately 1 in 5,000 live births.

SIGNS AND SYMPTOMS. After delivery, the infant has symptoms of respiratory distress and may need mechanical breathing assistance (ventilation).

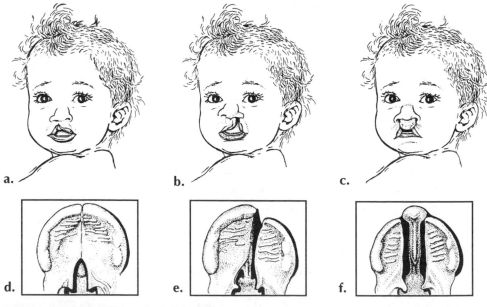

Figure 11.2. Cleft lip and cleft palate:

a. cleft lip notch
d. cleft in soft palate
b. unilateral cleft lip
e. unilateral cleft palate
c. bilateral cleft lip
f. bilateral cleft palate

TREATMENT. The abdominal organs are surgically placed in their proper positions and the hole in the diaphragm is closed. Even with immediate surgical repair, the death rate is approximately 50%, which is usually attributable to immature development of the infant's lungs. Intrauterine fetal surgery (surgical repair while the fetus is still in the uterus) has been used to successfully repair diaphragmatic hernia and allow more normal development of the fetal lungs. However, intrauterine surgery is still experimental.

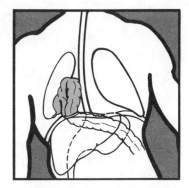

Figure 11.3. Diaphragmatic hernia: bowel is herniated into the chest cavity, crowding a lung

ESOPHAGEAL ATRESIA (EA) WITH AND WITHOUT TRACHEOESOPHAGEAL FISTULA (TEF)

When the esophagus and trachea do not form correctly into two fully separate structures during embryonic development, EA/TEF results. The incidence is approximately 1 in 32,000 live births. In esophageal atresia (EA), a portion of the esophagus is missing or closes abnormally, interrupting the normal passage of food and liquid from the mouth to the stomach.

Tracheoesophageal fistula (TEF) may or may not be present with EA. In TEF, abnormal pathways (called fistulas) are present between the esophagus and the trachea or one of the other large airways within the lungs, causing major feeding and breathing complications. Swallowed food may flow into the lungs, and gastric acids and other stomach secretions can enter the lungs from the stomach. In the most common type of EA/TEF, the upper esophagus ends in a closed pouch and the lower esophagus connects to the trachea, or other large air passage, through a fistula. This occurs in about 80% of cases (see figure 11.4).

SIGNS AND SYMPTOMS. Classic symptoms include coughing, choking, excessive drooling, breathing difficulty (respiratory distress, especially with feeding), and blue discoloration of the skin (cyanosis). If a fistula

connects the lungs with the lower esophagus and stomach, the stomach may fill with air, causing abdominal distention.

TREATMENT. EA/TEF is usually surgically repaired shortly after birth.

GASTROSCHISIS

Gastroschisis is similar to omphalocele (see page 142), except that the defect is in the abdominal wall away from the umbilicus, and the herniated abdominal structures spill freely from the abdomen. The incidence is approximately 1 in 6,000 live births.

SIGNS AND SYMPTOMS. Gastroschisis is visible at birth. It can be detected prenatally with ultrasound imaging.

TREATMENT. Gastroschisis is surgically repairable, often with good results.

HIRSCHSPRUNG DISEASE

Also known as congenital megacolon and aganglionic megacolon.

Hirschsprung disease is the absence of nerve fibers, called ganglions, within the muscular layer of a segment of the colon. Without ganglions the affected part of the colon cannot contract, and without muscular contractions (peristalsis) the feces or stool within the colon cannot be eliminated from the body. Feces collect in the colon above the aganglionic segment, causing the colon to become enlarged and eventually blocked. Hirschsprung disease runs in families and is probably a multifactorial defect. Some

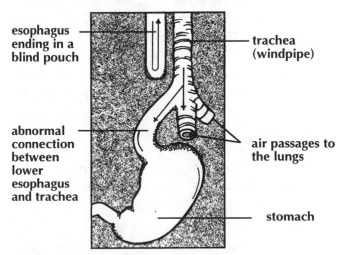

Figure 11.4. Esophageal atresia with tracheoesophageal fistula

researchers suggest it may follow an autosomal recessive pattern, but inheriting the mutant gene(s) may not always result in development of the disorder. The incidence is approximately 1 in 8,000 live births.

SIGNS AND SYMPTOMS. Infants and young children have long-term constipation, abdominal enlargement (distention) and discomfort, poor appetite, vomiting, and slowed growth.

TREATMENT. The aganglionic segment of the colon is surgically removed, and the remaining segments are joined (anastomosed).

IMPERFORATE ANUS
Also called anorectal malformation.

Imperforate anus is a general term that describes any defect of the anus and rectum in which the passage exiting the body is either missing or blocked because the rectum and anus failed to join properly during embryonic or fetal development. Imperforate anus is often classified as a high, intermediate, or low defect, depending on the exact location of the malformation.

SIGNS AND SYMPTOMS. The absence of bowel movement is the primary symptom of imperforate anus. The abdomen may show distention as time passes. Some cases are obvious on visual inspection of the anus.

TREATMENT. Imperforate anus malformations are corrected by surgery.

OMPHALOCELE

An omphalocele is the herniation (protrusion) of abdominal organs and structures through a defect in the umbilicus (belly button) and the base of the umbilical cord. This defect is the result of abnormal development during the embryonic and fetal periods. The herniated structures (usually the intestines, but sometimes the stomach and liver) are contained in a sac-like structure (the omphalocele), which protrudes from the abdomen and is covered by a thin, transparent tissue membrane. The presence of an omphalocele can make vaginal delivery difficult and traumatic for both the woman and infant. The incidence is approximately 1 in 4,000 live births.

SIGNS AND SYMPTOMS. Omphalocele is visible at birth, and can be detected prenatally with ultrasonography.

TREATMENT. The sac is kept moist and mouth feedings are withheld until the defect is surgically repaired, often with good results.

PYLORIC STENOSIS
Also called hypertrophic pyloric stenosis.

The incidence is approximately 1 in 250 live male births and approximately 1 in 1,000 live female births. It occurs more frequently in Whites than in Blacks. Pyloric stenosis is a narrowing of the pylorus, the circular muscle at the far end of the stomach that opens and closes as needed to empty food into the small intestine. In pyloric stenosis this opening is narrow because of marked enlargement of the pyloric muscle fibers, which obstruct the opening and make it difficult or impossible for the stomach contents to empty into the intestine.

SIGNS AND SYMPTOMS. Typically, at around three to four weeks of age, the infant begins vomiting, which becomes increasingly forceful and projectile as time goes by. Unless pyloric stenosis is corrected, the child develops dehydration, malnutrition, and severe chemical imbalances.

TREATMENT. Pyloric stenosis is treated by surgically enlarging the opening of the pylorus.

DISEASES AND DISORDERS
APPENDICITIS

The veriform appendix (appendix) is a pouch-like structure that is attached to the cecum (the first part of the large intestine in the lower right quadrant of the abdomen). Appendicitis is the inflammation of the appendix. It is usually seen in children, but it can occur in infants and adults. Most cases are thought to be caused by food or waste material that becomes trapped in the appendix, causing swelling and decreased blood supply to the tissues, which results in cell death (necrosis). Infection can develop, and the appendix can rupture and spread its infected contents throughout the abdominal cavity, causing peritonitis, a severe and potentially life-threatening complication.

SIGNS AND SYMPTOMS. Appendicitis can cause loss of appetite, nausea and vomiting, fever, and abdominal pain that at first is felt throughout the abdomen, then localizes to the right lower quadrant. Jarring movement can increase abdominal pain and discomfort and the probability of appendix rupture.

TREATMENT. The appendix has to be surgically removed, ideally before it ruptures. Antibiotics may be given before surgery to help reduce the infection, especially when appendix rupture is suspected. If the appendix has ruptured, prolonged hospitalization is often required to treat the resulting inflammation and infection within the abdominal cavity.

CELIAC DISEASE

Also known as celiac sprue; nontropical sprue; adult, childhood, or infantile sprue; glutin-induced enteropathy.

Celiac disease runs in families, suggesting a genetic connection that follows a dominant inheritance pattern, although inheriting the gene(s) may not always result in the development of the disease. It occurs at higher incidence among people of northern European ancestry.

Celiac disease is thought to result from either an allergic reaction to gluten (a protein found in grains such as wheat, barley, and oats) or an inflammatory reaction of the immune system. Glutin ingestion damages the mucosa of the small intestine in people with celiac disease, impairing the ability of the intestinal wall to digest and absorb nutrients.

SIGNS AND SYMPTOMS. After children have advanced to a diet that includes grains, at around 6 to 18 months of age, symptoms begin. These include abdominal swelling (distention), diarrhea, irritability, and signs of malnutrition, including thin arms and legs, weight loss, slow growth, anemia, and vitamin deficiencies. The subsequent lack of vitamin K leads to a decrease in the body's blood-clotting ability. The stool of affected people is usually very fatty and foul-smelling because of the malabsorption of food substances.

TREATMENT. A lifetime glutin-free diet is the mainstay of treatment. Routine health evaluations should be received because people with celiac disease may have a higher risk of developing gastrointestinal cancers.

CHOLELITHIASIS AND CHOLECYSTITIS

Cholelithiasis is the formation of gallstones within the gall bladder. Cholecystitis, inflammation of the gall bladder, results from blockage of the flow of bile out of the gall bladder by a stone in a bile duct. Most gallstones occurring in the U.S. population are cholesterol stones. The probability of developing gallstones is increased in people who are obese, use tobacco, take estrogen, have cirrhosis, or have any disorders that cause an increased destruction of red blood cells. People with family members who have gallstones may be at slightly higher risk, although not necessarily because of a direct genetic connection. Gallstones may not cause symptoms unless they interfere with or obstruct the flow of bile from the gall bladder or through the bile ducts, causing cholecystitis.

Other causes of cholecystitis include tumor or infection of the gall bladder. Cholecystitis causes swelling within the walls of the gall bladder and results in decreased blood flow and tissue death (necrosis). This process can end in the rupture of the gall bladder and subsequent spread of infection and inflammation throughout the abdomen (peritonitis).

SIGNS AND SYMPTOMS. Symptoms of cholecystitis include indigestion and belching after meals, especially if meals are high in fat; pain in the upper right side of the abdomen that often radiates to the back and right shoulder; and nausea and vomiting. Jaundice (yellow skin) may also occur.

TREATMENT. The treatment of choice is surgical removal of the gall bladder, but some nonoperative approaches are also available.

CIRRHOSIS

This chronic disease causes massive scarring within the liver, which decreases the liver's ability to function and distorts its appearance and structure. As the liver is slowly destroyed, new cells are regenerated but become trapped within bands of scar tissue and cannot function. Eventually the liver becomes a distorted, shrunken, hardened mass. These structural changes interfere with the flow of nutrient-rich blood from the intestines through the liver and cause blood to back up in the vessels surrounding the entire GI tract. Two major causes of cirrhosis are alcoholism and chronic hepatitis.

SIGNS AND SYMPTOMS. Symptoms occur only after major liver damage has occurred and include fever, severe fatigue and weakness, loss of appetite, nausea, vomiting, malnutrition, weight loss, abdominal pain (sometimes concentrated in the upper right abdomen), and jaundice (yellowish skin). Other symptoms include anemia, easy bruising, low blood sugar levels, the collection of fluid within the abdomen and dependent body parts, and bleeding within the GI tract. Profound liver failure may result in sudden mental deterioration, coma, and death.

TREATMENT. Cirrhosis cannot be cured, but the liver damage can be slowed and even halted; if not, cirrhosis is fatal. Treatment includes eliminating the cause when possible, getting adequate nutrition and rest, and avoiding alcohol and other agents that are harmful to the liver. Surgery to create a detour of blood around the liver from the GI tract is sometimes necessary to reduce the risk of life-threatening bleeding complications. Liver transplantation may be considered.

COLORECTAL CANCERS (CANCERS INVOLVING THE COLON AND/OR RECTUM)

Colorectal cancers are usually seen in people over 50 years of age and occur almost equally in men and women. It is the most common cancer in the United States when men and women are totaled together and is the second leading cause of cancer deaths after lung cancer. It is seen less frequently among people whose diets are low in animal fats and proteins and high in fresh fruits and vegetables (for example, among the Japanese, Finns, Africans, and in some Seventh Day Adventist and Mormon groups in the United States).

Risk factors other than diet include family history, colorectal polyps, ulcerative colitis or Crohn disease, or the genetic disease intestinal (familial) polyposis. There have been recent major advances in understanding the genetics of colon cancer.

SIGNS AND SYMPTOMS. Changes in bowel habits, such as changes in the consistency of the stool (diarrhea, constipation, or narrow, ribbon-like stool), the presence of mucus and/or blood in the stool, abdominal cramping or bloating, a feeling of incomplete bowel emptying after bowel movements, or unexplained weight loss and fatigue, are symptoms of colorectal cancers. Symptoms may not occur until the disease is advanced.

TREATMENT. Surgical removal of colorectal cancers is highly effective if the cancer is diagnosed early. Radiation therapy and chemotherapy may be used along with surgery. Because symptoms appear late in the disease, routine screenings for colorectal cancer are vitally important and should begin at age 50, or at age 40 if there is a family history.

DIVERTICULOSIS AND DIVERTICULITIS
Also known as diverticular disease.

A diverticulum is an outpouching or herniation of the inner mucosal lining through the muscle layer of the GI tract (see figure 11.5). Although diverticuli (the plural of diverticulum) can occur at any point along the tract, they usually occur along the lower segments of the colon (large intestine).

Diverticulosis is the presence of numerous diverticuli. Diverticulosis is more likely to occur after the age of 40, with risk increasing with age (seen in 10% of people over 40, in 50% of people over 60, and in 60% of people over 80). It may be associated with chronic constipation, overuse of laxatives, or a low-fiber diet. Some people with diverticulosis may have a congenital (present at birth) weakness within the muscle layer along some segments of the GI tract, which allows the diverticuli to outpouch.

SIGNS AND SYMPTOMS. Diverticulosis itself does not usually cause any symptoms, but the diverticuli can become inflamed and infected from trapped food and bacteria. This condition, called diverticulitis, usually causes cramping abdominal pain, fever, and changes in bowel patterns. Serious complications of diverticulitis include bleeding, bowel blockage, abscess formation, and rupture of the bowel, in which the inflammation and infection (peritonitis) can spread throughout the abdomen.

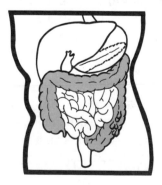

Figure 11.5. Diverticulosis of the bowel: note the presence of multiple diverticuli in the lower portion of the colon

TREATMENT. The only treatment needed for diverticulosis is adherence to a high-fiber diet that is non-irritating to the bowel, and the avoidance of food likely to become trapped in the diverticuli, such as popcorn, seeds, and nuts.

Treatment for diverticulitis often includes hospitalization so that intravenous fluids and antibiotics can be given while mouth (oral) feedings are stopped to allow the bowel to rest and heal. For people in whom diverticulitis recurs, surgical removal of the affected area of bowel may be indicated.

ESOPHAGEAL CANCER

Also known as cancer of the esophagus.

Esophageal cancer usually occurs in the lower part of the esophagus, although it can occur anywhere from the throat to the stomach. Usually seen in people over age 50, it affects more men than women, although the incidence among women is increasing. Tobacco use, chronic alcohol use, and a diet lacking in adequate amounts of fresh fruits and vegetables increase risk. Substances that cause chronic irritation of the esophagus, such as hot fluids or spicy foods, may increase risk as well. For unknown reasons, people of certain countries, including China and Iran, have much higher rates of esophageal cancer than the rest of the world population.

SIGNS AND SYMPTOMS. Often the first symptom of esophageal cancer is progressive difficulty in swallowing. Some people may have pain on swallowing. Other symptoms include coughing, persistent bad breath, spitting up of food, and a continuous loss of weight and strength. Eventually the cancerous tumor can totally block the esophagus.

TREATMENT. Surgery, chemotherapy, and/or radiation therapy can be used. The death rate from esophageal cancer is extremely high, and the long-term success of treatment is poor, because symptoms do not appear until very late in the course of the disease, and people often put off seeking health-care evaluation. Esophageal cancer can easily and rapidly spread into surrounding structures, including the lungs, heart, large blood vessels, and the lymphatic system (lymphatic vessels and lymph nodes). The only chance for cure is early, early detection. Any difficulty in swallowing, no matter how slight, should be checked immediately by a health-care provider.

GASTRIC CANCER

Also known as stomach cancer.

Stomach cancers are seen in more men than women and usually occur in people 40 years of age and older. The incidence is higher for the people of some countries, including Japan and Iceland. Risk factors associated with gastric cancer include the absence of

hydrochloric acid in the stomach (achlorhydria); chronic inflammation of the stomach (chronic gastritis); a diet high in pickled, salt-cured, smoked, or nitrite-processed foods; tobacco use; and family history.

SIGNS AND SYMPTOMS. Often symptoms do not appear until late in the disease, at which time the cancer has frequently spread (metastasized) to other areas of the body. Symptoms include indigestion, discomfort in the stomach area after eating, incomplete digestion of food, a loss of appetite, nausea and/or vomiting, weight loss, and anemia.

TREATMENT. Depending on how quickly the cancer is found and to what extent, if any, it has spread, treatment can include surgical removal of the entire cancer (the only complete cure), chemotherapy, and radiation therapy. With delayed diagnosis, the outcome is usually not favorable.

GASTRITIS

Gastritis is the inflammation of the mucosal lining of the stomach; it occurs when the protective layer of mucus within the stomach breaks down. It can occur in acute or chronic forms.

ACUTE GASTRITIS

This sudden and severe onset of symptoms usually lasts for two to three days. Acute gastritis can be caused by bacterial or viral infections, certain foods, too much food, certain medications such as aspirin or steroids, or excessive alcohol consumption. Often the cause is unknown.

SIGNS AND SYMPTOMS. Acute gastritis causes discomfort and pain in the abdomen, poor appetite, nausea and/or vomiting, and sometimes headache and fever.

TREATMENT. For acute gastritis all mouth (oral) feedings are stopped until the mucosa heals itself and symptoms subside. Foods are then gradually restarted, beginning with a bland diet, and advanced as tolerated.

CHRONIC GASTRITIS

This long-term, persistent, and/or recurring gastritis causes permanent damage to the stomach's mucosal lining. It can occur as a result of other disorders such as kidney, liver, or peptic ulcer disease; diabetes mellitus; or chronic alcohol use. Other contributing factors include the long-term ingestion of spicy and irritating foods, vitamin deficiencies, or long-term use of certain medications such as aspirin, ibuprofen, steroids, and some antibiotics. Infection of the stomach lining by the bacteria *Helicobacter pylori* is a common finding in chronic gastritis.

There are two types of chronic gastritis: type A affects the lining and glands of the upper stomach, and type B affects the lining and glands of the lower stomach. The likelihood of developing gastric cancer is increased after 10 years of chronic gastritis.

SIGNS AND SYMPTOMS. Anemia, poor appetite, and indigestion or burning in the middle-upper abdomen after meals can occur with chronic gastritis.

TREATMENT. Avoiding alcohol, caffeine, tobacco, and spicy foods, and using medications to reduce indigestion and heartburn are methods of treatment. Vitamin supplements may also be needed. Antibiotics to eradicate *Helicobacter pylori* infection may be indicated.

HEMORRHOIDS

Also known as "piles."

Hemorrhoids are swollen veins within the wall of the rectum. External hemorrhoids are visible on the anal area; internal hemorrhoids are located inside the anal opening. Approximately half of all people over age 50 have hemorrhoids, but some people develop them much earlier. Anything that increases pressure or gravity pull within the anal-rectal area can contribute to the occurrence of hemorrhoids, including prolonged periods of standing or sitting, pregnancy, and repeated straining during bowel movements because of chronic constipation. There may be a genetic susceptibility through the structural formation of the veins themselves.

SIGNS AND SYMPTOMS. Pain, itching, swelling, inflammation, and sometimes bleeding of the anal area are common symptoms. The formation of a blood clot (thrombosis) within the swollen vein can occur.

TREATMENT. Maintaining a high-fiber diet with adequate daily fluid intake helps regulate bowel elimination and prevent constipation; ointments, astringents, and anesthetics can help relieve symptoms. Lying down for frequent rest periods and soaking

the anal area in warm water (sitz baths) several times a day are also helpful. If these methods are not successful, more aggressive treatment may be used, such as injecting medication into the vein to close (sclerose) it or surgically removing the vein.

HEPATITIS

Hepatitis is inflammation of the liver. There are several types. In most cases hepatitis is caused by a virus, but some cases result from toxic or allergic reactions to certain medications, chemical agents such as metal compounds and solvents, or alcohol.

Hepatitis causes swelling, inflammation, and cell death within liver tissues. Fortunately, if the liver was previously healthy and not affected by preexisting disease or damage, it can regenerate and replace the destroyed cells. Occasionally the liver cannot rid itself of the viral infection and continues to carry live hepatitis virus for an extended period of time, sometimes for the life of the infected individual. People with this condition are called "hepatitis carriers." Hepatitis carriers may or may not continue to have symptoms, but they continue to be infectious to others. Some people may develop chronic hepatitis, in which there is progressive and continuous damage that the liver cannot overcome. People who become carriers or develop chronic hepatitis are at higher risk of developing liver cancer and cirrhosis.

The liver's functions include the breaking down of medications and other agents in the blood, cleansing impurities from the blood, forming many blood proteins and blood-clotting factors, controlling the levels of blood sugar and blood fat (lipids and cholesterol), and producing bile. These functions can be affected by hepatitis. Thus, medication given during hepatitis illness is given with caution, and the patient is monitored for signs of severe liver dysfunction, such as uncontrolled bleeding, abnormalities in blood sugar levels, or the buildup of toxic wastes within the blood. Severe liver dysfunction can lead to coma and death.

SIGNS AND SYMPTOMS. Regardless of the cause, the symptoms of all types of hepatitis are very similar. General symptoms include a loss of appetite and flu-like complaints such as headache, fever, fatigue, nausea, and vomiting. Some people develop a yellow discoloration to the skin (jaundice) accompanied by dark urine and pale-colored stools, pain in the upper right side of the abdomen, joint pain, and rash. Many people with hepatitis have no symptoms or have such mild symptoms they do not realize they have the disease.

HEPATITIS A

Also known as infectious hepatitis and epidemic hepatitis.

Hepatitis A is caused by the hepatitis A virus (HAV), which is transmitted through contaminated food and water, shellfish from contaminated water, and the oral ingestion of contaminated stool (feces) that can occur from poor sanitation and handwashing practices. Symptoms usually begin an average of 30 days after exposure to the virus, but the virus is found in the infected person's stool up to two weeks before the occurrence of jaundice, a telltale symptom of liver disease. The period during which people are still unaware that they have been infected is when the disease is most infectious to others. HAV usually runs its course without permanent liver damage or the development of fulminant hepatitis. Hepatitis A is not associated with chronic hepatitis or cancer of the liver.

HEPATITIS B

Also known as serum hepatitis.

Hepatitis B is caused by the hepatitis B virus (HBV). It is transmitted through infected body fluids, including blood, semen, vaginal secretions, and saliva. HBV is now classified as a sexually transmitted disease because it can be spread through intimate contact. (Unborn children can be infected with HBV from the infected mother through the placenta.) Symptoms can begin anytime from two to five months after exposure to the virus. Although the majority of people recover from HBV without permanent liver damage, about 1 in 10 develop chronic hepatitis or become hepatitis carriers. Hepatitis B can be a fatal disease if it progresses to fulminant hepatitis, or if, as the result of chronic hepatitis, it progresses to cirrhosis. Some limited success has been achieved in treating chronic hepatitis B infection with a drug called interferon that can kill some viruses.

HEPATITIS C

Formerly referred to as a non-A, non-B hepatitis.

Hepatitis C is caused by one of several hepatitis C viruses (HCV). These HCVs are currently the most common cause of post–blood transfusion hepatitis. HCV is transmitted through infected blood and blood products. Symptoms usually begin an average of 50 days after exposure to the virus. People infected with HCV have significant risk of developing permanent liver damage (cirrhosis) or liver cancer; some become hepatitis carriers. Limited success has been achieved in treating chronic hepatitis C infection with a drug called interferon, which can kill some viruses.

TOXIC HEPATITIS

This can be caused by a variety of medications, metals, or chemicals, including overdose of acetaminophen (i.e., Tylenol®), some antibiotics and anesthetic agents, isoniazid (medication used to treat tuberculosis), phosphorus, carbon tetrachloride, gold compounds, and alcohol. If the offending agent can be removed or discontinued promptly, permanent liver damage can be avoided. If long-term exposure to the offending agent has already occurred, however, the outcome may be the development of fulminant hepatitis and death.

FULMINANT HEPATITIS

This severe and widespread liver inflammation and cell damage is characterized by total liver failure, which usually leads to coma and eventual death in spite of aggressive medical treatment. Liver transplant may be considered.

TREATMENT. There are no medications to cure or treat hepatitis. While the disease runs its course, treatment includes plenty of rest, fluids, and nutritious food—a problem considering the loss of appetite. Substances that can irritate or stress the liver, such as alcohol, should be avoided.

The best treatment for all types of hepatitis is prevention. Good handwashing techniques before eating and after going to the bathroom can help prevent hepatitis A. A vaccine for hepatitis B is available to the general public and is very successful in providing long-term protection against hepatitis B. Practicing safe sex and using barrier devices such as condoms can also reduce the risk of contracting hepatitis B. All blood and blood products are screened for HBV and HCV to help decrease their spread through blood transfusions. People who suspect they have been exposed to any form of hepatitis should see a health-care provider immediately.

HIATAL HERNIA (HH)

Also called hiatus hernia.

The hiatus is the opening in the diaphragm that the esophagus passes through. In hiatal hernia the stomach pokes or herniates upward back through this hiatal opening into the chest cavity (the thorax) (see figure 11.6). There are two types of hiatal hernia. Most are type I or "sliding" hernias, in which the hiatus is enlarged due to muscle weakening within the diaphragm. Enlargement allows the lower esophagus and the upper portion of the stomach to slide in and out of the hiatus in response to body position changes or increases in abdominal pressure.

Type II hernias are also called "rolling" or "paraesophageal" hernias. In this type of hiatal hernia only a portion of the stomach bulges through the hiatal opening beside the esophagus. This type of hernia can cause bleeding or blockage of the GI tract, or it can cause no symptoms.

Hiatal hernias in general become more prevalent with age. Aging is thought to possibly weaken the muscle of the diaphragm, causing enlargement of the hiatal opening. Other causes can include injury to the chest and diaphragm and congenital malformations of the diaphragm.

SIGNS AND SYMPTOMS. In type I hiatal hernia there is heartburn caused by the reflux of stomach acid into the lower esophagus, difficulty swallowing, belching, and spitting up of undigested food. Many people with type I hiatal hernia have no symptoms. A symptom of type II hiatal hernia is a sense of fullness after eating only small amounts of food.

TREATMENT. Medication for heartburn, eating smaller and more frequent meals, not lying down for an hour or so after eating, and sleeping with the head of the bed slightly elevated can help alleviate symptoms. Surgery is sometimes indicated, more so with type II hernias because of the potential for bleeding or obstruction.

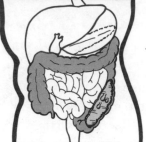

**Figure 11.7.
Polyps in the bowel**

INTESTINAL POLYPOSIS

Also called familial polyposis.

The incidence is approximately 1 in 10,000 people and is transmitted through an autosomal dominant inheritance pattern. Small tissue growths called polyps form on the intestinal wall within the colon and rectum (see figure 11.7). Polyp formation usually begins during early childhood to young adulthood, ages 10 to 25, with literally thousands of polyps forming by age 30. The type of polyp in this disorder is considered pre-malignant, and affected people have nearly a 100% chance of developing cancer of the colon before they reach age 50.

SIGNS AND SYMPTOMS. Intestinal polyposis can cause diarrhea and rectal bleeding.

TREATMENT. Treatment requires the surgical removal of the entire colon before cancer develops. People with a family history of intestinal polyposis should be screened by colonoscopy to identify whether they have this genetic disorder. DNA testing to identify people who have the polyposis gene before the onset of symptoms is available.

LIVER CANCER

Also known as hepatic cancer.

Liver cancer can occur as a primary cancer (originating in liver tissue) but more frequently occurs as a

**Figure 11.6.
Hiatal hernia:**

a. **normal stomach**
b. **type I "sliding" hiatal hernia**
c. **type II "rolling" or paraesophageal hernia**

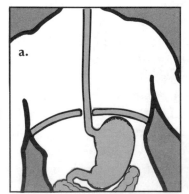
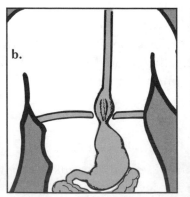
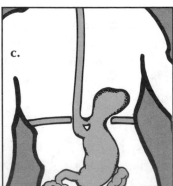

secondary cancer that has spread (metastasized) from another cancer site in the body. The liver has a vast blood supply, and cancer cells seem to multiply rapidly within it. Liver cancer is seen in men more than women, usually after 50 years of age.

Risk factors for liver cancer include chronic hepatitis B infection and cirrhosis. Long-term excessive alcohol use contributes to cirrhosis and is linked with liver cancer. Exposure to chemical toxins, such as vinyl chloride, also increases risk.

SIGNS AND SYMPTOMS. The upper right abdomen often becomes tender, and a mass may be felt. However, these symptoms often appear late in the disease, making the likelihood of early detection slim. Symptoms common to all cancers, such as fatigue, weight loss, and loss of appetite, occur as the cancer progresses.

TREATMENT. Surgery, chemotherapy, and radiation therapy can be used in combination to treat liver cancer. Unfortunately, in most people the cancer has already spread (metastasized) to other parts of the body (most often to the lung) before it is detected. Liver cancer is sometimes discovered during a search for metastases from other cancer sites in the body.

ORAL CANCERS

Oral cancers are cancers of the lip, mouth, tongue, and throat (pharynx). Oral cancers are usually seen in people 45 years of age and older and affect men more often than women, although the incidence among women is increasing. Unfortunately, more and more teens and young adults are developing oral cancers because of increased use of smokeless tobacco. Use of any type of tobacco, chronic use of alcohol, and family history of oral cancer increase the risk of developing oral cancers.

SIGNS AND SYMPTOMS. Sores on the lips or in the mouth that do not heal within two weeks, and pain, tenderness, or difficulty in chewing, swallowing, or moving mouth structures are symptoms of oral cancer. If the cancer involves the tongue or the base of the mouth, the probability that the cancer has spread (metastasized) before symptoms are noticed is great, because of the close proximity of numerous blood vessels and lymph nodes in these areas that can carry the disease to other parts of the body.

TREATMENT. When possible, the cancer is surgically removed. Other treatments include radiation therapy and/or chemotherapy. A cure is possible with early detection. Routine dental examinations increase the likelihood of early detection.

PANCREATIC CANCER

Cancer of the pancreas is seen in men more than women, usually in those over age 60, and more often in Blacks than in Whites. Tobacco use doubles the risk of pancreatic cancer. A diet high in fat may also increase risk. Some research supports the theory that people with diabetes mellitus, chronic pancreatitis, or chronic inflammation of the stomach (chronic gastritis) have an increased risk; in addition, evidence that supports a genetic predisposition to some types of pancreatic cancer has been reported.

SIGNS AND SYMPTOMS. Pancreatic cancer is called a silent cancer because symptoms very seldom occur early in the disease. A vague pain in the upper or middle abdomen that may radiate to the back appears as a late symptom in a significant number of people. Pain may increase at night and several hours after eating. Abnormalities in blood sugar regulation or the development of peptic ulcer disease can result from pancreatic damage and malfunction caused by the cancer. Loss of appetite, weight loss, and a yellow discoloration of the skin (jaundice) may also occur.

TREATMENT. The only cure for pancreatic cancer is the surgical removal of the entire cancer. This, unfortunately, is usually not possible because of the late onset of symptoms. At the time of diagnosis, most individuals have some degree of spread (metastasis), because this cancer grows and spreads rapidly. Radiation therapy and chemotherapy may be used as treatment. Surgery may relieve severe symptoms even though a cure may not be possible. The outlook is very poor, and most people live no more than a year and a half after diagnosis.

PANCREATITIS

This swelling and inflammation of the pancreas can occur when gallstones, tumors, or cysts block the pancreatic ducts that normally allow enzymes and juices to empty into the duodenum of the small intestine. Pancreatitis is also associated with excessive alcohol use, injury to the pancreas, peptic ulcer disease, and infection, and the overuse of acetaminophen, oral contraceptives, or steroids. The trapped pancreatic enzymes are forced into the pancreas's own tissues, and the pancreas begins digesting itself. The enzymes can erode completely through the pancreas and nearby blood vessels and other abdominal organs, causing severe bleeding, shock, peritonitis, and death.

ACUTE PANCREATITIS

Symptoms can occur once or in repeated episodes. The pancreas usually heals itself without permanent damage unless the cause is excessive long-term alcohol use, which permanently damages pancreatic tissue.

SIGNS AND SYMPTOMS. The major symptom is pain in the middle, upper abdomen that radiates to the back; other symptoms are nausea, vomiting, fever, and sometimes jaundice (yellow discoloration of the skin).

TREATMENT. The pancreas is rested by reducing or stopping mouth (oral) feedings and giving intravenous fluids until the inflammation subsides. Surgery to correct the cause may be effective, such as removing gallstones that are obstructing the common bile duct (the passageway connecting the gall bladder and pancreas to the duodenum).

CHRONIC PANCREATITIS

In chronic pancreatitis, pancreatic tissue is irreversibly destroyed over a long period of time.

SIGNS AND SYMPTOMS. People with chronic pancreatitis experience stools (bowel movements) that have a frothy and fatty appearance and an unusually foul odor; they also experience weight loss and vitamin deficiencies. Diabetes often results because the insulin-producing cells of the pancreas are damaged. Other symptoms are similar to those of acute pancreatitis.

TREATMENT. There is no cure for chronic pancreatitis. Treatment is aimed at preventing further pancreatic damage and includes avoiding alcohol and caffeine; eating a low-fat, bland diet; taking pancreatic enzymes by mouth with every snack and meal; taking vitamin supplements; and treating diabetes, if present.

PEPTIC ULCER DISEASE (PUD)

PUD is probably caused by a combination of both genetic susceptibility and environmental factors. It runs in families and is seen more frequently in people with type O blood. PUD occurs more often in young males than in young females, but in later years it occurs equally between the sexes. The presence of PUD is frequently associated with growth of a bacterium within the stomach called *Helicobacter pylori*. Although PUD is usually seen in adults, it can occur during childhood and even in infancy.

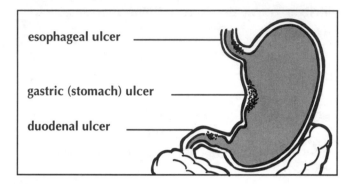

Figure 11.8. Sites of peptic ulcer disease

PUD is characterized by local tissue erosion that creates ulcers in the lining of the lower esophagus, the stomach, or the duodenum, resulting in (respectively) esophageal, gastric, and duodenal ulcers (see figure 11.8).

An ulcer can result from the excessive production of stomach acids and enzymes (although acid production is normal in some people with PUD) or from a weakness in the mucosal lining that normally protects these structures from being eroded or "self-digested." Long-term use of certain medications such as aspirin, ibuprofen, and corticosteroids, and long-term alcohol consumption, can weaken the mucosa and contribute to peptic ulcer formation. Once formed, an ulcer can erode completely through the mucosa and muscle layers of the structure involved.

SIGNS AND SYMPTOMS. Depending on the location of an ulcer, symptoms vary; however, pain described as gnawing or burning is common to all types. With gastric ulcers, pain is not usually relieved; it may increase with eating, and vomiting may occur. With duodenal ulcers, pain is relieved by eating but often reappears two to three hours later and during the night. Complications of PUD, including severe bleeding, can be life threatening. Other complications include slow, chronic bleeding that can cause anemia, and GI tract blockage caused by scarring from repeated ulcerations.

TREATMENT. Medications that neutralize and decrease the production of gastric acids are given to allow ulcers to heal. Treatment may also involve antibiotics to eradicate associated helicobacter infection. It is important to avoid tobacco, alcohol, caffeine, foods that cause discomfort, and stress. Stress itself has not been shown to cause PUD, but it can interfere with the healing of an ulcer and irritate existing ulcers. Surgical removal of an ulcer or affected portions of the GI tract may be necessary if the ulcer does not respond to medication or if severe bleeding (hemorrhage) occurs.

PERITONITIS

The peritoneum is the layer of tissue that lines the abdominal and pelvic cavities; peritonitis is the inflammation of the peritoneum and virtually all of the organs contained within those cavities. It is usually the result of infection or irritating substances such as bile or blood that have escaped into the abdominal cavity.

SIGNS AND SYMPTOMS. Peritonitis causes extreme abdominal tenderness and pain that becomes increasingly more severe and worsened by jarring movement. The abdomen becomes hard and rigid, and nausea, vomiting, and fever occur. Mental confusion and shock can develop alarmingly fast.

TREATMENT. Peritonitis can be life threatening and needs immediate medical attention. It is treated with intravenous fluids, antibiotic therapy, and surgery.

REGIONAL ENTERITIS

Also known as Crohn disease.

Crohn disease is classified as a chronic inflammatory bowel disease (IBD). The cause of Crohn disease is unknown, but it appears to result from both genetic and environmental factors, and usually becomes apparent during adolescence or young adulthood but may appear at any age. Aside from a family history of Crohn disease, having a family history of allergies and an ancestry from northern Europe may increase risk.

Crohn disease is characterized by patchy, ulcerated lesions (sores) that involve the entire thickness of the intestinal wall. The lesions can erode completely through the intestinal wall, creating passageways (fistulas) into the abdomen, other abdominal organs, or other parts of the bowel. The lesions often form abscesses and intestinal strictures that can lead to bowel blockage. Although Crohn disease can affect any part of the GI tract, it most commonly affects the junction of the small and large intestines located in the lower right section of the abdomen.

SIGNS AND SYMPTOMS. Crohn disease causes cramping abdominal pains that typically worsen with food intake (sometimes strongest in the right lower abdomen), malnutrition, weight loss, and repeated bouts of diarrhea. People with Crohn disease have episodic flare-ups and remissions of symptoms.

TREATMENT. Medications are used to reduce intestinal inflammation, prevent and treat bacterial infection, and slow the movement of the bowel. Mouth (oral) feedings may be stopped to rest the bowel during severe episodes, with nutritional and fluid needs met by intravenous feedings. Frequent rest periods, stress management, and a diet high in protein, calories, vitamins, and minerals with adequate fluid intake are important factors in long-term treatment. Long-term follow-up is important because people with Crohn disease have increased risk of developing colon cancer.

ULCERATIVE COLITIS (UC)

UC is a chronic inflammatory bowel disease that primarily affects the colon (large intestine) and the anus. The cause is unknown, but there are both genetic and environmental factors that contribute to its development. The disease usually becomes apparent during adolescence or young adulthood. Aside from a family history of UC, factors that may increase risk include a family history of allergies and a Jewish or northern European ancestry. UC is a lifelong disease with symptoms that come and go. The mucosal lining of the colon and rectum become inflamed and ulcerated. Permanent tissue damage and scarring of the affected areas can develop.

SIGNS AND SYMPTOMS. Recurrent episodes of severe diarrhea (as many as 10 to 20 episodes per day) that frequently contains pus and blood occur, as well as abdominal pain, poor appetite, weight loss, and fever. Hospitalization may be necessary. Nutritional deficiencies may result because of poor nutritional intake. Serious complications include GI hemorrhage and bowel perforation (rupture).

TREATMENT. Medications are used to reduce bowel inflammation, prevent and treat subsequent bacterial infection, and slow the movement of the bowel. Mouth (oral) feedings are often stopped to allow the bowel to rest and heal while nutritional and fluid needs are met with intravenous feedings. Substances that trigger symptoms, including alcohol and caffeine, are avoided. Adequate rest and stress reduction are also important. Although stress does not cause this disorder, it can aggravate it or cause a flare-up of symptoms. Surgical removal of the colon and rectum (total colectomy) is essential within 10 years of diagnosis of UC because of the high risk of colon cancer. It is this risk that makes long-term follow-up especially important.

SECTION 11
THE GASTROINTESTINAL SYSTEM

Check any of the following structural defects of the gastrointestinal system that were present at birth.

11.1 Cleft lip: document if the cleft was on the right, left, or both sides, if known, and indicate how it was treated. Cleft palate: indicate how it was treated.

11.2 Diaphragmatic hernia: indicate how it was treated.

11.3 Esophageal atresia (EA) or tracheoesophageal fistula (TEF): indicate how it was treated.

11.4 Gastroschisis: indicate how it was treated.

11.5 Hirschsprung disease: indicate how it was treated.

11.6 Imperforate anus (IA): indicate how it was treated.

11.7 Omphalocele: indicate how it was treated.

11.8 Pyloric stenosis (PS): indicate how it was treated.

11.9 Document any other structural defects present at birth and the treatment(s), if known.

Check any of the following diseases and disorders of the gastrointestinal system that are or were present.

11.10 Appendicitis: indicate age and treatment.

11.11 Celiac disease (also known as celiac sprue; nontropical sprue; adult, childhood, or infantile sprue; and glutin-induced enteropathy): indicate how it was treated.

11.12 Gallstones (cholelithiasis) with or without inflammation of the gall bladder (cholecystitis): indicate at what age and how it was treated.

11.13 Cirrhosis of the liver: indicate at what age symptoms began. Document the cause, if known, and any treatment, if known.

11.14 Colorectal cancers (colon and/or rectal cancer): indicate at what age the cancer occurred. Document whether the cancer was primary (began in the colon or rectum) or secondary (spread from a cancer site elsewhere in the body), if known. Document how the cancer was treated. If the colon or rectal cancer was a primary cancer, document any areas or organs of the body to which the cancer spread (metastasized), if known.

11.15 Diverticulosis or episodes of diverticulitis: document any treatment, if known.

11.10 Esophageal cancer: indicate at what age the cancer occurred. Document whether the cancer was primary (began in the esophagus) or secondary (spread from a cancer site elsewhere in the body), if known. Document how the cancer was treated. If the esophageal cancer was a primary cancer, document any areas or organs of the body to which the cancer spread (metastasized), if known.

11.17 Gastric cancer (cancer of the stomach): indicate age the cancer occurred. Document whether the cancer was a primary (began in the stomach) or secondary (spread from a cancer site elsewhere in the body), if known. Document how the cancer was treated. If the stomach cancer was primary cancer, document any areas or organs of the body to which the cancer spread (metastasized), if known.

CONTINUED

11.18 Gastritis: indicate at what age symptoms began. Document type, acute or chronic, and document any treatment, if known.

11.19 Hemorrhoids: document any treatments, if known.

11.20 Hepatitis: indicate the specific type(s): hepatitis A, also called infectious hepatitis; hepatitis B, also called serum hepatitis; hepatitis C; or others. Document at what age(s) the hepatitis occurred, and any treatments, if known.

11.21 Hiatal hernia (also called hiatus hernia): indicate whether type I (sliding hiatal hernia) or type II (rolling or paraesophageal hiatal hernia), if known. Document at what age symptoms began and any treatments, if known.

11.22 Intestinal polyposis (also known as familial polyposis): document at what age it was diagnosed and how it was treated.

11.23 Liver cancer (also called hepatic cancer): indicate at what age the cancer occurred. Document whether the cancer was primary (began in the liver) or secondary (spread from a cancer site elsewhere in the body), if known. Document how the cancer was treated. If the liver cancer was a primary cancer, document any areas or organs of the body to which the cancer spread (metastasized), if known.

11.24 Oral cancers (includes cancers of the lip, mouth, tongue, and throat): document the specific location of the cancer, if known. Indicate at what age the cancers occurred. Document whether the cancer was primary (began in the oral cavity) or secondary (spread from a cancer site elsewhere in the body), if known. Document how the cancer was treated. If the oral cancer was a primary cancer, document any areas or organs of the body to which the cancer spread (metastasized), if known.

11.25 Pancreatic cancer (cancer of the pancreas): indicate at what age the cancer occurred. Document whether the cancer was primary (began in the pancreas) or secondary (spread from a cancer site elsewhere in the body), if known. Document how the cancer was treated. If the pancreatic cancer was a primary cancer, document any areas or organs of the body to which the cancer spread (metastasized), if known.

11.26 Pancreatitis: indicate whether the occurrence was an acute episode only or in its chronic form. Indicate at what age(s) symptoms began. Document the cause and treatment(s), if known.

11.27 Peptic ulcer disease (PUD): document whether the ulcers were in the esophagus (esophageal ulcers), stomach (gastric ulcers), or the duodenum (duodenal ulcers). Indicate at what age symptoms began. Document treatments, if known.

11.28 Peritonitis: indicate at what age(s). Document the cause(s) of peritonitis, if known, and how it was treated.

11.29 Regional enteritis (also known as Crohn disease): indicate at what age symptoms developed. Document any treatment, if known.

11.30 Ulcerative colitis: indicate at what age symptoms developed. Document any treatment, if known.

11.31 Document any other diseases or disorders of the gastrointestinal system that are or were present, the age at onset, and treatment(s) that were received, if known.

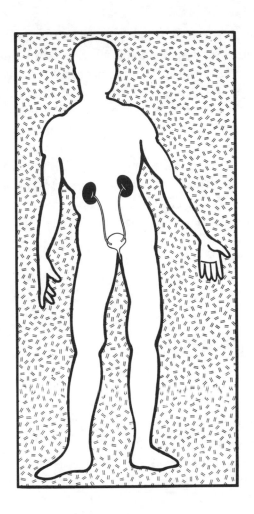

CHAPTER 12

THE URINARY SYSTEM

The urinary system, sometimes referred to as the genitourinary system, consists of the kidneys, ureters, bladder, and urethra. The purposes of this system are to form urine and to maintain both blood volume and blood composition, functions that are crucial for good health and well-being. Waste products that accumulate from body metabolism and the intake of medications and foods are filtered from the blood by the kidneys and eliminated through the urine. At the same time, the kidneys reabsorb blood components and other elements needed by the body, including water, sodium, chloride, potassium, glucose, and bicarbonate. The kidneys also maintain an appropriate acid-base (pH) balance within the blood, help regulate blood pressure, maintain adequate calcium levels, and stimulate red blood cell production.

STRUCTURES AND FUNCTIONS
KIDNEYS

The kidneys are bean-shaped organs that lie behind the slick lining of the abdominal and pelvic cavities (the peritoneum) in the flank (lower back) areas on either side of the spine. They are held in place by surrounding fibrous tissue (fascia); their upper portions are tucked under the two lowest ribs. A tough covering called the renal capsule encases and helps protect each kidney. An adrenal gland (part of the endocrine system) is located atop each kidney.

URINE FORMATION

Blood enters each kidney by way of a renal (kidney) artery that branches off the aorta. About 25% of the blood traveling through the aorta enters the renal arteries. In fact, the body's entire blood volume is circulated through the kidneys approximately

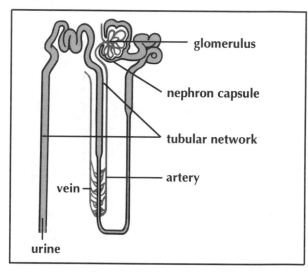

Figure 12.3. Nephron: pathway of urine formation: filtrate enters the nephron from the glomerulus and travels through the nephron's tubular network. The end product is urine

60 times in a 24-hour period. This is how the kidneys maintain balances in both volume and composition of the blood while they filter and eliminate wastes and unneeded elements.

Blood entering the renal artery is dispersed into smaller and smaller vessels called arterioles. Small clumps of vessels extend from the arterioles in structures called glomeruli. Each glomerulus is encircled by a nephron, the functioning unit of the kidney (see figure 12.3). Both glomeruli and nephrons have thin walls that are permeable to water and other blood components. Those elements cross freely from the blood into the nephron's collecting tubules. Blood components too big to cross through the glomerular walls into the nephrons include

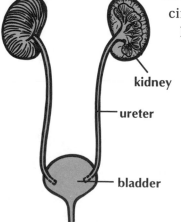

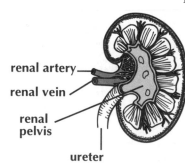

Figure 12.1. Structure of the urinary system

Figure 12.2. Blood flow through the kidneys

blood proteins and red blood cells. The fluid entering a nephron is not urine at this point but is referred to as filtrate, a fluid very similar in composition to blood plasma. The filtrate enters the nephron and travels through an extensive tubular network that empties into larger collecting tubules that, in turn, empty into the renal pelvis, the kidney's urine reservoir.

As the filtrate travels through this tubular system, water and other components needed by the body (e.g., sodium, calcium, chloride, potassium, glucose, and bicarbonate) are reabsorbed into nearby blood vessels; waste products (e.g., urea and acids) are added to the filtrate. The amount of water reabsorbed from the filtrate is regulated by a hormone called the antidiuretic hormone (ADH), which is secreted by the pituitary gland. The amount of ADH released by the pituitary gland depends on the concentration of the blood. If the blood is too concentrated, more ADH is released, causing the kidneys to reabsorb more water from the filtrate to dilute the blood. If the blood is too diluted, less ADH is released, causing the kidneys to reabsorb less water from the filtrate to make the blood more concentrated. The filtrate is so efficiently concentrated by the kidneys that the amount of urine produced is only about 1% of the total amount of filtrate moving through the nephrons. The filtrate changes in concentration and composition, and by the time it drains into the renal pelvis it has become urine.

Each kidney has approximately one million or more nephrons; each nephron functions independently from the others. This gives the kidneys an amazing amount of reserve; the kidneys can perform effectively with as little as 20% to 25% of their nephrons working properly. This is why people can live with only one kidney or part of one kidney, and why signs and symptoms of kidney disorders are often not apparent until a significant amount of kidney (renal) tissue is affected.

BLOOD PRESSURE REGULATION

Renin is a hormone produced by the kidneys. If blood flow through a kidney is reduced, the kidney releases renin into the bloodstream. When the renin reaches the liver, it triggers the production of angiotensin I, which travels via the bloodstream to the lungs where it converts to angiotensin II. Angiotensin II stimulates blood vessels throughout the body to narrow (constrict), increasing blood pressure and blood flow through the kidneys. Angiotensin II also stimulates the release of aldosterone, a hormone produced by the adrenal glands, which makes the kidneys reabsorb more sodium and water from the filtrate, increasing blood volume, blood pressure, and blood flow through the kidneys.

RED BLOOD CELL PRODUCTION

Another important hormone produced by the kidneys is erythropoietin, which stimulates red blood cells in the bone marrow to mature into adult cells. Because red blood cells are the carriers of oxygen in the blood, the kidneys release erythropoietin when they are not receiving enough oxygen.

CALCIUM BALANCE AND DISTRIBUTION

The parathyroid glands located in the neck produce parathyroid hormone (PTH), which, along with vitamin D (also considered a hormone), regulates the amount of calcium that is reabsorbed from the filtrate into the bloodstream by the kidneys. Although vitamin D is formed within the skin and liver, it is the kidneys that transform vitamin D into its "active" form. Active vitamin D allows calcium to be reabsorbed in the kidneys, absorbed into bone, and absorbed by the gastrointestinal tract to maintain normal blood calcium levels.

URETERS, BLADDER, AND URETHRA

When urine enters the renal pelvis it drains into the ureters, hollow muscular tubes that empty into the bladder. The bladder is a muscular, bag-like structure that expands to hold large amounts of urine. The urethra is the passage from the bladder to the outside of the body. The urethral opening is called the urethral meatus. In females the urethral meatus is in front of the vaginal opening; in males the urethral meatus is at the end of the penis. Rings of muscle called sphincters, which open and close at the base of the bladder and along the urethra, stay contracted or closed to hold the urine in the bladder until urination (voiding) is initiated. On urination, the bladder muscle contracts and the sphincter muscles relax and open to allow the urine to be expelled.

STRUCTURAL BIRTH DEFECTS

EPISPADIAS

This defect is characterized by an abnormal location of the urethral meatus. In males, the urethral meatus is located anywhere along the top surface of the penis instead of at the end. In severe cases the top of the urethra may be absent so that the urethra appears to be an open canal along the penis. In females, the urethral opening is more forward than normal. Epispadias occurs more in males than females. The risk of recurrence in subsequent offspring is thought to be low.

SIGNS AND SYMPTOMS. The abnormal location of the urethral meatus is visible at birth. Continual leakage of urine may or may not be present. On urination, the direction of the urine stream is deviated from the normal, straightforward stream.

TREATMENT. Epispadias can be surgically corrected. Male infants with epispadias are not circumcised because foreskin tissue may be used for repair.

EXSTROPHY OF THE BLADDER

This major defect involves the lower urinary tract and sometimes the male genitalia. It results from the failure of the lower abdomen and front wall

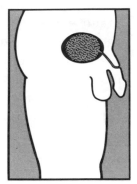

**Figure 12.4.
Epispadias**

of the bladder to completely close during embryonic development, leaving an open area in the lower abdomen. The back wall of the bladder protrudes through the opening, exposing the inside tissue of the bladder.

Exstrophy of the bladder occurs more in males than in females and is accompanied by other defects, including epispadias and nonfusion of the front pelvic bones (the pubic arch). Malformation of the penis may also occur. Risk of recurrence in a family with a history of extrophy of the bladder is higher than its occurrence in the general population.

SIGNS AND SYMPTOMS. This defect is visible at birth. Because the bladder is open and exposed, urine continuously leaks; preventing infection of the exposed tissue is a major concern.

TREATMENT. Surgical repair of the bladder is indicated at birth and is usually completed in stages. Efforts are made to repair the defect(s) and to provide urinary control and eventual sexual function.

HYPOSPADIAS

Hypospadias results from the incomplete development of the front part of the urethea. In males, the urethral meatus is located anywhere along the underside of the penis instead of at the end. In females, the meatus opens into the vagina. Hypospadias is fairly common and is the most common defect involving the penis (approximately 1 in 300 live male births). Hypospadias does seem to run in families, although the exact mode of transmission is unknown. Approximately 8% of male infants with hypospadias have fathers with the same defect. Risk of recurrence in subsequent offspring should be discussed with a genetic specialist or healthcare provider.

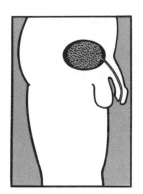

**Figure 12.5.
Hypospadias**

SIGNS AND SYMPTOMS. The abnormal location of the urinary meatus is visible at birth. The direction of the urine stream during urination is abnormal.

TREATMENT. Hypospadias can be surgically corrected. Male infants with hypospadias are not circumcised because foreskin tissue may be used for repair.

INFANTILE POLYCYSTIC KIDNEY DISEASE (IPKD)

IPKD is the presence at birth of cysts within one or both kidneys and often in other organs. IPKD follows an autosomal recessive inheritance pattern. Incidence is approximately 1 in 20,000 to 60,000 live births.

SIGNS AND SYMPTOMS. If both kidneys are cystic, there is typically very little amniotic fluid surrounding the affected fetus and no urine output after birth. If only one kidney is cystic, urine output is less than normal. Infants born with bilateral IPKD have poor lung development and the characteristic facial features of infants born with renal abnormalities: wide-set eyes, flat nose, and a "wizened" look. They may also have high blood pressure.

TREATMENT. Infants born with two (bilateral) cystic kidneys require kidney transplantation within a few months in order to survive. If only one kidney is cystic, it may require surgical removal.

KIDNEY (RENAL) AGENESIS

Bilateral kidney (renal) agenesis is the failure of the kidneys to form in the fetus. The fetus may survive until birth because the placenta performs the job of the fetal kidneys; however, some infants are stillborn. Bilateral kidney agenesis is suspected to be a multifactorial disorder. There is a 10% risk that other family members may have unevident (silent) genitourinary malformations (e.g., unilateral renal agenesis, horseshoe kidney, pelvic kidney).

SIGNS AND SYMPTOMS. Typically, very little amniotic fluid surrounds these fetuses because there are no kidneys to produce the urine that normally makes up most of the fluid. This lack of fluid in the uterus causes characteristic facial features in the newborn, including malformed low-set ears, wide-set eyes, flattened nose, a wizened "old man" look; arm and/or leg deformities; and underdevelopment of the lungs.

TREATMENT. There is no treatment for kidney agenesis; affected infants usually die shortly after birth due to underdeveloped lungs.

KIDNEY (RENAL) HYPOPLASIA

Kidney (renal) hypoplasia is the failure of one or both kidneys to form and develop completely during fetal life. The kidneys usually work to some degree, although not as well as healthy kidneys.

SIGNS AND SYMPTOMS. The degree and severity of symptoms varies, depending on the degree of normal kidney function that is present. High blood pressure is often present in childhood.

TREATMENT. Renal dialysis and eventual kidney transplantation may be needed if both kidneys are affected.

DISEASES AND DISORDERS
ADULT POLYCYSTIC KIDNEY DISEASE (APKD)

The incidence of APKD ranges from approximately 1 in 3,000 to 5,000 live births and is transmitted through an autosomal dominant inheritance pattern. Cysts form within both kidneys, slowly and progressively destroying healthy kidney tissue, ending in kidney failure and eventual death.

SIGNS AND SYMPTOMS. Because APKD progresses slowly, symptoms typically do not appear until people reach their 30s or 40s. The kidneys cease to function and enlarge to several times their normal size because of the cysts. The first symptom to appear may be pain in the flank—the area of the back where the kidneys are located. Approximately 75% of affected people have high blood pressure. Cysts are also likely to develop in other organs, including the liver, spleen, pancreas, lungs, and bladder, interfering with their functions as well. Researchers have noted an association between APKD and the presence of berry aneurysm in the blood vessels of the brain. This is a great concern, especially for those who have APKD-related high blood pressure, because rupture of the aneurysm can cause severe bleeding into the brain and sudden death.

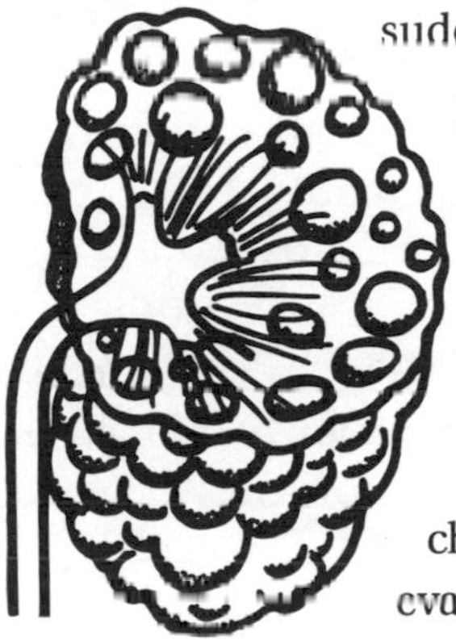

Figure 12.6. Polycystic kidney

TREATMENT. APKD-related high blood pressure is controlled primarily with medication; eventually, hemodialysis and kidney transplantation are necessary. People at risk for APKD should have frequent checkups that include ultrasound evaluation of the kidneys. Testing is now available to determine if a person does have the APKD gene.

ALPORT SYNDROME

Also known as hereditary nephritis.

Alport syndrome follows autosomal dominant and X-linked inheritance patterns. It is a form of nephritis (kidney inflammation) that causes a slow destruction of kidney tissue, eventually resulting in kidney failure. About half the people with Alport syndrome develop nerve deafness at some point in their lives, and some have defects of the eyes. Alport syndrome is thought to occur because the mutant gene(s) produces an abnormal protein that interferes with the normal development of membranes within the kidney and the inner ear.

SIGNS AND SYMPTOMS. Symptoms include high blood pressure and blood and protein loss through the urine. Renal failure can occur as early as adolescence; irreversible kidney damage is present by the mid-adult years.

TREATMENT. Dialysis and/or kidney transplantation are treatments available for Alport-related kidney disease.

BLADDER CANCER

Cancer of the bladder is seen more in men than in women; it usually occurs in people 50 years of age or older. Between 30% and 40% of cases are related to cigarette smoke inhalation, whether direct or second hand. Other risk factors include exposure to industrial or occupational toxins, including some chemical dyes, inks, leather, rubber, and petroleum products.

Bladder cancers can invade through the bladder wall or spread to other organs of the genitourinary system, including the ureters and kidneys.

SIGNS AND SYMPTOMS. One of the earliest symptoms is visible blood in the urine (hematuria) that is not accompanied by pain. Initially, the hematuria may come and go, but eventually it becomes continuous. Symptoms that may develop later in the course of the disease include pain and inflammation of the bladder, increased frequency of urination, and obstruction of urine flow through the ureters.

TREATMENT. Surgical removal of the cancer can be combined with radiation therapy and/or chemo-therapy. In severe cases, the entire bladder is removed and an alternate urinary outlet surgically constructed.

CONGENITAL NEPHROSIS

Also called congenital Finnish nephrosis.

Congenital nephrosis follows an autosomal recessive inheritance pattern and is seen in newborns and in infants before three months of age. Its highest incidence is among people of Finnish or Scandinavian descent.

Congential nephrosis is characterized by a change in the permeability of the glomeruli that causes the kidneys to function abnormally. The walls of the glomeruli usually do not allow blood protein (speci–fically albumin) to filter into the nephron; in congenital nephrosis they do, and large amounts of albumin are lost in the urine. When congential nephrosis is present

in the fetus, amniocentesis or maternal blood testing reveals elevated levels of alpha-fetoprotein (AFP).

SIGNS AND SYMPTOMS. Infants with congenital nephrosis are often small for gestational age, appear ruddy (red), and are very susceptible to infections. At delivery, the placenta appears large and swollen (edematous). Soon after birth it becomes apparent that the infant has protein in the urine, low blood protein levels, high blood levels of cholesterol and other fats (lipids), and swelling from accumulated fluid (edema) in the eyelids, genitals, abdomen, and dependent (positioned below the waist) areas of the body. Affected infants do not usually grow at expected rates and fall behind the norms.

TREATMENT. Standard treatment regimens for other types of nephrosis are not usually effective in con-genital nephrosis, and death usually occurs within the first few years of life unless a kidney transplant is performed.

Other forms of nephrosis run in families, but they are not usually as severe as congenital nephrosis.

CYSTINURIA

The incidence is approximately 1 in 10,000 live births; it is an autosomal recessive disorder. People with cystinuria lose large amounts of cystine and other amino acids (organic compounds that join to form proteins) through their urine, because their kidneys do not reabsorb these elements as they should.

SIGNS AND SYMPTOMS. Kidney stones (renal calculi) and bladder stones consisting mainly of cystine form readily because of the high concentration of cystine in the urine. There are three types of cystinuria, but all are inherited disorders and all involve the formation of urinary stones.

TREATMENT. Therapeutic approaches aim to prevent kidney stone formation and include measures to raise the alkalinity of the urine, altering the diet, drinking a high volume of fluids daily, and medication, such as penicillamine.

CYSTITIS

Cystitis is an inflammation of the bladder most commonly caused by infection. It is a lower urinary tract infection that occurs more in women than in men. In women, microorganisms usually gain entrance into the bladder by ascending from the outside of the body up the urethra. In men, cystitis is most often related to infection of a nearby structure, such as the prostate, or to bladder stones.

SIGNS AND SYMPTOMS. Cystitis causes pain on urination and a frequent, urgent need to urinate. Urine often has a strong, foul odor, appears cloudy, and may contain blood (hematuria). If fever and chills are present, the infection has probably progressed to the kidneys (pyelonephritis).

TREATMENT. Cystitis is treated with antibiotics and plenty of fluids to "flush out" the urinary system. Hygienic measures that help avoid recurrence in females include wearing cotton underwear and avoiding bubble baths. After a bowel movement, wiping should be in a front-to-back direction so as to avoid contaminating the urethra with the microorganisms normally present in the anal area. Other measures include drinking plenty of fluids, urinating regularly (e.g., every four hours), and avoiding feminine hygiene sprays and deodorants. Uncircumcised males should clean beneath the foreskin daily to discourage bacterial growth that could ascend the urethra and cause cystitis.

GLOMERULONEPHRITIS

This inflammation of the glomeruli is most often seen in children between the ages of 5 and 10 years. It is seen more in boys than in girls, and frequently occurs after recovery from an infection that occurred a few weeks earlier. Infections most often associated with postinfectious glomerulonephritis are streptococcal pharyngitis (strep throat) and impetigo. Multisystem diseases such as diabetes can also contribute to the occurrence of glomerulonephritis.

The precise cause of glomerulonephritis is unclear, but it is thought to be an immune response within the body that causes swelling and the accumulation of cellular debris (including white blood cells) within the glomeruli. This condition restricts the flow of blood through the glomeruli and reduces the output of urine, causing the kidneys to reabsorb more sodium and water in an attempt to improve blood flow through the kidneys. The retained water increases the volume of circulating blood within the blood vessels, increasing blood pressure and the work of the heart. Excess fluid moves into body tissues and causes swelling (edema);

fluid that moves into the lungs impairs respiratory function. The swelling that occurs within the glomeruli changes their permeability, allowing large blood components (proteins and red blood cells) to filter into the nephrons and be expelled through the urine. Glomerulonephritis occurs in acute (sudden and severe) and chronic (slow and long-lasting) forms.

ACUTE GLOMERULONEPHRITIS

SIGNS AND SYMPTOMS. Blood in the urine (hematuria), a decrease in the volume of urine output, high blood pressure, abdominal discomfort, irritability, and swelling (edema), all begin suddenly. Fever and headache may also be present. Protein can be seen in the urine on microscopic examination.

TREATMENT. People with acute glomerulonephritis are hospitalized so they get complete bed rest and can be monitored closely for complications such as heart or renal failure or fluid imbalances. During the most acute phase, severe high blood pressure is treated with medication, and dietary modifications may be instituted. Short-term hemodialysis may be indicated. Acute glomerulonephritis rarely recurs; most children recover completely from it, although a few develop chronic glomerulonephritis.

CHRONIC GLOMERULONEPHRITIS

Also referred to as chronic nephrotic syndrome.

SIGNS AND SYMPTOMS. The cause of this long-term inflammation and slow, progressive destruction of the glomeruli is often unknown. Kidney function decreases year after year, eventually resulting in complete kidney dysfunction and tissue deterioration.

TREATMENT. Measures to treat high blood pressure are instituted, and dietary modifications, including a low sodium, low potassium diet, are begun. Renal dialysis is required. Kidney transplantation may be performed.

KIDNEY (RENAL) CANCER

Cancer can form in any part of the kidney; it occurs more in males than in females, and in people 50 years of age or older. Tobacco use (including the smokeless kind) is a significant risk factor. Occupational or industrial exposure to toxins such as cadmium, lead, and phosphate may also increase risk. A family history of kidney cancer is significant.

SIGNS AND SYMPTOMS. Initially, kidney cancers may not produce symptoms. Blood in the urine (hematuria) may be continuous or intermittent, obvious to the eye or detectable only under a microscope. Hypertension (high blood pressure) may or may not be present. Symptoms of advanced cancer can include the presence of a tender or painful mass in the area of the affected kidney, loss of appetite and weight, fatigue, and anemia. Kidney cancer can spread (metastasize) to other parts of the body, including the brain, bones, lungs, liver, or to the other kidney.

TREATMENT. Depending on the presence and degree of metastasis, surgical removal of the affected kidney can be combined with radiation therapy and chemotherapy.

NEPHROGENIC DIABETES INSIPIDUS

This disorder is characterized by the inability of the kidneys to concentrate the filtrate (the fluid that eventually becomes urine) that enters the nephrons, resulting in excessive body water loss through the urine. The nephrons fail to reabsorb water because they do not respond to the antidiuretic hormone produced by the pituitary gland. Nephrogenic diabetes insipidus is a different disorder from diabetes mellitus.

Nephrogenic diabetes insipidus is transmitted through an X-linked recessive inheritance pattern. Thus, it primarily affects males; usually females are carriers only. Other causes of nephrogenic diabetes insipidus include chemical imbalance in the blood (such as low potassium or high calcium levels), kidney (renal) failure, and sickle cell anemia.

SIGNS AND SYMPTOMS. Extreme thirst is caused by the water lost in passing excessive amounts of urine. Severe dehydration, which can be fatal, can result.

TREATMENT. Adequate hydration must be maintained at all times by drinking plenty of fluids by mouth or through intravenous feedings. Medication may be used in some cases.

NEPHROSIS

Also called nephrotic syndrome, childhood nephrosis, minimal change nephrotic syndrome (MCNS), or idiopathic nephrosis.

Nephrosis occurs most frequently in young children, more often in boys than in girls. The cause is not usually known, and nephrosis can appear in previously healthy children. Some cases are associated with infection, systemic disease such as diabetes, chemical agents, some medications, or allergic reaction.

Nephrosis is characterized by the abnormal function of the kidneys caused by a change in the permeability of the glomeruli. The glomerular walls usually do not allow blood proteins (especially albumin) to filter across into the nephrons. When they do, large amounts of albumin are lost through the urine. One of albumin's important jobs is to help hold water within the blood vessels. Low albumin levels cause large amounts of water to leave the blood vessels and enter other body tissues. This shift in fluid causes swelling (edema) within the skin and other body tissues. Blood becomes concentrated, and the pituitary gland releases antidiuretic hormone (ADH) in an attempt to increase the blood volume by increasing water reabsorption by the kidneys. But the ADH only reduces the amount of urine being produced and worsens the swelling. The liver, in trying to replace some of the lost albumin, begins to process extra fat-protein compounds (lipoproteins, of which cholesterol is one). This liver activity causes another common finding in nephrosis: high fat levels in the blood.

SIGNS AND SYMPTOMS. Children with nephrosis may initially appear to be gaining weight due to normal growth, but eventually the swelling becomes obvious. Irritability, loss of appetite, nausea, vomiting, and diarrhea are frequent symptoms. The fluid that collects around the lungs can cause breathing difficulties.

TREATMENT. Hospitalization and bed rest are necessary during times of severe swelling (edema), along with dietary modifications and medication, including steroids. Steroid medications are usually continued (in lower doses) for weeks or months after the nephrosis has subsided. Nephrosis usually runs its course without causing permanent kidney damage, although some children develop chronic renal failure. Many children will continue to have recurrences of nephrosis years later.

PYELONEPHRITIS

This inflammation of one or both kidneys, usually caused by infection, is an upper urinary tract disorder. The microorganisms that cause the infection enter the kidneys by ascending the ureters from the bladder, or filter from the blood into the kidneys. People most at risk of having pyelonephritis are those who have recurrent lower urinary tract infections (bladder infections/cystitis), chronic urinary stones (urolithiasis), structural defects of the genitourinary system, diabetes, or nerve impairment (paralysis) of the bladder. Pregnant women are at increased risk because the enlarging uterus can "pinch" the ureters against other structures and obstruct the flow of urine from the kidneys. Early and complete treatment of all lower urinary tract infections (cystitis) can greatly reduce the occurrence of pyelonephritis.

Microorganisms enter the kidneys, causing inflammation and swelling. As the infection dissipates, the inflamed renal tissue is replaced by scar tissue. Collective scarring from repeated or chronic occurrences of pyelonephritis decreases the kidneys' ability to function; in time, complete renal failure may occur. Pyelonephritis occurs in both acute and chronic forms.

ACUTE PYELONEPHRITIS

SIGNS AND SYMPTOMS. Sudden and usually severe symptoms include fever, chills, pain in the area of the infected kidney(s), and discomfort in the lower abdomen. If pyelonephritis was caused by bladder infection (cystitis), the signs and symptoms of cystitis will be present as well (see page 160).

TREATMENT. Adequate daily intake of fluids is important to help flush out the urinary system while antibiotics are given to fight the infection.

CHRONIC PYELONEPHRITIS

SIGNS AND SYMPTOMS. Inflammation and infection continue for an indefinite period of time. There may be no overt symptoms unless an acute flare-up occurs. Generalized symptoms of chronic pyelonephritis include fatigue, headache, loss of appetite and weight, and high blood pressure. As scarring continues within the affected kidneys, signs and symptoms of kidney failure eventually become evident.

TREATMENT. When possible, the cause is removed (if urinary stones, for example) or surgically corrected (if a structural urinary system defect). If the infection cannot be eradicated from a nonfunctioning kidney, its removal may be indicated.

UROLITHIASIS

Urolithiasis is the development of stones (also called calculi) within the urinary system. They may be formed in the kidney (also known as renal calculi or nephrolithiasis), in the ureters (also known as ureterolithiasis), or in the bladder.

Urinary stones occur more in men than in women and usually affect people during early to mid-adulthood; specific geographic regions in the United States reflect a higher incidence of urinary stones than occurs in the population as a whole. The exact cause of urinary stones is often unknown. Size can vary from that of a grain of sand to an orange. Some genetic disorders that result in abnormal enzyme formation affect the composition of urine and have a high incidence of urinary stone formation. Cystinuria (see page 160) is a genetic disorder that causes the formation of multiple stones within the urinary system.

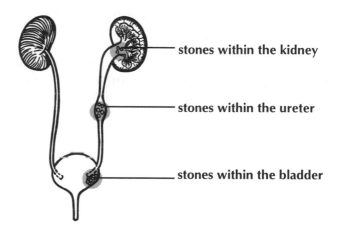

stones within the kidney

stones within the ureter

stones within the bladder

Figure 12.7. Urolithiasis

Other factors known to contribute to stone formation include not drinking enough fluids (inadequate hydration), inadequate urine elimination, prolonged bed rest, gout, recurrent urinary tract infections, parathyroid tumor, and surgeries that shorten the length of the intestinal tract. The composition of urinary stones varies, but most contain calcium, uric acid, phosphate, and/or oxalate.

SIGNS AND SYMPTOMS. Urinary stones may not cause symptoms until they become lodged in an area that obstructs the flow of urine, resulting in pain, inflammation, and infection with fever and chills. Urinary stones that begin to travel down a ureter to the bladder can cause intense pain, nausea, vomiting, blood in the urine (hematuria), and even shock. The pain in this instance often radiates from the flank area down to the genital area and thighs.

TREATMENT. The size and location of the stones determines treatment. Many small stones are eventually passed spontaneously in the urine. Lithotripsy is a nonsurgical technique that is sometimes used; it crumbles stones with ultrasound waves so the resulting stone fragments can pass from the body in the urine. Stones may also be removed with the use of a scope, which is a flexible tube that is passed from the outside of the body through the urethra into the bladder, permitting visualization of the inside of the urethra and bladder. Use of a scope allows certain treatments to be performed without surgery. However, sometimes surgery is required. The best measure is prevention by drinking adequate amounts of fluid daily and making dietary modifications. Medication may also be prescribed.

About 50% of people who have urinary stones will have a recurrence at some point in their lives.

WILMS TUMOR
Also known as nephroblastoma.

Wilms tumor is the most common malignant (cancerous) tumor of the urinary tract in children. It develops in one or both kidneys, and in some families it appears to follow an autosomal dominant inheritance pattern. Although Wilms tumor is usually diagnosed by the age of three or four, it is thought to originate during embryonic development from abnormal renal tissue. It is sometimes associated with the occurrence of genitourinary structural defects. This malignancy grows very rapidly, and if malignant cells escape from the kidneys' tough outer layer (the capsule), it can spread easily to other parts of the body, including the lungs, bone, liver, and brain.

SIGNS AND SYMPTOMS. A nontender abdominal mass and increased abdominal circumference (girth) are the two most common symptoms of Wilms tumor. Other symptoms can include high blood pressure, nausea, loss of appetite, weight loss, fatigue, hematuria (blood in the urine), and anemia.

TREATMENT. Surgical removal of the tumor(s) and affected renal tissue is combined with chemotherapy and/or radiation therapy.

INSTRUCTIONS: To be sure your health-care provider has all the information needed to plan and individualize your health care, answer the following questions after you read Chapter 12, The Urinary System. Write your answers in Section 12 of the *GENETIC CONNECTIONS*™ *HEALTH HISTORY FORM*, which you will find at the back of this book. Use a separate *HEALTH HISTORY FORM* for each family member.

SECTION 12
THE URINARY SYSTEM

Document any of the following structural defects of the urinary system that were present at birth.

12.1   Epispadias: indicate how it was treated.

12.2   Extrophy of the bladder: indicate how it was treated.

12.3   Hypospadias: indicate how it was treated.

12.4   Kidney (renal) agenesis.

12.5   Kidney (renal) hypoplasia: indicate how it was treated.

12.6   Document other structural defects present at birth and treatment(s), if known.

Check any of the following diseases and disorders of the urinary system that are or were present.

12.7   Adult polycystic kidney disease (APKD): indicate at what age symptoms began and how the disease was treated.

12.8   Alport syndrome: indicate at what age symptoms began and how the disease was treated.

12.9   Bladder cancer: indicate at what age the cancer occurred. Document whether the cancer was primary (began in the bladder) or secondary (spread from a cancer site elsewhere in the body), if known. Indicate how the cancer was treated. If the bladder cancer was a primary cancer, document the areas or organs of the body to which the cancer spread (metastasized), if known.

12.10   Congenital nephrosis (also called Finnish nephrosis): indicate how it was treated.

12.11   Cystinuria: indicate at what age it began. Document the specific type of cystinuria, if known, and treatment(s), if known.

12.12   Cystitis: indicate at what age(s) cystitis occurred, and document any treatment, if known.

12.13   Glomerulonephritis: indicate at what age(s) glomerulonephritis occurred and how it was treated.

12.14   Infantile polycystic kidney disease (IPKD): indicate how it was treated.

12.15   Kidney (renal) cancer: indicate whether it occurred in the right, left, or both kidneys. Indicate at what age the cancer occurred. Document whether the cancer was primary (began in the kidneys) or secondary (spread from a cancer site elsewhere in the body), if known. Indicate how the cancer was treated. If the kidney cancer was a primary cancer, document any areas or organs of the body to which the cancer spread (metastasized), if known.

12.16   Nephrogenic diabetes insipidus: indicate how it was treated.

12.17   Nephrosis: indicate at what age(s) nephrosis occurred and how it was treated.

12.18   Pyelonephritis: indicate at what age(s) pyelonephritis occurred, and document any treatments, if known.

12.19   Urolithiasis, or urinary stones (calculi) that developed in the kidneys, ureters, or bladder: document any treatment, if known.

12.20   Wilms tumor (a cancerous tumor of the kidneys): indicate at what age it was diagnosed and how it was treated. Document any areas or organs of the body to which the cancer spread (metastasized), if known.

12.21   Document any other diseases or disorders of the urinary system that are or were present, age at onset, and treatment(s) that were received, if known.

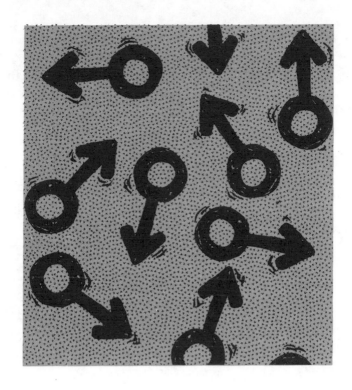

CHAPTER 13

THE MALE REPRODUCTIVE SYSTEM

The male reproductive system consists of both external and internal structures. The external structures are the penis and scrotum; the internal structures are the testes (testicles), epididymides, vas deferens, and the accessory glands. The accessory glands comprise the seminal vesicles and the prostate and bulbourethral glands (also called Cowper's glands).

The male reproductive system produces sperm, provides a method for depositing sperm into the female reproductive tract, and produces testosterone, the primary male hormone necessary for the development and maintenance of male sex characteristics.

INTERNAL STRUCTURES AND THEIR FUNCTIONS

THE TESTES

The testes, also called testicles, are the male gonads—the glands that produce sperm (male reproductive cells) and testosterone. The right and left testes are housed in a pouch-like structure called the scrotum, which holds the testes away from the body because sperm cannot survive for long at normal body temperatures.

THE EPIDIDYMIDES

Connected to the upper back portion of each testis is a structure called the epididymis (the plural form is epididymides). The epididymides receive sperm from the testes and store the sperm while they mature.

THE VAS DEFERENS

The vas deferens is a tube, or passageway, that connects each epididymis with the urethra. Sperm are transported from the epididymides through the vas deferens to the urethra. The urethra is the passageway from the bladder to the outside of the body, which opens at the end of the penis. Both urine and seminal fluid exit the body through the urethra.

THE ACCESSORY GLANDS

Fluids from the accessory glands are secreted into the vas deferens at various points to mix with the sperm and form seminal fluid (semen). These glandular secretions play an important role in the reproduction process by protecting and nourishing the sperm and allowing them to move freely.

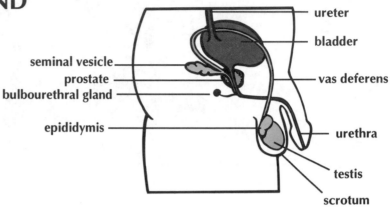

Figure 13.1. The male reproductive system

STRUCTURAL DEFECTS

CRYPTORCHIDISM

Also called cryptorchism and undescended testicles.

Cryptorchidism is the failure of one or both testes to descend into the scrotum. Usually only one testis is involved. The undescended testis may remain in the abdomen or within the groin area. The testes normally descend into the scrotum after week 36 of fetal life. In those infants whose testes are not descended at birth, most will have descended testes by one year of age. Cryptorchidism appears more frequently within some families, and an autosomal dominant inheritance pattern has been suggested. It also occurs with some genetic and/or chromosomal syndromes.

SIGNS AND SYMPTOMS. The health-care examiner checks by hand for the presence of both testes within the scrotum. If cryptorchidism is present, the scrotal pouch feels empty.

TREATMENT. Hormones can be used to stimulate the testis to descend, or surgery may be performed to correct placement. To give the testis a chance to descend on its own and to protect its sperm-producing capability, treatment is usually begun between a boy's first and second birthdays.

Undescended testes have a higher incidence of testicular cancer. Although correcting their placement may not necessarily reduce this risk, the cancer will be easier to identify should it occur. Thus, it is very important that males with a history of cryptorchidism examine their testicles every month throughout their lives so that testicular cancer may be diagnosed and treated early.

DISEASES AND DISORDERS

BENIGN PROSTATIC HYPERPLASIA (BPH)

Also referred to as benign prostatic hypertrophy.

BPH is characterized by prostate gland enlargement because of an increase in the number of prostate cells. BPH is not a cancerous condition. It occurs primarily in men over age 50; its prevalence increases with age, and it is seen worldwide. The exact cause of BPH is unknown but may be related to the hormonal changes that occur with normal aging. As many as 75% of men over the age of 75 have some symptoms of BPH.

SIGNS AND SYMPTOMS. As the prostate enlarges, it compresses the lower portion of the bladder and the upper urethra, hindering the flow of urine from the bladder. Symptoms of BPH include difficulty in starting a urine stream, a decrease in the force of the urine stream, which often requires straining to keep flowing, frequent night urination, incomplete emptying of the bladder, an urgent need to urinate, and blood in the urine (hematuria). General symptoms include abdominal discomfort, loss of appetite, and fatigue. Severe BPH that totally obstructs the urethra must be treated immediately because urine must drain from the bladder.

A complication of BPH is permanent kidney damage caused by recurrent urinary tract infections and/or the chronic backup of urine within the ureters and kidneys. Any urine remaining in the bladder after urination can become stagnant and harbor bacteria that can travel up the ureters to the kidneys, causing urinary tract infection. Repeated infections can lead to permanent kidney damage and failure if BPH is not treated.

TREATMENT. The health-care provider may decide that no treatment, except for frequent reexaminations, is necessary. Treatment options include medication, open surgery, or the surgical removal of enough prostate tissue to widen the urethral pathway (transurethral resection of the prostate, called TURP). Whereas open surgery requires an incision, with TURP the surgeon goes through the urethra with special equipment to "shave" tissue from the prostate, and there is no outside incision. BPH can also be treated with hormones to shrink prostate tissue, thereby improving the outflow of urine.

CANCER OF THE PROSTATE

Also known as prostatic cancer.

In the United States, prostate cancer is the most common cancer among men, after skin cancers. It is seen most often in men over age 50; risk increases with age. African American men have the highest incidence in the world. There are increased incidences in the populations of some geographic regions, including North America and northwestern Europe, and a decreased incidence in others, including Africa, Central and South America, and the Near East. The lowest incidence is in Japan.

Prostate cancer frequently runs in families, suggesting a genetic influence. High-fat diets have also been proposed as a factor. Men exposed to cadmium (such as welders, electroplaters, and battery producers, among others) have a higher incidence of prostate cancer. Other environmental factors may also be involved.

The prostate gland encircles the lower portion (neck) of the bladder and the urethra. When it enlarges as a result of cancer or benign hyperplasia (see above), it compresses the bladder neck and urethra, causing interference or change in urination patterns.

SIGNS AND SYMPTOMS. Changes include difficulty starting and maintaining a flow of urine, pain on urination, having to urinate more frequently than usual (because the bladder is not being emptied completely), and frequent night urination. A constant sense of urgency to urinate may also be present. Prostate cancer grows slowly but can spread to the lymphatic system (lymph nodes and lymphatic vessels), the bones, and other organs. If the cancer has spread, other symptoms may include back and/or hip pain, thigh pain, blood in the urine, anemia, loss of appetite and weight, and fatigue.

TREATMENT. Surgical removal of the prostate can be combined with radiation therapy and/or chemotherapy (including hormone therapy to suppress the production of male hormones). Although the majority of people recover from prostate surgery without complication, some men experience sexual impotence and loss of bladder control. Cryosurgery (freezing) techniques are being investigated. It is important for men over age 50 to have a rectal examination during their annual physical examination because the examiner often can feel cancerous changes of the prostate in its early stages. Annual screening of blood PSA levels should also be included. Prostate-specific antigen (PSA) levels in the blood elevate as prostate tissue grows, whether due to cancer or benign enlargement. An annual PSA blood level test allows comparison of PSA levels from year to year and thus helps identify prostate cancer early. PSA levels can also be useful in evaluating prostate tumor growth and the tumor's response to treatment. Men with a family history of prostate cancer should be examined yearly (by rectal exam and blood PSA levels) beginning at age 40. If discovered early, a complete cure for prostate cancer is possible.

The cells of the prostate need the male hormone testosterone to grow, and so does prostate cancer. Because testosterone is produced within the testes, surgical removal of the testes, in a procedure called orchiectomy, may be indicated. Without testosterone the cancer will shrink, reducing pain and the obstruction of urine flow. Another method of counteracting or reducing testosterone levels includes administering drugs that indirectly interfere with the production of testosterone within the testes. Side effects of suppressing male hormone production can include hot flashes and breast enlargement.

CANCER OF THE TESTIS

Also known as testicular cancer.

Occurring primarily in young men between the ages of 18 and 40 years, this is perhaps the most common form of cancer in young males, although overall it is a fairly rare disorder. Testicular cancer occurs more often in Whites than in Blacks. The exact cause is unknown. One of the biggest risk factors is a history of undescended testis (cryptorchidism). Even if the undescended testis had been repositioned into the scrotum, it has a higher risk of developing cancer. Another risk factor is any abnormality of the genital system, including hypospadias (see page 158). Abnormalities of the sex chromosomes, including Klinefelter syndrome or hermaphroditism (having male and female sex characteristics and organs), may increase the risk as well. Other suspected risk factors include injury or previous infection of the testis (orchitis).

Testicular cancer has a very high cure rate if found and treated early. The majority of tumors are discovered by the men themselves or their partners. All men, including teenagers, should perform testicular self-examination (TSE) every month so that unusual masses or lumps can be examined by a health-care provider immediately.

SIGNS AND SYMPTOMS. Enlargement of the testis and scrotum and a painless lump within the scrotum are common symptoms. Testicular cancer is usually limited to one testis. Testicular cancer can also spread to other organs such as the lymph nodes or lungs.

TREATMENT. Depending on the specific cancer type, surgical removal of the affected testis can be combined with radiation therapy and/or chemotherapy to treat testicular cancer. Because post-treatment complications may include loss of ejaculation and/or sterility, men who want children in the future may want to discuss with their health-care provider storing sperm in a sperm bank before treatment begins. Stored sperm can later be used for artificial insemination. New nerve-sparing techniques used during surgical treatment of testicular cancer may prevent the nerve damage that causes loss of ejaculation.

EPIDIDYMITIS

Epididymitis is the inflammation of one or both epididymides caused by injury, infection, the spread of a urinary tract or prostate infection, or irritation from chemical agents, such as urine. (Straining on urination because of a narrowed or blocked urethra can force urine to back up into the vas deferens and the epididymis.) Bilateral epididymitis can result in sterility.

SIGNS AND SYMPTOMS. Scrotal pain and swelling and groin tenderness can occur and may be accompanied by fever. Untreated infection can lead to tissue death within the epididymides and testes; the infection may continue to spread throughout the entire body and result in septicemia or sepsis, a very serious complication.

TREATMENT. Epididymitis is treated with rest, elevation of the scrotum, application of cold or ice to the scrotum, and medications, including antibiotics.

ORCHITIS

Orchitis is the inflammation of one or both testes (usually both) from infection or injury. Infection in the urinary tract or the blood can enter the testes and cause orchitis. Men who contract mumps after puberty can develop orchitis as a complication.

SIGNS AND SYMPTOMS. Pain and swelling of the scrotum and pain in the groin area(s) occur with orchitis and are sometimes accompanied by nausea and vomiting. If both testes are involved, sterility can result. Epididymitis often accompanies orchitis.

TREATMENT. Rest, elevation of the scrotum, application of cold or ice packs to the scrotum, and medication can control pain and swelling; antibiotics are used to control the infection. Postpubertal men who are exposed to the mumps virus but lack immunity against it can be given gamma globulin (a natural protective protein antibody) to reduce the severity of the mumps infection should it develop, thereby reducing the risk of orchitis (and resultant sterility).

PROSTATITIS

Prostatitis is the inflammation of the prostate gland from infection. It can also be associated with enlargement of the prostate from benign prostatic hyperplasia. Prostatitis occurs in both young and adult men. Complications of prostatitis can include abscess formation, spread of infection throughout the bloodstream (sepsis or septicemia), or obstruction of the flow of urine.

SIGNS AND SYMPTOMS. Prostatitis can cause pain in the genitoanal area, difficulty urinating, increased urinary frequency, a constant urgent need to urinate, pain in the lower back, and a discharge from the urethra. With acute infection, fever and chills may occur.

TREATMENT. Antibiotics are given to treat bacterial infection; discomfort is controlled by soaking the genital area in warm water and taking pain medication. Adequate rest is recommended, as is preventing constipation by drinking plenty of fluids and using stool softeners to avoid irritating the prostate and causing painful straining.

INSTRUCTIONS: To be sure your health-care provider has all the information needed to plan and individualize your health care, answer the following questions after you read Chapter 13, The Male Reproductive System. Write your answers in Section 13 of the *GENETIC CONNECTIONS™ HEALTH HISTORY FORM,* which you will find at the back of this book. Use a separate *HEALTH HISTORY FORM* for each family member.

SECTION 13
THE MALE REPRODUCTIVE SYSTEM

Document any structural defects of the male reproductive system that were present at birth and treatments, if known.

13.1   Cryptorchidism: document treatments, if known.

13.2   Document other structural defects and treatments, if known.

Check any of the following diseases and disorders of the male reproductive system that are or were present.

13.3   Benign prostatic hyperplasia (BPH): indicate at what age symptoms began. Document treatment(s), if known.

13.4   Cancer of the prostate: indicate at what age the cancer occurred. Document whether the cancer was primary (began in the prostate) or secondary (spread from a cancer site elsewhere in the body), if known. Indicate how the cancer was treated. If the prostate cancer was a primary cancer, document any areas or organs of the body to which the cancer spread (metastasized), if known.

13.5   Prostatic specific antigen (PSA): document test dates and results.

13.6   Cancer of the testis: indicate whether the right, left, or both testes were affected and at what age. Document whether the cancer was primary (began in the testis) or secondary (spread from a cancer site elsewhere in the body), if known. Document how the cancer was treated. If the testis cancer was a primary cancer, document any areas or organs of the body to which the cancer spread (metastasized), if known.

13.7   Epididymitis: indicate at what age(s) the epididymitis occurred. Document the cause and treatment, if known.

13.8   Orchitis: indicate at what age(s) orchitis occurred. Document the cause and treatments, if known.

13.9   Prostatitis: indicate at what age(s) prostatitis occurred. Document the cause and treatments, if known.

13.10   Document any other diseases and disorders of the male reproductive system that are or were present, the age at onset, and treatment(s) that were received, if known.

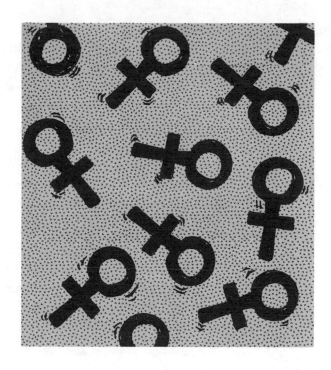

CHAPTER 14

THE FEMALE REPRODUCTIVE SYSTEM

The female reproductive system consists of both external and internal structures. The external structures include the labia majora and minora and the clitoris; the internal structures include the ovaries, fallopian tubes, uterus, cervix, and vagina. The female breasts, also known as the mammary glands, are considered accessory organs of the female reproductive system.

The female reproductive system provides egg cells (ova), houses and supports the fetus after an egg is fertilized, and produces the female hormones estrogen and progesterone. Estrogen and progesterone are necessary for the development and maintenance of female sex characteristics, the maintenance of pregnancy, and the regulation of the female reproductive (menstrual) cycle.

The female reproductive cycle encompasses the maturation and release of an egg from an ovary (ovulation), the changes that occur to prepare the lining of the uterus for the implantation of a fertilized egg, and the shedding of the uterine lining (menstruation) when a fertilized egg is not implanted. All these events and changes within the female reproductive system are regulated by the cyclical highs and lows of estrogen and progesterone levels and hormones released by the pituitary gland (see pages 184-85).

Menarche is the onset of menstruation, and thus the start of the female reproductive cycle. Menarche occurs in most females between the ages of 11 and 17. Menopause is the other end of the spectrum, the cessation of menstruation and the female reproductive cycle. Although menopause can occur as early as 35 or as late as 58, menopause occurs in most women between the ages of 48 and 52. Menopause has occurred when a woman has had no menstrual periods for one year. It results from the cessation of hormone production by the ovaries.

INTERNAL STRUCTURES AND THEIR FUNCTIONS

THE OVARIES

The ovaries are the female gonads; these glands and the more than one million immature egg cells they house are present in females when they are born. The ovaries also produce the hormones estrogen and progesterone. Cyclical changes in the levels of these two hormones, and hormones released from the pituitary gland, stimulate an immature egg cell to mature and break out from an ovary approximately every 28 days, an event called ovulation. Each ovary lies in close proximity to a fallopian tube.

THE FALLOPIAN TUBES

The fallopian tubes are hollow passages that open into the upper uterus. At the end of each tube, finger-like projections move back and forth, trying to sweep up and capture the egg as it falls from the ovary, to start it on its journey down the tube. An egg is usually within a fallopian tube when it is fertilized by a sperm.

THE UTERUS

In its nonpregnant state, the uterus is a hollow, pear-shaped organ that lies within the pelvic cavity. During pregnancy the uterus grows to an enormous size to house and support the growing fetus. The uterus contains three layers of muscle that forcefully contract during labor and delivery to thin and dilate (open) the cervix, propel the infant through the birth canal, and prevent excessive loss of blood after childbirth.

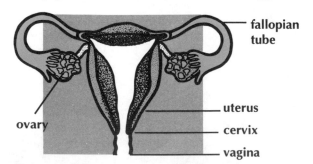

Figure 14.1. Internal reproductive structures

THE CERVIX

The cervix is the lower portion of the uterus, the passageway between the uterus and the vagina. During labor, the cervix "thins" and dilates (opens) to become a circular opening that measures approximately 10 cm in diameter (about 4 inches) to allow passage of the fetus from the uterus into the vagina (birth canal).

THE VAGINA

The vagina is the muscular birth canal between the cervix and the outside of the body. The main characteristic of both the cervix and the vagina is the ability to stretch and expand during childbirth, making vaginal delivery possible.

THE BREASTS

The breasts, or mammary glands, consist of fat, fibrous, and glandular tissues. The glandular tissue is arranged into a network of lobes and ducts that exit through the nipple. Hormonal changes that occur after childbirth stimulate the production of milk from special cells in the glandular lobes; the milk travels through the network of ducts that exit through the nipple.

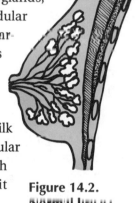

Figure 14.2. Normal breast

DISEASES AND DISORDERS

BREAST CANCER

Breast cancer is second only to lung cancer in causing cancer-related deaths in American women. It occurs in all races and ethnic groups and can occur in men, although this is rare. Japanese women living in Japan have a lower incidence than women—including Japanese women—who live elsewhere. The risk of breast cancer increases with age, especially after menopause.

Although all women have some risk of breast cancer (estimates are that 1 in 9 women will have breast cancer), women whose mother, sister, or daughter had breast cancer before age 40 have a much higher risk. Breast cancers in women under 40 are most likely genetically caused. It is suspected that as many as 10% of breast cancers are inherited by means of one or more

mutant genes. These cancers tend to follow an autosomal dominant inheritance pattern, so that people who inherit the mutant gene(s) have an increased risk of developing breast cancer themselves and a 50% chance of passing the mutant gene(s) to their offspring. Researchers have recently discovered that chromosome 17 is one location for such a gene, and they are attempting to identify the gene itself. Once it is identified, a blood test could be used to test for this breast cancer gene. Women whose family histories suggest an inheritable form of breast cancer should talk with their health-care provider about self-screenings and information on testing.

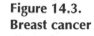

Figure 14.3. Breast cancer

Nonhereditary breast cancers usually occur after age 50 and still account for the majority of breast cancers. They are called nonhereditary because at this time they are not known to be associated with a specific gene mutation. However, because the cause is not known, their occurrence within families is significant.

Risk factors associated with breast cancer, aside from family history, include exposure to high doses of radiation (e.g., radiation therapy or exposure to nuclear radiation) during childhood or adolescence; the onset of menstrual periods before the age of 12 and/or the onset of menopause after age 55; never bearing children; and not bearing a child until after age 30. Fibrocystic breast disease is a risk factor only if microscopic examination of a tissue sample shows abnormal changes within the breast tissue cells. A diet high in fat has been suspected as a risk factor of breast cancer, but studies have been varied in their findings. It is also suspected that long-term female hormonal stimulation has something to do with its development.

SIGNS AND SYMPTOMS. Breast cancer grows as a mass (single or multiple) within the breast, often but not always in the upper outer portion of the breast. The cancer mass(es) may initially be small and can be moved with the fingers, and is usually nontender. Later it becomes hard and nonmovable as it becomes fixed to the underlying tissues. Pain can occur in late stages.

Other noticeable late symptoms include new asymmetry (unevenness) of the breasts, the retraction (inversion) of a nipple, dimpling (like an orange peel) along the skin of the breast, or drainage from the nipple. General signs of significant cancer involvement and/or spread (metastasis) include loss of appetite and weight, and fatigue.

To increase the probability of discovering breast cancer in the early stages when it is most treatable, women should perform monthly breast self-examinations and see their health-care provider at least once a year. Breast tissue actually extends into the axilla (armpit), as do some of the lymph nodes; this area should be checked thoroughly during monthly breast self-examination. The American Cancer Society, the National Cancer Institute, and other professional health organizations recommend the following guidelines for breast cancer screening:

- At all ages, have a health-care provider examine the breasts by hand once a year.
- Beginning at age 40, have a mammogram every one to two years.
- From age 50 on, have a mammogram every year.

These are general guidelines; personal or family history may warrant screenings beginning at age 35 or younger. A mammogram can detect masses even before they can be felt, and therefore it is a very important screening tool.

TREATMENT. A breast lump should be examined by a health-care provider right away. Tests such as needle aspiration or biopsy, or the surgical removal of the mass (lumpectomy), can determine if the lump is cancerous.

The success rate of breast cancer treatment has improved greatly, but, as with all cancers, the earlier the cancer is discovered the better the outcome. A combination of surgical removal of the cancerous mass(es) with or without the surrounding tissue, removal of the entire breast (mastectomy), radiation therapy, chemotherapy, and hormone therapy is usually used.

CERVICAL CANCER

Also known as cancer of the cervix.

All women have some risk of having cancer of the cervix. In the United States, Hispanic and Black females have a higher incidence than White females. Cancer of the cervix is most often seen in women over age 30, but is being diagnosed in younger women as well.

Abnormal changes in the tissue cells of the cervix, called dysplastic changes or dysplasia, are seen among women of all ages, even teenagers. These cell changes can be precancerous or forerunners of cervical cancer. The Papanicolaou test, better known as a Pap test or Pap smear, identifies abnormalities in cervical cells, including dysplastic changes, cancer *in situ* (which is cervical cancer that involves only the outer layer of cells), and invasive cancer (which involves deeper tissues of the cervix). Although dysplastic changes in cervical cells are seen even among teenagers, the average age at which cancer *in situ* is diagnosed is 35, and the average age at diagnosis of invasive cancer is 45. Fortunately, the incidence of invasive cervical cancer is decreasing, probably in part because women are more educated about health care and receive annual Pap tests that allow early diagnosis and treatment of precancerous (dysplastic) and early cancer (cancer *in situ*) lesions.

Risk factors associated with cancer of the cervix include sexual intercourse before age 20, multiple sex partners, childbearing at an early age, and having 10 or more pregnancies. The female children of women who took the drug diethylstilbestrol (DES) to prevent miscarriage or preterm labor have a higher incidence of cervical cancer and cervical abnormalities than the general female population. Women whose mothers took DES during pregnancy should alert their health-care provider and be screened regularly for cervical cancer. If diagnosed early, cervical cancer is treatable, even curable. For that reason, routine Pap tests have greatly reduced the incidence of, and therefore the number of deaths from, invasive cervical cancer in the United States.

Cigarette smoke, first-hand and second-hand, has been noted as a risk factor for cervical cancer. Although the exact relation is unclear, it is speculated that cigarette smoke lowers the body's resistance to disease, which may in turn increase the risk of cancerous changes within body tissues. Some sexually transmitted diseases (STDs) are suspected of increasing the risk of cervical cancer, specifically some types of human papillomavirus that cause genital warts. Having intercourse with a man who has a history of sexually transmitted disease or prostate cancer may also increase risk.

Nutritional deficiency of vitamins A, C, folic acid (a B-complex vitamin), and beta-carotene increase risk because these elements are thought to contribute to the body's resistance to all cancers.

SIGNS AND SYMPTOMS. Cervical cancer often has no signs or symptoms, but painless bleeding from the vagina between menstrual periods, bleeding after sexual intercourse or trauma to the cervix, or unusual vaginal discharge can occur. If invasive cervical cancer spreads to nearby organs and throughout the body, fatigue, loss of appetite and weight, and anemia occur.

TREATMENT. Cervical cancer can be treated by destroying cancerous cervical tissue by freezing it (cryosurgery), vaporizing it with lasers, burning it with electrical current (cauterization), or surgically removing it. In more advanced cancers, hysterectomy (surgical removal of the uterus and cervix) and the removal of some surrounding structures may be necessary in combination with radiation therapy and/or chemotherapy.

ENDOMETRIAL CANCER

Also known as cancer of the uterus and uterine cancer.

In the United States, endometrial cancer affects White and Hawaiian females more often than Black females and is seen most often between the ages of 60 and 74. Most endometrial cancers begin within the endometrium, the inner lining of the uterus. Endometrial cancer can spread to the muscle layer of the uterus (the myometrium), surrounding tissues and organs, and throughout the body. Fortunately, many endometrial cancers have a slow rate of growth, which provides better opportunity for successful treatment.

Some factors associated with increased risk of endometrial cancer center on long-term stimulation by and/or exposure to the hormone estrogen. These factors include never bearing children, onset of menopause after age 55, long-term use of estrogen replacement therapy during and after menopause, and obesity. Obese women often have higher levels of estrogen than same-aged women of healthy body weight. Other risk factors include diabetes mellitus and high blood pressure, although the relation between these two disorders and endometrial cancer is not clearly understood.

Factors that *decrease* the risk of endometrial cancer include having more than four pregnancies and using birth control pills or menopause treatments that contain progesterone in addition to estrogen; progesterone seems to balance or oppose the risk associated with the use of estrogen alone.

SIGNS AND SYMPTOMS. Endometrial cancer may not cause symptoms in early stages. Vaginal bleeding between menstrual periods in premenopausal women, vaginal bleeding at any time after menopause, other abnormal vaginal discharge, and low back and/or pelvic pain can occur.

TREATMENT. Most often a combination of therapies is used, including surgical removal of the uterus, cervix, ovaries, and surrounding structures; radiation therapy; chemotherapy; and hormone therapy.

The key to successful treatment is early detection. Women should have a gynecological examination that includes both a manual (by hand) pelvic examination and a Pap (Papanicolaou) test annually to increase the probability of early diagnosis. A Pap test (the microscopic examination of cells scraped from the cervix) cannot detect all endometrial cancers, but the examination of endometrial cells taken from within the uterus can. To increase the chance of early diagnosis, endometrial tissue sampling may be included in the routine gynecological examination of women at risk of endometrial cancer.

The American Cancer Society recommends that "women of any age who are or have been sexually active, or who have reached age 18, should have an annual Pap test and pelvic examination. After three or more consecutive satisfactory annual examinations, the Pap test may be performed less frequently at the discretion of [their] physician."

ENDOMETRIOSIS

Endometriosis is seen in more Whites than in Blacks, and occurs most frequently during the third and fourth decades of life.

Endometriosis is characterized by deposits of tissue that resemble the inner lining of the uterus but are located outside the uterus. These clumps of tissue, called implants, can be attached to the abdominal wall, ovaries, colon, intestines, or other structures. Endometrial implants have also been known to occur in distant organs such as the lungs or the brain. Regardless of their location, the implants respond to the cyclical hormone changes of the menstrual cycle just as the inner lining of the uterus does. Every month the tissue grows and thickens and bleeds during menstruation. The blood becomes trapped within the abdominal/pelvic cavities or in the tissues and/or organs to which the implants are attached, resulting in pain, inflammation, and eventual scar formation (adhesions). The scarring can interfere with the function of other organs or cause complications such as bowel obstruction or blockage of the fallopian tubes.

The exact cause of endometriosis is not known, but increased risk is associated with both a family history and never bearing children. Endometriosis regresses during pregnancy because hormone levels are different. Since there are no menstrual periods during pregnancy, the implants do not bleed and may temporarily dry up. Menopause also causes endometriosis to regress; therefore, it is usually not seen in postmenopausal women.

SIGNS AND SYMPTOMS. The symptoms of endometriosis vary. The severity of symptoms does not always correlate with the severity and/or extent of the disorder. Common symptoms include painful intercourse, unusual vaginal bleeding, and unusually severe menstrual pain and cramping that typically begin a few days before the onset of menstruation. Low back pain, low pelvic pain, nausea, and diarrhea often accompany menstrual periods. On the other hand, some women have very few or no symptoms. Infertility occurs in almost half the women who have endometriosis, perhaps due to implants within the fallopian tubes or formation of scar tissue that obstructs the tubes. There may be unknown factors associated with endometriosis that also contribute to infertility.

TREATMENT. Hormone therapy, including the use of birth control pills or a male-type hormone, can be prescribed to dry up the implants. The implants can also be surgically removed by cautery (burning) or laser (evaporation) techniques performed through a small abdominal incision or puncture with the use of a laparoscope, an instrument the examiner uses to see the inside of the abdomen. In some instances, dam-

aged ovaries or fallopian tubes can be reconstructed to increase fertility. In many cases infertility can be treated or corrected to allow successful pregnancy. As a final resort, surgical removal of the uterus and ovaries can be performed if future childbearing is not a concern or if the symptoms become too severe.

FIBROCYSTIC BREAST DISEASE (FBD)

Also known as chronic cystic mastitis and mammary dysplasia.

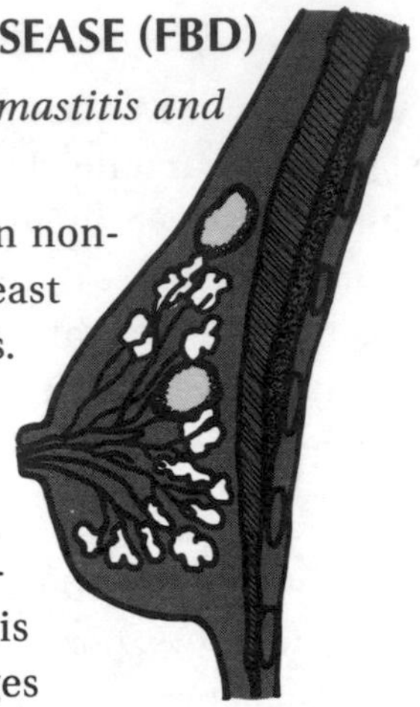

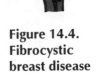

FBD is the most common noncancerous disorder of the breast in women aged 20 to 50 years. The exact cause of the disease is unknown. However, because symptoms fluctuate with the menstrual cycle, researchers suspect that FBD is affected by the normal changes in hormone levels that occur during the cycle period. For example, symptoms usually peak during the week or so before the

Figure 14.4. Fibrocystic breast disease

onset of menstruation, are somewhat relieved after menstruation, and build again during the next premenstrual period. After menopause the disease usually dissipates unless the woman is taking supplemental hormones (primarily estrogen).

In FBD, normal breast tissue thickens (becomes fibrous) and causes masses or lumps, usually in both breasts. Fluid-filled cysts can also form; hence, the term "fibrocystic." It is important to correctly differentiate FBD from other disorders, including breast cancer, so that appropriate treatment can be started. Mammogram (x-ray of breast tissue), needle aspiration (drawing fluid from one of the cysts with a thin needle), and manual breast examination (feeling the consistency of the breasts by hand) can help healthcare providers correctly identify FBD. If results are questionable, a biopsy of one or more of the breast masses can confirm a diagnosis.

SIGNS AND SYMPTOMS. FBD masses are generally round, tender, even painful at times and easy to move with the fingers. In some women the mass(es) can be clearly felt; in others, the breasts take on a lumpy or nodular feel, without any singularly identifiable masses. The masses fluctuate in size throughout the menstrual cycle, creating a sense of fullness and tenderness that is most noticeable right before menstruation.

Women with FBD should examine their breasts every month so they will recognize any changes or new masses. Women whose FBD shows cellular changes (seen on microscopic examination) have a slightly higher risk of having breast cancer. All women with FBD should have routine checkups and—depending on the woman's age—mammograms.

TREATMENT. Women with FBD are often instructed to take vitamin E and thiamine (a B vitamin), reduce sodium intake, avoid foods and liquids that contain caffeine (some over-the-counter medications, coffee, tea, and chocolate, especially dark and sweet chocolate), and wear a supportive bra. Mild pain relievers can control pain, and mild diuretics can reduce fluid retention during peak times of discomfort. Cysts can be drained by needle aspiration, but often the fluid reaccumulates.

OVARIAN CANCER

Also called cancer of the ovaries.

Ovarian cancer is seen in more White and Hawaiian females than Black or Hispanic females in the United States. With the exception of Japan, which has a low incidence, industrialized countries tend to have higher incidence rates than nonindustrialized countries. The risk of ovarian cancer increases with age, with most cases appearing after age 50. It is estimated that 1 in 70 women will have ovarian cancer. Although ovarian cancer is not the most common female reproductive system cancer, it is among the most deadly.

Women with a personal history of breast cancer or who have a mother, sister, or daughter with breast or ovarian cancer have a higher risk of ovarian cancer. Some forms of ovarian cancer are suspected to be genetically determined or heritable cancers. In some families the disease seems to follow a modified dominant inheritance pattern. Women who have either breast cancer or ovarian cancer have a higher risk of having the other.

Another risk factor is never bearing children, whether by choice or because of infertility, which indicates that the development of ovarian cancer may be influenced by hormones. Possible risk factors include high-fat diets, exposure to cigarette smoke, and alcohol ingestion.

Factors that appear to *reduce* the risk of ovarian cancer include pregnancy and the use of combination-type birth control pills.

SIGNS AND SYMPTOMS. Ovarian cancer usually grows rapidly yet often causes no symptoms until it invades surrounding tissues or spreads to other parts of the body. Symptoms may be vague and seem to involve the gastrointestinal tract, including a sense of fullness, an increased abdominal circumference, gas, and low abdominal cramping. Other symptoms include abnormal menstrual periods and pelvic discomfort.

TREATMENT. Usually, a combination of treatments is used, consisting of surgical removal of one or both ovaries and/or the uterus and surrounding structures, radiation therapy, chemotherapy, and hormone therapy. Treatment is most successful if the cancer is discovered early. Routine gynecological pelvic examinations can increase the chance of early diagnosis because sometimes the examiner can feel the ovarian mass (tumor). The Pap test is very important in diagnosing cervical and even some endometrial cancers, but it does *not detect* ovarian cancer. Women over 40 should have annual gynecological examinations. More frequent examinations may be necessary for women with a family history of ovarian or early breast cancer.

PELVIC INFLAMMATORY DISEASE (PID)

PID is the inflammation and infection of one or more internal organs of the female reproductive system, including the uterus, fallopian tubes, and ovaries. Inflammation of the uterus is also known as endometritis (not to be confused with endometriosis). The microorganisms that cause PID usually enter through the vagina and ascend upward through the cervix into the uterus and the fallopian tubes, causing the fallopian tubes to become inflamed and infected (salpingitis). These microorganisms can move beyond the fallopian tubes to inflame and infect the ovaries (oophoritis). The inflammation and infection may extend throughout the pelvic and abdominal cavities, causing peritonitis, a severe illness.

PID can be caused by a variety of microorganisms. Chlamydia, a sexually transmitted disease, causes a significant number of cases. PID can also be caused by microorganisms from the anal area or the urinary tract. PID can also occur as a complication of child-birth, miscarriage (spontaneous abortion), elective/medical abortion, or other surgical procedures involving the female reproductive structures.

Other risk factors associated with PID include using an intrauterine birth control device (IUD) and having multiple sex partners.

SIGNS AND SYMPTOMS. Mild, vague symptoms of fatigue and loss of appetite, or acute symptoms such as nausea and vomiting, fever and chills, severe pelvic or abdominal pain, low back pain, and vaginal dis-charge can occur. Scarring that develops in affected organs can block and/or distort the fallopian tubes, resulting in infertility, increased probability of ectopic (tubal) pregnancy, and long-term abdominal dis-comfort.

TREATMENT. PID can be treated with antibiotics to eliminate the infection (if bacterial) and other medica-tions to reduce inflammation and decrease pain. Hospitalization is sometimes required. If the cause of PID is a sexually transmitted disease, sexual partners may also need treatment to prevent reinfection. Scarred tissue or organs sometimes require surgical removal.

INSTRUCTIONS: To be sure your health-care provider has all the information needed to plan and individualize your health care, answer the following questions after you read Chapter 14, The Female Reproductive System. Write your answers in Section 14 of the *GENETIC CONNECTIONS™ HEALTH HISTORY FORM,* which you will find at the back of this book. Use a separate *HEALTH HISTORY FORM* for each family member.

NOTE: Section 14 of the *HEALTH HISTORY FORM* also contains an obstetric history chart for you to record all pregnancies and their subsequent outcomes. Fill in the information requested for EACH pregnancy, regardless of the outcome. Begin by listing the first pregnancy as pregnancy number 1, the second as pregnancy number 2, etc., proceeding in order of occurrence.

SECTION 14
THE FEMALE REPRODUCTIVE SYSTEM

14.1 Age at menarche (start of menstrual periods).

14.2 Age at menopause (cessation of menstrual periods). Document any treatment received for menopause or symptoms.

14.3 List any structural defects of the female reproductive system present at birth, and treatment(s), if known.

Check any diseases and disorders of the female reproductive system that are or were present.

14.4 Breast cancer: document whether the right, left, or both breasts were involved and the age at which the cancer was diagnosed. Document whether the breast cancer was primary (began in the breast) or secondary (spread from a cancer site elsewhere in the body), if known. Indicate how the cancer was treated. If the breast cancer was a primary cancer, document any areas/organs of the body to which the cancer spread (metastasized), if known.

14.5 Cervical cancer (cancer of the cervix): indicate age at which the cancer was diagnosed. Document whether the cancer was primary (began in the cervix) or secondary (spread from a cancer site elsewhere in the body), if known. Indicate how the cancer was treated. If the cervical cancer was a primary cancer, document any areas/organs of the body to which the cancer spread (metastasized), if known.

14.6 Endometrial cancer (cancer of the uterus): indicate at what age the cancer was diagnosed.

Document whether the cancer was primary (began in the lining of the uterus) or secondary (spread from a cancer site elsewhere in the body), if known. Indicate how the cancer was treated. If the endometrial cancer was a primary cancer, document any areas/organs of the body to which the cancer spread (metastasized), if known.

14.7 Endometriosis: indicate at what age symptoms began. Document any treatment(s), if known.

14.8 Fibrocystic breast disease (FBD): indicate at what age symptoms began. Document any treatment(s), if known.

14.9 Ovarian cancer (cancer of an ovary): document whether the right, left, or both ovaries were involved. Indicate the age at which the cancer was diagnosed. Document whether the cancer was primary (began in an ovary) or secondary (spread from a cancer site elsewhere in the body), if known. Document how the cancer was treated. If the ovarian cancer was a primary cancer, document any areas/organs of the body to which the cancer spread (metastasized), if known.

14.10 Pelvic inflammatory disease (PID): indicate at what age(s) PID occurred. Document the cause and treatment, if known.

14.11 Document other diseases and disorders of the female reproductive system that are or were present, the age at onset, and treatment(s) that were received, if known.

CONTINUED

OBSTETRIC (CHILDBIRTH) HISTORY

(INSTRUCTIONS APPEAR ON PRECEDING PAGE)

Column A: Document both the age that this pregnancy occurred, and the year.

Column B: Check here if this pregnancy delivered at term (after week 37 of pregnancy) regardless of whether the infant was born live. Also include here post-term deliveries (after week 42 of pregnancy), but document in Column J that the infant's condition was post-term.

Column C: Check here if this pregnancy delivered an infant that was preterm (before week 37 of pregnancy) regardless of whether the infant was born live.

Column D: Check here if this pregnancy terminated in miscarriage (spontaneous abortion), which is defined as delivery occurring before week 20 of pregnancy; also check here if therapeutic or elective abortion was performed before week 20 of pregnancy.

Column E: Indicate here how many infants this pregnancy produced (1 for single births, 2 for twins, etc.).

Column F: Indicate here the number of live infants the pregnancy delivered regardless of whether death occurred at any time after birth.

Column G: Indicate here whether the pregnancy was delivered by vaginal birth or cesarean section, marking "V" for vaginal births and "C/S" for cesarean section births.

Column H: Indicate here the sex of the infant(s) delivered from this pregnancy, marking "M" for male infants, "F" for female infants, and "U" for infants of unknown gender.

Column I: Indicate here the birth weight of the infant(s) delivered, using the symbols for pounds (#) and ounces (oz) or kilograms (kg) and grams (gm). (See page 51 for weight conversion charts.)

Column J: Indicate here the condition of the infant(s) at birth; for example, healthy or ill. If ill, list the cause or type of illness, if known, and include any other information you feel is important or unusual.

Column K: Document here any health disorders or complications that occurred during this pregnancy, including:

- medical conditions such as hypertension; pregnancy-induced hypertension (either preeclampsia or eclampsia, previously known as toxemia); diabetes mellitus; gestational diabetes; blood Rh factor incompatibility (between the woman's and the infant's blood); incompatibility between the woman's blood group (A, B, AB, or O) and the infant's blood group; maternal infections; and other medical disorders or conditions;

- bleeding complications such as threatened miscarriage (referred to also as threatened spontaneous abortion), incomplete miscarriage, missed miscarriage, gestational trophoblastic disease (also known as hydatidiform mole or molar pregnancy), ectopic pregnancy, incompetent cervix, placenta previa, or abruptio placentae;

- labor and delivery complications such as premature (early) rupture of membranes, labor of more than 24 hours or less than 3 hours, difficulty in labor due to a small maternal pelvis and/or larger than usual infant or abnormal presentation of the infant (breech, shoulder, transverse, or face presentation).

Also document other health disorders or complications that occurred during the pregnancy.

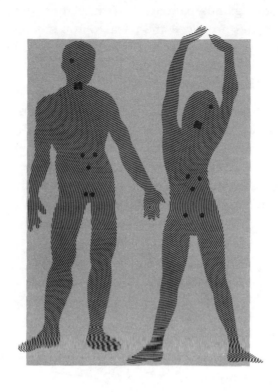

CHAPTER 15
THE ENDOCRINE SYSTEM

T he endocrine or glandular system consists of the pituitary gland, thyroid gland, parathyroid glands, pancreas, adrenal glands, and gonads (the testes and ovaries). Hormones produced and released into the bloodstream by these endocrine glands, together with the nervous system, regulate and control essential body functions by maintaining internal balance (homeostasis) and normal growth and development within the body.

A large portion of endocrine system activity is regulated by the nervous system through a structure called the hypothalamus, the part of the brain stem that controls the automatic functions of the body. The hypothalamus receives information from practically all areas of the brain and uses that data to direct many body functions. It regulates endocrine system activity by releasing chemical substances called "releasing factors," which travel through the bloodstream to the pituitary gland, where they direct either the manufacture, storage, or release of pituitary hormones.

STRUCTURES AND FUNCTIONS
THE PITUITARY GLAND

Although only about half an inch in diameter, the pituitary gland (also called the hypophysis) releases hormones that direct the activity of body organs and tissues. It also releases hormones that direct other endocrine glands to release their hormones. The pituitary gland lies under the brain, next to the brain stem. It is divided into front (anterior) and back (posterior) portions, called lobes; each lobe produces specific hormones (see figure 15.1).

The anterior lobe of the pituitary gland releases six hormones of great importance to normal body function and growth:

- adrenocorticotropic hormone or corticotropin (ACTH) stimulates growth of the adrenal glands and their release of hormones;

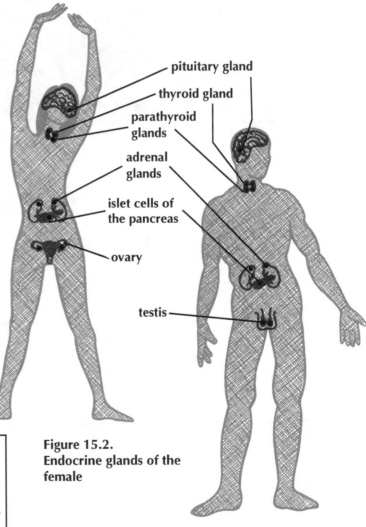

pituitary gland

thyroid gland

parathyroid glands

adrenal glands

islet cells of the pancreas

ovary

testis

**Figure 15.2.
Endocrine glands of the female**

**Figure 15.3.
Endocrine glands of the male**

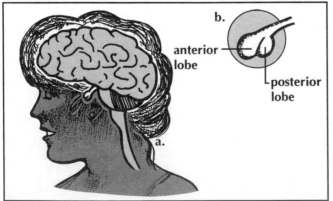

b.

anterior lobe

posterior lobe

a.

**Figure 15.1. The pituitary gland:
a. location of the pituitary gland
b. anterior and posterior lobes of the pituitary gland**

- thyroid-stimulating hormone (TSH) stimulates growth of the thyroid gland and its release of hormones;
- growth hormone (GH) or somatotropin stimulates normal growth and development of body tissues;
- follicle-stimulating hormone (FSH) stimulates the ovaries and testes to produce mature reproductive cells (egg and sperm) and the ovaries to release the hormone estrogen;
- luteinizing hormone (LH) stimulates the ovaries to release egg cells during ovulation, as well as both the ovaries and testes to release their sex hormones;
- prolactin (PRL) stimulates the female breasts to produce milk for breastfeeding (lactation).

The posterior lobe of the pituitary gland releases two important hormones that are produced by the hypothalamus but are stored in and released from the pituitary gland:

- antidiuretic hormone (ADH) directs the kidneys to reabsorb more water and sodium from the urine;
- oxytocin causes the uterus to contract during and after childbirth and stimulates the release of milk from the breast for breastfeeding (lactation).

THE THYROID GLAND

The thyroid gland is located at the front of the neck in front of the windpipe (trachea) right below the Adam's apple. The thyroid gland needs iodine to produce the hormones triiodothyronine (T_3) and thyroxin (T_4). The release of T_3 and T_4 is directed by a pituitary gland hormone called thyroid-stimulating hormone (TSH). Thyroid hormones are needed for normal body growth and metabolism.

Another hormone, calcitonin (or thyrocalcitonin), which is thought to increase the amount of calcium excreted in the urine, is released from the thyroid in response to high calcium levels within the blood. Calcitonin is also thought to keep calcium within the bone, thereby maintaining bone strength.

THE PARATHYROID GLANDS

Four parathyroid glands, each about the size of a grain of rice, are located behind the thyroid gland, to which they are also often attached. The parathyroid glands produce and release parathyroid hormone (PTH), which regulates calcium and phosphorus levels in the blood and their use by the body. Low levels of calcium in the blood trigger the release of PTH, which causes calcium to move from bone tissue into the bloodstream. PTH also increases reabsorption of calcium from the kidneys and absorption of calcium from the intestines.

THE PANCREAS

The pancreas is located in the upper portion of the abdomen behind the stomach. Because it plays a major role in the digestion of food, it is considered to be a structure of the gastrointestinal system. However, some cells within the pancreas called islets of Langerhans or islet cells perform endocrine functions. Islet cells produce several hormones, including insulin, glucagon, and somatostatin. These hormones maintain normal blood levels of glucose, the major energy fuel used by the body.

Rising levels of glucose in the blood trigger the islet cells to release insulin. Insulin allows the glucose to enter body cells, where it is immediately used for energy or stored for later use, thereby lowering blood glucose levels.

Glucagon does just the opposite of insulin. It increases blood glucose levels in response to low levels. Glucagon causes the liver to produce glucose and release some of its stored glucose into the bloodstream.

Somatostatin decreases blood glucose levels by inhibiting the release of hormones that increase glucose levels, including glucagon.

THE ADRENAL GLANDS

One adrenal gland is located atop each kidney (see figure 15.4). Each adrenal gland has two parts that produce and release hormones: the outer layer, called the adrenal cortex, and the center, called the adrenal medulla. Some adrenal gland hormones are essential throughout one's life.

The adrenal cortex produces three types of corticosteroid (steroid) hormones: glucocorticoids, mineralocorticoids, and androgens.

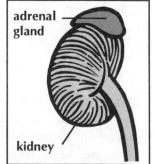

Figure 15.4. Location of the adrenal gland in relation to the kidney

GLUCOCORTICOIDS. Cortisol, the primary hormone in this group, helps cells use (metabolize) sugars, starches, fats, and proteins for energy and growth. Cortisol also plays a big role in the body's response to injury and stress, reduces tissue inflammation, and fights infection. The release of cortisol and other glucocorticoids of the adrenal cortex are regulated by adrenocorticotropic hormone, which is released by the pituitary gland.

MINERALOCORTICOIDS. The primary hormone in this group is aldosterone, which increases the amount of sodium reabsorbed into the bloodstream by the kidneys and absorbed by the intestines. Aldosterone also increases the amount of potassium that is eliminated from the body, helping to maintain fluid volume and chemical balance within the blood and throughout the body. Aldosterone is released from the adrenal cortex, usually when a chemical called angiotensin II is present in the blood; these work together to increase blood volume, blood pressure, and blood flow through the kidneys.

ANDROGENS. Androgens are converted to testosterone, the primary male hormone, and estrone, an estrogen, the primary female hormone. Androgens have a major effect on the nature of secondary sex characteristics, such as the shape and contour of the body, the pattern and distribution of body hair and body fat, and voice changes. Their relative ratio is reversed in males and females; males have more testosterone and females have more estrone. If the ratio is disturbed, a female may have masculinization of features, such as the growth of facial hair and diminished menstruation, and a male may have feminization of features, such as breast enlargement and a female pattern of body fat distribution.

The adrenal medulla produces and releases two hormones known as catecholamines, epinephrine (adrenaline) and norepinephrine. Amounts of these hormones are continually released into the bloodstream to help the nervous system perform its tasks. When the body is stressed, as for example during times of fear or excitement, the nervous system directs the adrenal medulla to release large amounts of catecholamines, which prepare the body to handle the stress. The catecholamines stimulate the heart to beat faster and stronger, the pupils to dilate, blood pressure to rise, the brain to become more alert, and more stored glucose to be released from the liver for energy. Catecholamines are also produced in small amounts by the nervous system.

THE GONADS

Ovaries produce the hormones estrogen and progesterone. Their functions are discussed in Chapter 14, The Female Reproductive System. The testes produce the hormone testosterone, the functions of which are discussed in Chapter 13, The Male Reproductive System.

DISEASES AND DISORDERS
ADDISON DISEASE

Also known as adrenocortical insufficiency or adrenocortical hypofunction.

Addison disease is caused by absent or decreased production of hormones by the adrenal cortex (the outer portion) of the adrenal glands. Two of the adrenal cortex (adrenocortical) hormones, cortisol and aldosterone, are essential. Although it is uncommon, Addison disease can be life threatening unless it is discovered and treated. It can develop at any point in life as a result of the destruction of adrenal gland tissue by the body's own immune system, from infections within the adrenal glands, such as tuberculosis, or from shrinkage (atrophy) of the adrenal glands for unknown reasons. Addison disease (and Addisonian crisis) can develop abruptly in people following the surgical removal (for whatever reason) of their adrenal glands if hormone replacement is not begun. Abnormality of the hypothalamus or pituitary gland can cause Addison disease if the pituitary gland's release of adrenocorticotropic hormone is reduced, because this hormone stimulates the production of the hormones of the adrenal cortex, primarily the production of cortisol. Addison disease that is present at birth is called congenital adrenal hypoplasia, a condition in which the adrenal glands are underdeveloped and nonfunctional.

SIGNS AND SYMPTOMS. Addison disease is characterized by muscle weakness and fatigue, loss of appetite and weight, abdominal pain, nausea, vomiting, diarrhea, difficulty concentrating, and depression. Body hair may become thin, and the skin may darken. Internally, fluid and chemical imbalances cause low blood pressure, low blood sugar levels, dehydration of body tissues, and dangerously high blood potassium levels. The body's ability to respond to stress or to fight infection is impaired. Severe, abrupt onset of these symptoms is called an Addisonian or adrenal crisis; it can cause low blood pressure to become so severe that shock and even death may result. Addisonian crisis can be precipitated by physical and emotional stress, including infection and exposure to temperature extremes. Hospitalization is required during these episodes.

TREATMENT. Medications that replace the adrenal cortex hormones are prescribed for life. Once treatment is begun, the symptoms of Addison disease usually dissipate.

CONGENITAL ADRENAL HYPERPLASIA (CAH)

Also known as adrenogenital hyperplasia, adrenocortical hyperplasia, and adrenogenital syndrome.

CAH is a group of genetic disorders caused by specific defects in enzymes needed for the formation of cortisol (the primary glucocorticoid hormone) by the cortex (outer layer) of the adrenal gland. CAH appears in infancy and occurs in various forms. As a group these defects are transmitted through an autosomal recessive inheritance pattern.

Low or absent blood levels of cortisol cause the pituitary gland to increase its release of adrenocorticotropic hormone (ACTH) in an attempt to raise the amount of cortisol. ACTH is the hormone that stimulates growth of the adrenal glands and their release of hormones. The high levels of ACTH cause the adrenal glands to overgrow (hypertrophy), which affects the gland's production of its other hormones, aldosterone and androgen (testosterone). The production of aldosterone may be excessive, normal, or decreased, affecting the body's balance of water and critical blood components such as sodium and potassium. The production of androgens usually increases, causing genital masculinization in female infants and genital enlargement in male infants. But no matter how much ACTH the pituitary gland releases, cortisol levels do not increase because the enzyme defect does not allow the cortex of the adrenal glands to form cortisol.

SIGNS AND SYMPTOMS. In female newborns, it may be difficult to tell whether the external genitalia are male or female. The clitoris can be enlarged and appear like a penis, and the labia are often enlarged and **fused**, resembling a scrotum. Fortunately, internal reproductive organs are not usually affected. Male infants have enlarged external genitals. If CAH is untreated, both boys and girls have premature puberty with the development of secondary sex characteristics (pubic hair, breast development, deepening voice) at extremely early ages.

When infants who have the type of CAH involving low aldosterone are undiagnosed, life-threatening episodes of diarrhea, vomiting, dehydration, and shock typically occur around one month of age. Quick recognition and initial treatment of CAH is critical for the survival of these infants. Because of excessive male hormone levels in children with CAH, accelerated bone growth makes untreated children tall for their age initially, but when bone growth stops at an early age because of early puberty, they remain short of stature when they become adults.

TREATMENT. Cortisol is taken by mouth daily throughout life. Other hormone replacement may be needed if aldosterone production is also low or absent. Female infants can undergo surgical correction of genital abnormalities and thereby achieve normal reproductive development and function. If treatment of CAH is begun early, the child can attain normal physical growth and development.

During pregnancy, presumptive prenatal (before birth) therapy is started, which consists of giving the mother cortisol-like hormones that cross the placenta, enter the fetal bloodstream, and prevent masculinization of females. Therapy is discontinued if testing reveals the fetus is male or an unaffected female.

CUSHING SYNDROME

Also called hypercortisolism.

Cushing syndrome is caused by excessive production of hormones by the adrenal cortex, the outer layer of the adrenal glands. Cortisol (the major glucocorticoid) is the primary hormone present in excessive amounts, although other adrenal cortex hormones, including aldosterone and androgens, may also be elevated.

Cushing syndrome is seen more in females than in males. The most common cause is the excessive release of adrenocorticotropic hormone (ACTH) from the pituitary gland (called Cushing disease), which in turn stimulates the adrenal cortex to release excessive hormones. Pituitary gland tumors often are the cause of the excessive release of ACTH. Other causes of Cushing syndrome include tumors elsewhere in the body that secrete ACTH, or tumors within the adrenal glands themselves. Cushing syndrome can develop in people who take excessive amounts of ACTH or steroid medication (i.e., cortisone) to treat disorders such as rheumatoid arthritis or to suppress the immune system before and after organ transplantation.

SIGNS AND SYMPTOMS. Excessive amounts of adrenal cortex hormones (primarily cortisol) result in the physical features seen in Cushing syndrome. These features include heavy fat distribution around the abdomen and trunk of the body, the back of the neck and between the shoulder blades, and a round face often described as a "moon" face. The arms and legs usually appear thin and wasted because the body is forced to break down protein and muscle tissue for energy. Excessive androgen release increases facial and body hair, and many people develop acne. The skin becomes thin and fragile, develops stretch marks, and bruises very easily. Other symptoms include the development of high blood sugar (diabetes mellitus); the retention of water and sodium, which contributes to high blood pressure and potential congestive heart failure; and calcium loss from the bones, which increases the risk of bone fractures. People with Cushing syndrome are more prone to infections, and wounds heal more slowly than usual. They may have mood swings, depression, fatigue, confusion, and impotence or cessation of menstruation.

TREATMENT. Tumors of the pituitary or adrenal gland may be surgically removed or treated with radiation therapy. Medications that interfere with the production of ACTH or cortisol may be used. If Cushing syndrome is caused by excessive hormone therapy in the treatment of other disorders, dosage will be adjusted to achieve hormone balance. Once treatment has begun, symptoms of Cushing syndrome usually dissipate.

DIABETES INSIPIDUS

Diabetes insipidus (DI), not to be confused with diabetes mellitus, is caused by low or absent levels of antidiuretic hormone (ADH), which is normally re-leased by the posterior (back) lobe of the pituitary gland. Since ADH directs the kidneys to reabsorb more sodium and water from the urine to maintain adequate blood volume and composition, lack or insufficiency of ADH causes excessive loss of body sodium and water through the urine.

Diabetes insipidus can have several causes. One form of primary DI is a genetic disorder transmitted through an X-linked recessive inheritance pattern that becomes apparent in infancy. Other forms follow an autosomal dominant inheritance pattern. Secondary or nongenetic forms of DI usually develop slowly, occur in adults and children, and may be caused by head injury or infections or tumors of the pituitary gland. The surgical removal of, or surgery close to, the pituitary gland can also result in DI.

SIGNS AND SYMPTOMS. Extreme thirst and the production and elimination of excessive amounts of dilute urine, as much as 20 quarts a day, occur. Sleep is interrupted by repeatedly having to urinate. Dehydration that results can cause flushed, dry skin and dry mouth, low blood pressure, and the development of shock that can lead to coma.

TREATMENT. ADH preparations can be taken by intramuscular injection or by nasal spray to attain normal kidney function and normal concentration of urine. To prevent dehydration, the individual should drink daily the amount of fluid lost through the urine. Some people with DI produce small amounts of ADH on their own; in those cases oral medication can help their kidneys respond better to the small amount of ADH produced.

DIABETES MELLITUS (DM)

Insulin is needed for glucose to move into the body's cells. DM is caused either by a lack of insulin production by the islet cells of the pancreas or the inability of the body to use the insulin produced. When insulin attaches to receptor sites located on cell walls (membranes), glucose enters through the cell wall to be used immediately for energy or stored for later use. Since glucose (blood sugar) is the body's primary energy source, getting it into the cells is crucial. Without available or usable glucose, cells are forced to break down fats and proteins (including muscle tissue) to meet their energy needs; this process can lead to ketoacidosis, a potentially life-threatening disorder.

Two different types of DM exist. Their exact cause is unknown, but genetic factors seem to play a role.

INSULIN-DEPENDENT DIABETES MELLITUS (IDDM)

Also known as type I DM.

Once called juvenile-onset diabetes, it is usually seen in people younger than 30 years of age, but there are exceptions. People with IDDM take insulin to survive. IDDM is caused when the pancreas does not produce insulin, perhaps as a result of an attack on the insulin-producing cells of the pancreas by the body's own immune system that may possibly be triggered by an infection. The symptoms of IDDM develop quickly after more than 90% of the insulin-producing cells of the pancreas are destroyed. About 10% of people with diabetes have IDDM. Uncontrolled IDDM can cause ketoacidosis, a condition that leads to coma and death if untreated. Ketoacidosis occurs when the body is forced to break down (metabolize) fats and proteins for energy because there is no insulin to make glucose (blood sugar) usable. This leads to a buildup of dangerous byproducts that alter the chemical balance of the blood. Ketoacidosis causes dehydration of tissues and results in dry, flushed skin; dry mouth; and low blood pressure. Breathing becomes deep and rapid, the breath has a fruity odor, and the person becomes increasingly stuporous and unresponsive.

NONINSULIN-DEPENDENT DIABETES MELLITUS (NIDDM)

Also known as type II DM.

Once called adult-onset diabetes, it is usually seen in people aged 40 years or older, but there are exceptions. In NIDDM insulin is not required for survival even though it is often used for its treatment and management. Instead, medications called oral hypoglycemics are frequently used. In NIDDM, the pancreas produces some insulin, but either not enough is produced to meet the body's demands, or the body resists or is unable to use the insulin, perhaps because of an abnormality in or absence of the insulin receptors on cell walls that ordinarily allow glucose (blood sugar) to enter the cell.

About 90% of people with DM have this type; although ketoacidosis can occur, it is extremely rare. Instead, people with NIDDM can develop a very dangerous condition called nonketotic hyperosmolar coma, which is characterized by exceptionally high

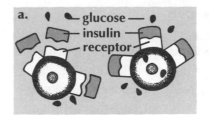
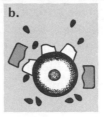

Figure 15.5.

a. insulin attaches to receptors on cell wall allowing glucose to enter cell

b. diabetes mellitus may be caused by decreased production of insulin by the islet cells of the pancreas, or abnormal insulin receptor sites on the cell walls

blood sugar levels and severe dehydration. Approximately 50% of people who develop this condition die.

SIGNS AND SYMPTOMS. The symptoms are the same for both types of DM and are related to the body's inability to use glucose for energy. High blood sugar levels, sugar in the urine on laboratory examination, weight loss, and excessive thirst, hunger, and urination are classic symptoms of DM. Other symptoms include weakness and fatigue, changes in vision, and an increased susceptibility to infection that can cause problems with wound healing. Impotence and menstrual cycle changes are not uncommon. Symptoms indicating the presence of advanced or long-term DM include vision loss, tingling or numbness of extremities (fingers, toes, hands, feet, arms, and legs), high blood pressure, poor circulation, and other signs of cardiovascular disease and renal (kidney) disease.

TREATMENT. IDDM is always treated with insulin injections; NIDDM is only sometimes treated with insulin. NIDDM can be treated with oral medication that stimulates the pancreas to boost its insulin production or acts to improve the ability of the cells to use insulin. Otherwise, treatment and management of DM is the same, regardless of the type. The goal is to maintain blood glucose levels close to the normal range at all times, decreasing the risk of long-term complications such as loss of vision and blindness, early cataract formation, periodontal disease, and kidney and nerve damage.

Diet, exercise, and weight control are important components of diabetes management. Reducing intake of sugars and fats and exercising regularly help the body use insulin, decrease blood sugar and blood fat levels, reduce stress, and help control blood glucose levels. Weight loss is encouraged for people with DM who are overweight; sometimes weight loss is all that is necessary to correct NIDDM. Successful management of DM requires a lot of self-discipline and compliance with diet, exercise, and medication regimens. People with DM also have to learn to adjust their management regimens during times of illness, increased stress, and travel. DM is a lifelong disorder, but with appropriate management people with DM can lead long and healthy lives.

GIGANTISM AND ACROMEGALY

Also known as giantism.

This disorder is due to an excess production of GH (growth hormone or somatotropin) by the pituitary gland causing accelerated growth of body tissues. Gigantism and acromegaly are most often caused by hormone-secreting pituitary gland tumors. Some syndromes that have gigantism as a feature (symptom) may be hereditary.

SIGNS AND SYMPTOMS. Excess growth hormone causes a child to grow to eight feet or so before growth of the arms and legs halts. The growth of other body structures is proportional to height. Acromegaly is caused by excess GH that occurs after the long bones of the arms and legs have completed their growth. Bones then grow in an outward direction, causing the hands and feet to become large and wide, and the forehead, brow, nose, and lower jaw to enlarge and appear to be disproportionate to the rest of the head. Teeth often become widely separated as the jaw bone enlarges. Complications of gigantism and acromegaly include diabetes mellitus, high blood pressure, enlargement of the heart and other body organs, and heart failure. Neurologic symptoms such as headaches or vision disturbances can occur if a pituitary tumor begins to press on the brain or other nervous system structures.

TREATMENT. If a pituitary gland tumor exists it may be surgically removed or treated with radiation therapy. Medication may also be given to interfere with the production of GH.

GOITER

Goiter is the enlargement or overgrowth of the thyroid gland. Goiters have many causes; they vary greatly in size, consistency (smooth or lumpy), and symmetry. Thyroid enlargement can occur because an inadequate amount of hormone is produced by the thyroid gland or because an overactive hypothalamus or pituitary gland causes excessive release of thyroid-stimulating hormone, which in turn stimulates growth of the thyroid gland.

Goiters can occur with or without associated hypothyroidism or hyperthyroidism. *Simple* or *endemic* goiter is caused by an inadequate dietary intake of iodine, which the thyroid gland needs to produce its hormones. In the United States table salt is fortified with iodine (iodized), and the incidence of simple goiter has been reduced significantly. Some foods such as cabbage and turnips can interfere with the formation of thyroid hormones despite an adequate dietary intake of iodine. *Toxic* goiters are associated with hyperthyroidism, for instance, as in Graves disease.

SIGNS AND SYMPTOMS. Enlargement of the neck may occur on one or both sides of the windpipe (trachea) in the area of the Adam's apple. Large goiters can compress the windpipe and interfere with breathing.

TREATMENT. Treatment can include iodine supplements, surgical removal of the goiter, and treatment of hypothyroidism or hyperthyroidism depending on the cause. Surgical treatment should be considered only if the goiter is unsightly (for cosmetic purposes), interferes with breathing or swallowing, or if there is a nodule (tumor) within the goiter in which a cancer cannot be excluded.

GRAVES DISEASE

See Hyperthyroidism, page 191.

HYPERPARATHYROIDISM

Parathyroid hormone moves calcium out of bone and into the bloodstream, and increases the amount of calcium reabsorbed by the kidneys and absorbed by the intestines. In hyperparathyroidism, the over-production of parathyroid hormone results in elevated blood levels of calcium. Hyperparathyroidism is seen in more females than males and usually occurs after 40 years of age.

Most cases of hyperparathyroidism are caused by a noncancerous tumor within one of the parathyroid glands. Other causes include abnormal overgrowth (hyperplasia) of the parathyroid glands and some genetic syndromes. An excessive intake of vitamin D can cause a secondary form of hyperparathyroidism. Hyperparathyroidism does occur at higher incidences in some families, suggesting a genetic predisposition in those cases. People who have undergone radiation therapy to the head or neck have a higher incidence of hyperparathyroidism than the general population. People with hyperparathyroidism have an increased risk of stomach or intestinal ulcers (peptic ulcer disease) and permanent kidney damage.

SIGNS AND SYMPTOMS. Some people have no symptoms at all, while others have mood swings, depression, headaches, and fatigue. The movement of calcium from bone to the blood over a period of many years demineralizes and weakens bones, causing fractures to occur easily (even without injury) and bone pain. High blood calcium levels cause muscle weakness, abnormal heart rate, kidney stones, nausea, appetite loss, vomiting, and abdominal discomfort.

TREATMENT. The abnormal parathyroid gland can be surgically removed. Reducing the intake of foods high in calcium and phosphorus, including milk and milk products, is recommended. Medications that increase the kidneys' excretion of excess blood calcium and prevent the movement of calcium from bone tissue are also used. Severe hyperparathyroidism can become life threatening and require hospitalization.

HYPERTHYROIDISM

Also known as thyrotoxicosis.

Hyperthyroidism is caused by excessive production of thyroid hormone, which increases the body's functions and metabolic rate to above-normal levels. Hyperthyroidism occurs in more females than males, usually developing between the ages of 30 and 50 years.

The cause of hyperthyroidism is usually unknown but frequently is seen in association with Graves disease, also called toxic diffuse goiter. Features of Graves disease include hyperthyroidism, goiter, and bulging eyes (exophthalmia). Graves disease is suspected to be a disorder of the immune system. It occurs more frequently in some families, which suggests an inheritable genetic predisposition in those cases.

Other causes of hyperthyroidism, although rare, include cancer tumors within the body (i.e., thyroid or ovaries) that secrete thyroid hormone into the blood-stream, or disorders of the hypothalamus or pituitary gland that increase the release of thyroid-stimulating hormone (TSH) from the pituitary gland, which then stimulates excessive growth of the thyroid gland and leads to goiter formation and increased release of thyroid hormone.

SIGNS AND SYMPTOMS. The increase in the body's metabolism causes anxiety, agitation, shakiness, and increases in heart rate, blood pressure, and body temperature. Weakness and shortness of breath, particularly with activity, also occur. Other common symptoms include weight loss despite a good appetite, intolerance of heat, and difficulty sleeping. Skin texture can become thin, smooth, and moist from increased sweat gland activity, while hair often becomes thin and silky. The increased strain and work on the heart is a major concern for people with hyperthyroidism.

Thyroid crisis or thyroid storm is an extreme life threatening episode of hyperthyroidism symptoms, which requires hospitalization. Death, although uncommon, can occur.

TREATMENT. Treatment is determined by age and the severity and cause of the hyperthyroidism. Medication that interferes with the formation of thyroid hormone can be taken. Sometimes a radioactive iodine mixture is taken by mouth to destroy the thyroid gland completely. Part or all of the thyroid gland may be surgically removed (thyroidectomy). A complication of some treatments is the eventual development of hypothyroidism.

HYPOPARATHYROIDISM

This rare disorder is caused by low or absent production of hormone by the parathyroid glands. Sometimes this is caused by the accidental surgical removal of the parathyroid glands during surgical removal of the thyroid gland and other neck surgeries. It can also be caused when the parathyroid gland tissue is destroyed by the body's own immune system. Heredity may play a role in the occurrence of hypoparathyroidism in some instances. Hypoparathyroidism causes low calcium and high phosphorus levels in the blood.

Pseudohypoparathyroidism is a hereditary disorder in which the parathyroid produces adequate amounts of parathyroid hormone but the tissues that usually react to that hormone (intestines, kidneys, and bone tissue) do not.

SIGNS AND SYMPTOMS. Muscle irritability, including twitching, jerking, spasms, numbness, and tingling of the fingers and toes and around the mouth can occur. Severe cases can cause seizures. Spasms (tightening and narrowing) of the airways within the throat and lungs and heart rate irregularities can be fatal complications. Long-term or chronic hypoparathyroidism can contribute to cataract formation and abnormal skin, nail, and tooth growth.

TREATMENT. The symptoms of hypoparathyroidism can be alleviated by adhering to a diet high in calcium and vitamin D, taking calcium and vitamin D supplements, avoiding foods that contain phosphorus (including milk and milk products), and taking medications to help eliminate excess phosphorus from the body. Treatment is continued for life.

HYPOTHYROIDISM

This low (or nonexistent) production of thyroid hormone by the thyroid gland is seen in females more than males and may be present at birth (congenital) or acquired later, usually between the ages of 30 and 60 years.

Hypothyroidism has many causes, including abnormal thyroid development or formation, the surgical removal of the thyroid gland, damage to the thyroid gland caused by inflammation and/or infection, and diets deficient in iodine (although this is a rare cause in the United States because most table salt contains iodine). Treatment of an overactive thyroid or thyroid cancer with radioactive iodine which destroys thyroid tissue can result in thyroid underactivity (hypothyroidism) years later. In a few cases hypothyroidism is caused by a genetic enzyme disorder that prevents the thyroid gland from forming thyroid hormone.

Hypothyroidism can also be caused by disorders of the hypothalamus or the pituitary gland. This type of hypothyroidism is not usually associated with goiter formation.

Without the thyroid hormone, many body systems fail to grow or develop normally. Once abnormal growth or mental impairment has occurred it cannot be reversed, but treatment may prevent future damage. Congenital hypothyroidism may not become a problem for some children until they are teenagers if the thyroid is able to produce enough thyroid hormone to meet the body's demands for growth and development. Eventually, however, the child requires more hormone than the thyroid can produce. This type of hypothyroidism is not associated with mental impairment because the nervous system (brain) has usually completed its development by the time the hormone is no longer meeting the body's needs.

SIGNS AND SYMPTOMS. Untreated congenital hypothyroidism (cretinism) causes short stature (dwarfism), distinct facial features (a puffy, short, wizened face with wrinkled, wide-set eyes and a large tongue), a protruding abdomen (often with an umbilical hernia), sparse and brittle body hair, dry skin, and varying degrees of mental impairment. If treatment for congenital hypothyroidism is begun within the first few months of life, the child's physical and mental growth and development should be normal. Fortunately, in the United States newborn screening for congenital hypothyroidism is required by law.

Symptoms of acquired hypothyroidism, which are characterized by a slowing down of the body's functions and metabolic rate, include a loss of energy, slowing of the heart rate, decrease in body temperature with an intolerance to cold, a dulling of mental processes, and a slowing of the gastrointestinal tract, which contributes to constipation. Other symptoms include thinning and dryness of hair and nails, pale complexion, weight gain, and dry skin. Goiter formation may occur in some forms of hypothyroidism.

A condition of hypothyroidism called myxedema occurs when hypothyroidism becomes worse and mucus-type fluids collect within the fatty layer of skin, causing thickened, wax-like skin; puffy, droopy, and expressionless facial features; and large-appearing hands and feet. Mental abilities can slow considerably. In rare cases, myxedema advances to coma because of extreme slowing down of body functions, and it can be life threatening.

TREATMENT. As soon as congenital hypothyroidism of newborn infants is diagnosed, it is treated with medication that replaces the thyroid hormone within the body. Thyroid medication is taken for life.

People with acquired hypothyroidism take oral thyroid medication; symptoms usually resolve within several months, and medication is continued throughout life.

PHEOCHROMOCYTOMA

Pheochromocytoma is a rare adrenal gland tumor that grows out of the inner tissue of the gland, the adrenal medulla. These tumors are seen most often in people 25 to 50 years of age; the majority are noncancerous (benign) and usually occur on just one adrenal gland, although approximately 10% of people with pheochromocytoma have tumors on both. Approximately 10% of pheochromocytomas are located away from the adrenal glands along nerve tissue fibers in other areas of the body such as the head, neck, chest, or abdomen. All pheochromocytomas are overgrowths of adrenal medulla tissue; therefore, they produce and release epinephrine (adrenaline) and norepinephrine, the same hormones produced and released by the adrenal medulla. Pheochromocytomas occur at higher incidences in some families and can be transmitted as an autosomal dominant disorder. Pheochromocytomas are associated with some genetic syndromes and are sometimes associated with a particular thyroid cancer (medullary cell carcinoma).

SIGNS AND SYMPTOMS. Sudden episodes of high blood pressure, a pounding, usually slow but occasionally racing heart rate, sweating, shakiness, and mental agitation occur—either for apparently no reason or in response to physical or emotional stress. Other symptoms include headache, blurred vision, dizziness, ringing in the ears, and shortness of breath. Severe episodes can be fatal if they cause heart rhythm abnormalities, stroke (cerebral vascular accident), or kidney failure.

TREATMENT. Treatment is the surgical removal of the tumor. Hospitalization is necessary to stabilize blood pressure and other body systems before surgery. Hormones produced by the adrenal cortex (the outside tissue of the adrenal glands) are essential and are produced only by the adrenal cortex. Therefore, if the entire adrenal gland must be removed, adrenal cortex hormone replacements must be taken throughout life.

RICKETS, VITAMIN D RESISTANT

See page 223.

THYROID CANCER

Cancer of the thyroid gland is uncommon. The type that occurs most often is papillary carcinoma of the thyroid gland. It occurs in females more than males. It can occur in childhood but usually presents itself in young adulthood to middle age. It can spread via the lymphatic system (usually to the lymph nodes in the neck, which usually does not affect the long-term prognosis if treated).

The 10-year survival rate of people with papillary carcinoma is about 90%. Follicular cancer is a less common form of thyroid cancer which occurs in older people and has a tendency to spread more easily.

Risk of some types of thyroid cancer is increased in people whose head and neck areas have been exposed to radiation therapy. At one time radiation therapy was used in the treatment of acne and enlarged tonsils, adenoids, and thymus glands.

A very uncommon form of thyroid cancer is called medullary carcinoma of the thyroid gland. It occurs at a higher incidence in some families, which may indicate a genetic connection in those cases.

SIGNS AND SYMPTOMS. A hard, nontender lump or mass, usually single, can be felt in the thyroid gland. Growth of the tumor may be slow or rapid.

TREATMENT. All or part of the thyroid gland can be surgically removed (thyroidectomy). Radiation therapy, chemotherapy, and/or radioactive iodine therapy are also used.

THYROIDITIS

This inflammation of the thyroid gland has various causes. Bacterial or viral infection of the thyroid gland, although quite uncommon, can cause thyroiditis. Thyroiditis may cause the thyroid gland to temporarily increase its release of thyroid hormone, causing transient hyperthyroidism.

The most common type of thyroiditis is a long-term (chronic) disorder called Hashimoto thyroiditis or Hashimoto disease. It is thought to be an autoimmune disorder; for some unknown reason the body produces antibodies that attack and destroy its own thyroid tissue. Hashimoto thyroiditis may be associated with genetic factors.

SIGNS AND SYMPTOMS. Thyroid gland enlargement and tenderness, difficulty swallowing, and fever occur with thyroiditis.

Hashimoto thyroiditis causes nontender goiter formation and hypothyroidism (low hormone production by the thyroid gland).

TREATMENT. Bacterial thyroiditis can be treated with antibiotics; viral infections are treated with medications that reduce inflammation while the infection runs its course. Hashimoto thyroiditis is treated with thyroid hormone, which may also help reduce the size of the enlarged thyroid (goiter). Part of the thyroid gland itself can be surgically removed (partial thyroidectomy).

SECTION 15
THE ENDOCRINE SYSTEM

15.1   Document any structural defects of any of the glands that make up the endocrine system: the pituitary gland, the thyroid gland, the parathyroid glands, the islet cells of the pancreas, the adrenal glands, the ovaries, and the testes.

Check any of the following diseases and disorders of the endocrine system that are or were present.

15.2   Addison disease: indicate the age symptoms began. Document the cause and treatment, if known.

15.3   Congenital adrenal hyperplasia: document treatment, if known.

15.4   Cushing syndrome: indicate the age symptoms began. Document the cause and treatment(s), if known.

15.5   Diabetes insipidus: indicate the age symptoms began. Document the cause and treatment, if known.

15.6   Diabetes mellitus: document the type as either insulin-dependent diabetes mellitus (IDDM), also known as type I diabetes, or non–insulin-dependent diabetes mellitus (NIDDM), also known as type II. Indicate the age symptoms began and the treatment(s), if known.

15.7   Gigantism and/or acromegaly: document the cause and treatment(s), if known.

15.8   Goiter(s): indicate the age it became apparent. Document the cause and treatment, if known.

15.9   Hyperparathyroidism: indicate the age that symptoms began. Document the cause and treatment(s), if known.

15.10   Hyperthyroidism or Graves disease: indicate the age symptoms began. Document the cause and treatment, if known.

15.11   Hypoparathyroidism: indicate the age symptoms began. Document the cause and any treatment(s), if known.

15.12   Hypothyroidism: indicate the age symptoms began. Document the cause and treatment, if known.

15.13   Pheochromocytoma: indicate age when the tumor was discovered. Document where the tumor was located and treatment(s), if known.

15.14   Thyroid cancer: indicate the age when the cancer was diagnosed. Document whether the cancer was primary (began in the thyroid gland) or secondary (spread from a cancer site elsewhere in the body), if known. Indicate how the cancer was treated. If the thyroid cancer was a primary cancer, document any areas/organs of the body to which the cancer spread (metastasized), if known.

15.15   Thyroiditis or Hashimoto disease: indicate the age symptoms began. Document the cause and treatment(s), if known.

15.16   Document other diseases or disorders of the endocrine system that are or were present, age at onset, and treatment(s) received, if known.

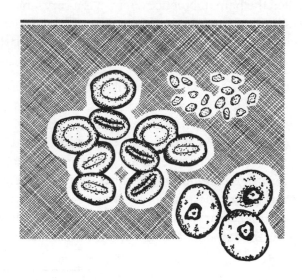

CHAPTER 16

THE BLOOD AND IMMUNE SYSTEMS

The blood is called the hematopoietic system. It is a very large organ, unusual in that it has a liquid form. The blood consists of a yellowish, water-based fluid called plasma that contains the blood cells, blood proteins, blood clotting factors, sodium, potassium, calcium, and glucose (blood sugar).

Blood transports hormones and other regulatory substances throughout the body; transports oxygen from the lungs and delivers it to body tissues; transports carbon dioxide waste from the tissues to the lungs for removal from the body; delivers nutrients absorbed from the intestines of the gastrointestinal system to tissues of the body; and delivers waste elements from body tissues to the kidneys to be filtered into the urine for removal from the body. It also keeps the body free of infection and forms blood clots to maintain blood vessel integrity and prevent harmful blood loss. The structures of the hematopoietic system include the bone marrow and the cellular components of the blood—the blood cells.

THE BLOOD
STRUCTURES AND FUNCTIONS

BONE MARROW

The cellular components of the blood are the red blood cells (RBCs), called erythrocytes; white blood cells (WBCs), called leukocytes; and platelets, called thrombocytes. These blood cells are continuously produced by bone marrow, the soft, pulpy substance in the center of each bone. Each type of blood cell is produced at a different rate because each type survives a different length of time before it must be replaced. When the body requires more blood cells, healthy bone marrow can step up production to meet the demand. Bone marrow can be considered a body organ because the blood cells it produces play crucial roles in both the blood and immune systems.

Bone marrow can be active or inactive. Active bone marrow produces blood cells. Infants have active bone marrow in almost every bone, but adults have active bone marrow only in flat bones such as the skull, shoulder blades, sternum (breastbone), ribs, and hips. If an adult needs more blood cells, however, inactive bone marrow in other bones can become active and begin producing additional blood cells very quickly.

RED BLOOD CELLS (RBCs)

The RBCs (erythrocytes) are round, flat, very flexible structures that can bend and contort to squeeze through the tiniest of the blood vessels—the capillaries. RBCs contain hemoglobin, an iron-rich protein that gives the cells their red color. Hemoglobin

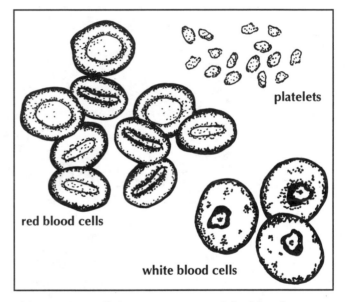

Figure 16.1. Cellular components of the blood

binds with both oxygen and carbon dioxide so these two gaseous compounds can be transported by the RBCs throughout the body. RBCs pick up (bind with) oxygen when circulating throughout the lungs. They then release this oxygen from their hemoglobin as they travel through capillaries. The released oxygen crosses through the capillary wall and enters body tissues; in turn, carbon dioxide (a waste product of cell activity) crosses from the tissues through the capillary wall into the capillary, where it is picked up (bound) by the hemoglobin of the RBCs. RBCs release the carbon dioxide when recirculating throughout the lungs, where it is eliminated from the body with exhaled air.

RBCs are the most prevalent blood cells and survive approximately three to four months. When the kidneys are not getting enough oxygen, they produce and release a hormone called erythropoietin, which stimulates the bone marrow to speed up its RBC production. More RBCs mean more oxygen can be delivered by the blood to the kidneys and other organs.

Certain elements and compounds must be available for the formation of functional, mature RBCs, including the minerals iron, copper, cobalt, and nickel, and the vitamins B12, folic acid, and pyridoxine (vitamin B6). A lack of these substances can decrease the number of RBCs formed and cause various forms of anemia.

WHITE BLOOD CELLS (WBCs)

White blood cells (leukocytes) are the fighter cells of the body, the unseen soldiers that amass quickly into organized armies to protect the body from invading microorganisms and other foreign substances. The WBCs are the working arm of the immune system (see page 201). Each of the three types of WBCs has a specific role in protecting the body from infection. Although the types of WBCs are different from each other, they work together and direct each other's activities to give the body maximum protection. Some WBCs destroy invading microorganisms by releasing chemical enzymes; some by surrounding, engulfing, and digesting invaders and other foreign substances; and some by forming antibodies that build immunity to certain diseases. An abnormality in any one type of WBC can result in a compromised defense (immune) system, making the body vulnerable to infection and disease.

The three types of WBCs are granulocytes, monocytes, and lymphocytes.

GRANULOCYTES

Granulocytes contain pouches of enzymes that give them a grainy or granular appearance. When granulocytes encounter foreign invading microorganisms, they release these powerful enzymes to render the invader helpless or to destroy it. The three types of granulocytes are neutrophils, eosinophils, and basophils. The neutrophils, the most prevalent granulocyte, are called phagocytic cells because they can engulf, digest, and kill invading microorganisms, a process called phagocytosis (see figure 16.2). Neutrophils leave the blood and enter body tissues to fight and engulf infectious agents in areas where infec-

tion, inflammation, or injury has occurred. Eosinophils and basophils participate in allergic and stress reactions in the body.

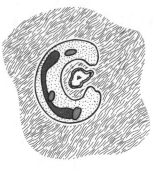

Figure 16.2. Phagocytosis–a WBC engulfing a foreign intruder cell

MONOCYTES

These relatively large WBCs circulate in the blood for a short while and then move into body tissues. There they become powerful macrophages—cells that are exceptionally good at engulfing bacteria and other microorganisms as well as dead or injured body cells. Some macrophages concentrate where they are most likely to encounter foreign invading substances: the liver, spleen, lymph nodes, lungs, kidneys, and gastrointestinal tract. Monocytes also help trigger the action of the lymphocytes, another group of white blood cells.

LYMPHOCYTES

The lymphocytes provide the body with specific immunity and protection against infectious disease. Two types of lymphocytes, B cells and T cells, are discussed on page 201.

PLATELETS

Platelets (thrombocytes) are cell fragments that clump and stick together to begin the formation of blood clots. Platelets seal up small tears within blood vessels and protect the body by controlling blood loss.

CLOTTING FACTORS

Clotting factors are protein substances that circulate in the blood and help form blood clots. The blood's ability to clot is an important protective mechanism that enables injured blood vessels to be repaired, thus stopping or controlling bleeding. The first step in blood clot formation is thought to be performed by the platelets, which in turn trigger the clotting factors into action. The 12 known clotting factors are identified as Factors I through V, and Factors VII through XIII. Abnormalities or the absence of one or more clotting factors can interfere with the body's ability to control bleeding. Hemophilia A, for example, is a genetic disorder caused by a deficiency of Factor VIII, which results in easy bruising, severe bleeding following injury, and spontaneous bleeding.

THE IMMUNE SYSTEM

The immune system is a vastly complex defense system that seeks out, recognizes, neutralizes, and destroys foreign invaders of the body's internal environment. These invaders include microorganisms (bacteria, viruses, protozoa, fungi, and parasites), as well as body cells that become damaged or diseased, body cells that have undergone cancerous (malignant) change, and other foreign substances such as pollen and insect venom. A normally functioning immune system enables the body to fight, control, or limit the severity of infection, and it aids in the body's recovery from infection. Thus, the major result of a nonfunctioning immune system is susceptibility to infection—even by agents which normally do not pose a threat to healthy people.

The immune system is thought to communicate or work in some way with the nervous system to perform its tremendous task. People are exposed to millions and millions of microorganisms every day, and a competent, fully functional immune system is very important to well-being and good health. The immune system forms fighter cells and antibodies to match almost every foreign cell and substance it comes in contact with, and it reproduces those specific fighter cells or antibodies in great numbers whenever that foreign cell or substance reenters the body.

Another important function of the immune system is its ability to cause inflammation. The classic signs of inflammation are redness, warmth, swelling, pain, and loss of function in the affected area. Inflammation usually results from injury; although inflammation is uncomfortable, its purpose is to protect the body from further injury and infection by walling off the damaged, injured area and kicking the immune system cells into action.

RECOGNIZING SELF FROM NONSELF

For the immune system to function normally, the white blood cells (WBCs) must be able to distinguish body cells, called *self*, from foreign substances and microorganisms, called *nonself* or antigens. WBCs determine whether an element they bump into is self or nonself by reading the protein markers located on the outside walls (membranes) of all cells, including the walls of the WBCs themselves. When a WBC encounters a cell or substance, it compares its own markers to those of the encountered cell. If the markers do not match, the WBC views the invader as nonself, attacks it, and calls other WBCs into action.

People have specific self markers on each of their bodies' cells which are determined by genes located on chromosome 6; these markers, which characterize tissue type, are called human leukocyte antigens (HLA). When tissues or organs are surgically transplanted from one person to another, the tissue types of the donor and recipient are usually closely matched to prevent the recipient's immune system from viewing the transplanted tissue as nonself and attacking it.

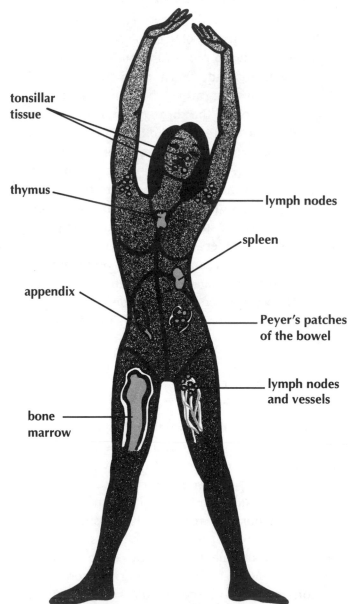

tonsillar tissue

thymus

appendix

bone marrow

lymph nodes

spleen

Peyer's patches of the bowel

lymph nodes and vessels

Figure 16.3. Sites where lymphoid (immune system) tissue is located within the body

THE IMMUNE SYSTEM STRUCTURES AND FUNCTIONS
CELLULAR COMPONENTS
LYMPHOCYTES

Lymphocytes, a type of white blood cell, are major operatives in the immune system. The major types of lymphocytes are B cells and T cells.

B CELLS. B cells produce antibodies. When B cells encounter an invading microorganism such as a bacterium or virus, they encircle it, read the markers on its outside walls, and transform themselves into large cells called plasma cells and memory cells. The plasma cells are truly factories that produce and secrete the protective protein substances called antibodies that fit against the markers on invading cells or microorganisms (antigens) much like interlocking puzzle pieces. When the antibodies lock on to invading cells or microorganisms (antigens), they render the invaders helpless. These antigen-antibody complexes (interlocked antibodies and invaders) attract other WBCs to the area to destroy the invaders. The memory cells remember the microorganism, and the next time the body is exposed to that type of microorganism the memory cells quickly stimulate the production of the specific antibodies that prevent reinfection.

An example of this process can be seen with measles infection. Once infected with the measles virus, the body is immune from future infection by the measles virus because the immune system's B cells have already produced antibodies against it, and its T cells—having previously reacted to this virus—quickly squelch the virus if it ever enters the body again.

T CELLS. T cells release chemicals that regulate immune system responses by directing and regulating much of the activity of the other WBCs. T cells play a vital role in protecting the body from viral and parasitic infections.

The three major types of T cells are helper/inducer, killer/effector, and suppressor cells. Each performs specific duties.

The majority of T cells are helper/inducers, which assist and direct the activity of all other WBCs such as B cells, killer T cells, and macrophages (the largest of the phagocyte cells that stem from monocytes).

Killer/effector T cells recognize and destroy nonself cells, such as invading microorganisms, as well as self cells that have been infected with a virus or become cancerous (malignant). Killer/effector T cells rush to the site of infection, destroy invading microorganisms, and release chemicals that call other WBCs into action. Killer/effector T cells must be suppressed by medication before and after organ transplant so they do not attack the transplanted organ.

Suppressor T cells help to slow down or turn off immune system responses (WBC activity) so that WBCs do not overreact or keep going in a destructive fashion after an infection has been eradicated from the body.

PHAGOCYTIC CELLS

The phagocytic WBCs, which engulf and digest nonself microorganisms and debris, are divided into neutrophils (one of the granulocytes), and monocytes, also called macrophages (see page 199).

In addition to these cells, the immune system contains an entire system of cells that are closely related to but different from macrophages. These cells are specially equipped to present foreign substances or antigens (nonself substances) to the antibody-producing and other immunocompetent cells. These cells, often called the professional antigen presenting cells of the body, have antigen (nonself) receptors on their surfaces, as well as a high concentration of self markers, which ensure that antigens are presented to the T and B lymphocytes. This is important to ensure that the foreign quality of antigens is recognized, as well as to ensure that the body does not direct destructive immune functions against its own components.

COMPLEMENT SYSTEM

The complement system is a group of protein components in the blood that help fight infection. Complement components are activated when they encounter an antibody attached to a foreign microorganism (an antigen-antibody complex) or when they encounter a foreign microorganism directly. Once activated, the individual complement components kick each other into action in a domino-like sequence and act to coat invading microorganisms, making it easier for phagocytic WBCs to engulf them. They also call other WBCs to an area of infection and/or attach themselves to the outside wall (membrane), effectively punching holes in the surface of each invading cell or microorganism to destroy it.

THE LYMPHATIC SYSTEM

The lymph nodes, the lymphatic vessels, and lymph make up the lymphatic system. The lymphocytes (B cells and T cells) are the primary blood cells of the lymphatic system; they travel throughout the lymphatic vessels and blood vessels in search of foreign microorganisms and other invaders.

LYMPH NODES

Small, bean-shaped lymph nodes are scattered throughout the body and are connected by the lymphatic vessels (see figure 16.4). Groups or chains of lymph nodes are concentrated in the areas of the neck, chest, underarm (axilla), abdomen, and groin. Lymph nodes contain large numbers of lymphocytes (B cells and T cells) as well as macrophages (large phagocytes) that trap and destroy invading microorganisms and other debris to confine infection to a local area. When infection is present, the lymph nodes in the area become enlarged as the number of lymphocytes increase to help fight the infection. Depending on their location, some enlarged lymph nodes can be felt or even seen.

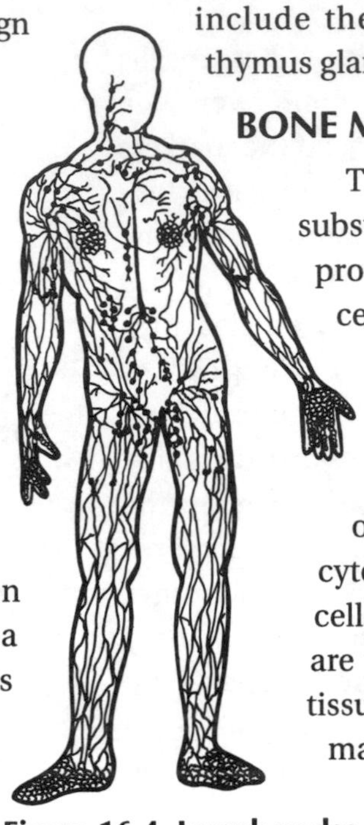

LYMPHATIC VESSELS

The lymphatic vessel network is a lot like the blood vessel network in that it extends to all areas of the body and terminally connects to the large veins that return blood to the right side of the heart.

LYMPH

Lymph is a fluid similar to blood plasma that flows within the lymphatic vessels. The primary blood cells in lymph are the lymphocytes. Lymph circulates around the cells of the body collecting microorganisms and other debris, then drains into the lymphatic vessels. There the lymph circulates and passes through the lymph nodes, which contain masses of lymphocytes (B cells and T cells) and macrophages that clean out the debris and destroy the microorganisms before they infect other parts of the body. Lymph, and the lymphocytes it contains, eventually empty into the bloodstream. Lymphocytes circulate throughout the body, reenter the lymphatic system with lymph fluid,

Figure 16.4. Lymph nodes and lymphatic vessels

recirculate, and reenter the bloodstream. The cycle repeats continuously to protect the body from invaders.

OTHER COMPONENTS

Other structures are considered components of the immune system because they either produce, house, or assist in the development of WBCs. These include the bone marrow, spleen, and the thymus gland.

BONE MARROW

The bone marrow is the soft, pulpy substance in the center of each bone that produces red blood cells, white blood cells, and platelets (see page 198).

THYMUS

The thymus gland sits behind the sternum (breastbone); it is the organ in which immature lymphocytes mature into adult, functioning T cells. In the thymus, developing T cells are made to not attack the body's own tissue by being taught to use the "self" markers located on cell wall surfaces to recognize foreign substances.

WBCs are also housed in the liver, walls of blood vessels, tonsils, adenoids, lungs, and small patches of tissue in the intestines (Peyer's patches) to help trap and destroy invading microorganisms and other foreign substances.

SPLEEN

The spleen is located in the upper left abdomen. As blood circulates through the spleen, lymphocytes and phagocytic WBCs engulf old blood cells, debris, bacteria, and other foreign substances. The spleen also stores a large number of RBCs for release into the bloodstream as needed.

THE IMMUNE SYSTEM AND DISEASES

Diseases with causes related to the immune system include autoimmune, immune complex, hypersensitivity, and immune deficiency disorders. In autoimmune disorders, the immune system attacks the body's own tissues. Diabetes mellitus and rheumatoid arthritis are autoimmune disorders.

In immune complex (or immunocomplex disorders), antigen-antibody complexes become trapped within small blood vessels or body tissues, causing inflammation and disease, such as systemic lupus erythematosus or immune complex glomerulonephritis.

Hypersensitivity disorders are caused by the immune system's inappropriate response to antigens that should not ordinarily trigger a response. One type of antigen is called an allergen. The immune system response triggered by an allergen is called an allergy. Some common allergies are hay fever, extrinsic asthma, and a potentially life-threatening allergic reaction called anaphyllaxis. These reactions are largely attributable to a specialized part of the antibody system that perhaps was originally developed to defend against large parasites.

Immune deficiency (or immunodeficiency) disorders result from a faulty or deficient immune system response. An immune deficiency disorder can have a genetic cause (for example, Wiskott-Aldrich syndrome), or an acquired cause (for example, acquired immunodeficiency syndrome or AIDS). Immune deficiencies, whether genetic or acquired, may be the most common basis of serious, life-threatening disease in humans.

Genetically determined immune deficiencies may involve the deficient or abnormal development or function of T cells, B cells, or macrophages; deficient production of antibodies; deficient development of the complex complement system; or deficient function of phagocytic and inflammatory processes. Primary immune deficiencies occur as frequently as all the leukemias and lymphomas combined.

Secondary immune deficiencies can occur naturally in premature babies, newborn infants, in the elderly, and as a function of many infections, especially those caused by viruses and parasites. Secondary immunodeficiencies can also result from any of the following: drug treatments for many cancers and autoimmune diseases, metabolic disturbances, and chemical dependency to alcohol and other drugs.

BLOOD DISEASES AND DISORDERS

ANEMIA

Anemia itself is not a disease; it is a symptom of disease that can be caused by genetic or environmental factors. Environmental factors can include infection, injury, and chemicals. Anemia caused by unknown factors is called idiopathic anemia.

In anemia, the number of RBCs or the amount of hemoglobin produced by the body is too low. Anemia can also be caused by slow or rapid blood loss or increased destruction of RBCs. RBCs contain hemoglobin, which transports oxygen from the lungs to all tissues of the body. Lack of hemoglobin or RBCs results in a lack of oxygen available to body tissues, which causes many of the symptoms of anemia.

SIGNS AND SYMPTOMS. Regardless of the type or cause of anemia, general symptoms include the following: fatigue; intolerance to physical exertion and cold; shortness of breath; paleness of skin, nailbeds, and gums; headaches; increased heart rate; or a pounding sensation in the chest (palpitations). Chest pain and heart failure caused by severe anemia can be fatal.

Hemoglobin released into the bloodstream while RBCs are destroyed is converted to bilirubin. If anemia is due to excessive destruction of RBCs, bilirubin will accumulate in the blood, causing jaundice (yellow discoloration of the skin).

APLASTIC ANEMIA

In this anemia, the bone marrow does not produce enough RBCs. Aplastic anemia may be idiopathic (have no known cause) or be caused by agents toxic to the bone marrow that suppress the bone marrow's ability to produce blood cells. Such agents include certain antibiotics and antiseizure medications, chemotherapy medications, radiation therapy, and chemicals such as benzene. Severe aplastic anemia can also occur as a complication of viral infections such as hepatitis. Aplastic anemia is a serious, potentially life-threatening disease.

Bone marrow produces all types of blood cells—RBCs, WBCs, and platelets. When the bone marrow's production of RBCs drops due to aplastic anemia, its production of WBCs and platelets often drops as well.

Decreased production of all types of blood cells is a condition called pancytopenia, a life-threatening condition. Lack of WBCs weakens the body's ability to fight infection, and lack of platelets increases the risk of spontaneous or uncontrollable bleeding. If aplastic anemia does not respond to treatment, the resulting infection and bleeding can cause death within a year.

Aplastic anemia can develop slowly or abruptly, depending on the cause. Exposure to a toxic agent or infection frequently causes a rapid onset of symptoms, while unknown (idiopathic) causes frequently result in a gradual onset of symptoms.

SIGNS AND SYMPTOMS. Aplastic anemia causes general symptoms of anemia (see page 203), which are often accompanied by infection and bleeding.

TREATMENT. The underlying cause is removed or treated when possible. Transfusions of RBCs, WBCs, platelets, and other blood components may be given. Medications (or other substances) to suppress the immune system and to stimulate the bone marrow to recover and begin producing RBCs may be used. Bone marrow transplantation is a life-saving treatment for severe aplastic anemia, if a compatible donor is available.

FOLIC ACID DEFICIENCY ANEMIA

Folic acid (also known as folate) is one of the B-complex vitamins and is necessary for the formation of RBCs. Lack of folic acid usually results from an inadequate intake of dietary folic acid but can also result from an inability of the body to either absorb folic acid from the gastrointestinal tract or to use it once it is absorbed. Chronic alcohol use, intestinal malabsorption disorders such as celiac disease, and some medications can interfere with folic acid absorption. Folic acid is found in raw fruits and vegetables, some organ meats, and yeast, but it can be destroyed by overcooking.

SIGNS AND SYMPTOMS. Folic acid deficiency causes general symptoms of anemia (see page 203), sore mouth and tongue, loss of appetite and weight, indigestion, and diarrhea or constipation.

TREATMENT. Because the most common cause is an inadequate intake of dietary folic acid, increasing the intake of raw fruits and vegetables is usually recom-

mended. Folic acid supplements may be taken by mouth unless a malabsorption disorder exists, in which case the supplements are given by injection. An adequate dietary intake of vitamin C, which converts folic acid into the active form used by the body, is also important.

GLUCOSE-6-PHOSPHATE DEHYDROGENASE DEFICIENCY

Also called G6PD deficiency.

The incidence is approximately 1 in 10 live births among African American males and approximately 1 in 50 live births among African American females. The deficiency follows an X-linked inheritance pattern. This most common enzyme deficiency in the world usually occurs in dark-skinned populations, including Asian, Mediterranean, and African populations. The deficiency of the G6PD enzyme leads to the destruction of red blood cells during certain situations. Infection, the eating of certain foods (such as fava beans), or the taking of certain medications (such as sulfa products) can cause severe red blood cell destruction, resulting in profound and possibly fatal anemia.

SIGNS AND SYMPTOMS. People with G6PD deficiency typically have no symptoms until they either get an infection or ingest a triggering food or medication. Then, headache, fatigue, shortness of breath (especially on exertion) may follow, as well as yellowing of the skin (jaundice) caused by the massive destruction of red blood cells.

TREATMENT. People with G6PD deficiency are taught to avoid triggering substances. A fetus that inherits G6PD deficiency from either parent is at special risk; even if the pregnant woman does not have G6PD, any triggering substances she ingests may cross the placental membrane and cause fetal anemia or death.

HEMOCHROMATOSIS

Also called hereditary hemochromatosis.

Incidence is 10 times greater in males than females. Approximately 600,000 to one million Americans have hemochromatosis; 20 to 23 million are suspected of being carriers. It is an autosomal recessive disease.

Hemochromatosis causes excessive amounts of dietary iron to be absorbed into the body. Iron is essential for life, but in excessive amounts it is toxic. Excess iron slowly accumulates in the liver, pancreas, heart, and other organs, leading to tissue damage and organ failure. People with hemochromatosis do not usually have symptoms until after age 30.

SIGNS AND SYMPTOMS. Liver failure with cirrhosis, diabetes, heart failure, and arthritis can occur and be accompanied by nonspecific symptoms such as fatigue, weight loss, backache, and abdominal discomfort. Bronze or yellow skin (jaundice) and liver enlargement are signs of associated liver damage. Malignant liver tumors occur in about one third of people who have symptoms. Carriers of the hemochromatosis gene accumulate higher amounts of iron than unaffected people but do not have the iron buildup or organ damage seen in people who have hemochromatosis.

TREATMENT. Treatment includes phlebotomy—a procedure that involves the removal of a specified amount of blood to draw off excess iron. Initially, one to two phlebotomies per week for up to two years are performed to get iron levels within a normal range; then approximately four to six maintenance phlebotomies per year are performed for life. Agents that bind or chelate with iron may also be used to help rid it from the body. Although there is no special diet, vitamins and iron supplements should *not* be used. Food labels must be read carefully so iron-fortified or iron-supplemented foods can be avoided.

HEMOPHILIA A

Also called Factor VIII deficiency and classical hemophilia.

The incidence is approximately 1 in 10,000 live male births and is transmitted through an X-linked inheritance pattern. It is estimated that one third of occurrences are the result of new gene mutation in the egg or sperm. Hemophilia A is caused by deficiency of a protein called Factor VIII, an important element in the process of normal blood clotting. Without adequate amounts of this factor, uncontrolled bleeding is a major concern. The severity of bleeding varies among affected people. Severe bleeding (hemorrhage) into vital organs such as the brain or the lungs can be fatal.

SIGNS AND SYMPTOMS. The first sign of hemophilia may occur when circumcision causes excessive and/ or prolonged bleeding. As the child grows, the tendency to bruise (even with slight bumping) becomes apparent. With the development of standing and walking, bleeding into joints such as the knees causes swelling and pain that can eventually cause permanent joint damage. Although simple skin cuts can usually be controlled by applying pressure and ice, spontaneous internal bleeding is life threatening. Severe, spontaneous bleeding within the brain is often fatal.

TREATMENT. Factor VIII concentrate or other blood products that contain Factor VIII are given intravenously. This factor can now be produced by genetic engineering. Factor VIII produced in this way is a nonblood product that poses no risk of transmitting blood-borne diseases such as hepatitis or human immunodeficiency virus (HIV). People with hemophilia are taught to administer intravenous Factor VIII at home, which allows them better management of their disease and more independence while significantly reducing their health-care costs. DNA testing is available to identify people with the gene.

HEMOPHILIA B

Also called Christmas disease.

The incidence is approximately 1 in 30,000 to 50,000 live male births and is transmitted through an X-linked inheritance pattern. Hemophilia B occurs less frequently than hemophilia A, accounting for roughly 15% of occurrences of hemophilia as a whole. Hemophilia B is caused by a deficiency of clotting Factor IX.

SIGNS AND SYMPTOMS. Symptoms of hemophilia B are similar to those of hemophilia A (see above), but may not be as severe.

TREATMENT. Clotting Factor IX or other blood products containing adequate amounts of Factor IX are given intravenously. DNA testing is available to identify people with the gene.

HEMOLYTIC ANEMIA

Hemolysis is a term used to describe the premature destruction of RBCs; hemolytic anemia occurs as a result of hemolysis. Hemolytic anemia can be caused by a variety of disorders in which the destruction of RBCs (hemolysis) occurs more rapidly than the bone marrow can replace them. Blood Rh-factor incompatibility between a pregnant woman and her fetus (see page 34), mismatched blood transfusion, exposure to certain chemicals, hypersensitivity to medication (e.g., an antibiotic), or a misguided attack by the body's own immune system on the red blood cells can cause hemolytic anemia. Genetic disorders that render the RBCs weak or fragile and prone to destruction, thereby resulting in hemolytic anemia, include hereditary spherocytosis, sickle cell anemia, and thalassemia.

SIGNS AND SYMPTOMS. General symptoms of anemia (see page 203) and jaundice (yellow discoloration of the skin) occur. Severe hemolytic anemia can cause oxygen deprivation, heart failure, and death.

TREATMENT. Treatment begins with finding the cause of the RBC destruction (hemolysis) and correcting or treating the cause when possible. Surgical removal of the spleen may be helpful in certain cases, as in those caused by hereditary spherocytosis. Other treatments include blood transfusions, and medications to suppress the immune system and to stimulate bone marrow production of RBCs.

HEREDITARY SPHEROCYTOSIS

The incidence is 1 in 4,500 to 5,000 live births in people of northern European descent and is transmitted through an autosomal dominant inheritance pattern. It is the most common hereditary hemolytic anemia among Whites. A defect in the outer membrane of the red blood cells makes them unstable and therefore easily damaged (especially as they travel through the spleen) and destroyed.

SIGNS AND SYMPTOMS. Anemia results from the destruction of red blood cells; the severity varies and typically becomes more pronounced with illness.

TREATMENT. Removal of the spleen reduces the destruction of red blood cells and usually helps correct the anemia. However, this may not be necessary in very mild cases.

IRON-DEFICIENCY ANEMIA

Iron enters the body primarily through dietary intake of meat and green, leafy vegetables. Iron is used to produce hemoglobin, an important element in RBCs. Excess iron is stored in the liver, spleen, and bone marrow for release as needed. Iron-deficiency anemia results from an inadequate amount of iron available for hemoglobin production. This may occur because of a long-term lack of dietary iron along with a depletion of stored iron, conditions most often seen among young children and the elderly. Iron deficiency anemia in adults is frequently caused by blood loss from gastrointestinal tract bleeding, cancer, peptic ulcers, or heavy, prolonged, or frequent menstrual periods. Poor absorption of iron by the gastrointestinal tract can also cause iron-deficiency anemia.

SIGNS AND SYMPTOMS. General symptoms of anemia (see page 203) occur. If the iron deficiency was caused by a rapid, significant loss of blood, the general symptoms are more severe. Additional symptoms seen in chronic, long-term iron deficiency anemia can include misshapen nails; a smooth, tender tongue; and unusual dietary cravings for nonfood items such as dirt, clay, laundry starch, and hair.

TREATMENT. The cause of the iron deficiency is corrected or treated when possible, and the body's supply and stores of iron are restored with oral supplements, which are usually taken for about a year to fully restore the body with iron. Injections of iron may also be recommended.

SICKLE CELL ANEMIA

Sickle cell anemia is the most common of the hemoglobin diseases. The incidence among African Americans is approximately 1 in 625 live births. Incidence among Mexican Americans is approximately 1 in 1,000 to 1,500 live births. Although this disorder is most common in people of African or Mediterranean descent, it has occurred in Whites.

People who inherit the sickle cell gene from only one parent have the sickle cell trait, which means they are carriers. Prevalence of the sickle cell trait (carriers) among African Americans is estimated to be as high as 1 in 12, while the estimated prevalence among Africans is as high as 4 in 10. Some scientists believe the sickle cell trait is an evolutionary advantage that is more common among people who live in regions where malaria is prevalent: the malarial parasites cannot survive in red blood cells that have the sickle cell trait.

Red blood cells carry oxygen throughout the body. In sickle cell anemia, the red blood cells, which normally have a round, flexible shape, buckle or collapse into a sickle or crescent shape. These sickled red blood cells can clump together to congest and clog small blood vessels and organs. These clogged vessels obstruct the delivery of oxygen to tissues fed by those vessel(s), resulting in pain and tissue death (infarction). Because the sickled cells are also easily destroyed, increased red blood cell destruction contributes to lifelong anemia.

Sickle cell crisis is a general term that describes the sudden and severe occurrence of symptoms caused by massive numbers of sickling red blood cells. Sickling can be triggered by physical stress such as infection, dehydration, or decreased circulating blood oxygen; sometimes sickle cell crisis occurs for no apparent reason. The crisis usually begins suddenly and severely, with joints of the body becoming swollen, warm to the touch, and extremely painful from the clumping of sickled red cells within them. Clumping can also occur and cause pain in abdominal organs or bone, and cause tissue death within internal organs such as the liver, spleen, kidneys, and retinas of the eyes. If it occurs in the brain, clumping can lead to coma and/or stroke. Other forms of sickle cell crisis include the development of aplastic anemia, in which the bone marrow fails to produce red blood cells, and hemolytic anemia as a result of massive red blood cell destruction.

SIGNS AND SYMPTOMS. Infants typically do not have symptoms until four to six months of age because the fetal hemoglobin that stays in the blood until this age resists sickling. Children then become irritable and pale, experience growth delay and infections, and may have painful swelling of the tissues of the hands and feet (dactylitis). The spleen and liver may be enlarged, and blood count analysis reveals chronic, profound anemia. The severity of symptoms and the frequency of crisis varies greatly from person to person. Sickle cell anemia itself does not affect mental capacity (unless stroke has occurred during crisis), and most people have normal intelligence. People who are carriers of the sickle cell trait usually do not have symptoms of sickle cell crisis. However, in certain environments and situations (i.e., high altitudes with low oxygen concentrations, such as during air travel and in mountainous terrains) a carrier can have mild symptoms.

TREATMENT. There is no cure, but measures can be taken to reduce or prevent episodes of crisis. Children require a well-balanced, nutritious diet and a steady intake of fluids, especially during the summer, to prevent dehydration. Families are encouraged to avoid

people with known infection because children with sickle cell anemia have less resistance against illness. Antibiotics may be prescribed on a continuous basis beginning as early as six months of age to help prevent infection. Immunizing children against childhood communicable diseases is necessary to prevent infections that could trigger sickle cell crisis and/or a fatal infection. Children should be taught ways to handle both emotional and physical stress to help minimize episodes of crisis.

Although physical exercise is encouraged, some activities should be avoided. For example, long-distance running can cause dehydration, which could initiate crisis; contact sports (e.g., football) could cause injury, even rupture, to an enlarged spleen.

Children need to receive regular health-care evaluations to monitor their anemia and to detect complications. Their eyes should be checked closely, because death of retinal tissue can cause permanent vision loss. Sickle cell crisis is a life-threatening emergency that requires hospitalization, where the pain can be managed and the body rehydrated with fluids. Blood transfusions may be required, but only in select cases. Sickle cell screening is included in newborn screening programs in some states. DNA testing can identify people with the sickle cell gene.

THALASSEMIA

Thalassemia occurs worldwide, but is primarily seen in people of Mediterranean, Southeast Asian, Middle Eastern, or African descent. Incidence in the United States varies among ethnic groups; overall U.S. incidence is increasing because of increasing numbers of Southeast Asian immigrants.

Thalassemia encompasses a group of anemias in which a specific defect is present in hemoglobin, the oxygen-carrying substance in red blood cells. Alpha- and beta-thalassemias are included in this group. Depending on whether the thalassemia mutation is inherited from one or both parents, there is an extreme variance in severity. As with sickle cell anemia, carriers may have some resistance to malaria, which may explain its prevalance among certain populations.

SIGNS AND SYMPTOMS. Signs of anemia such as pale color, listlessness, poor eating, delayed growth, and susceptibility to infections occur. Cooley anemia, also called thalassemia major or Mediterranean anemia, is the most severe form of the beta-thalassemias. Death will occur without ongoing blood transfusions. Children with severe anemia also have liver and spleen enlargement, bone pain with frequent fractures, and heart enlargement with susceptibility to heart failure and infections, both of which are common causes of death.

Physical features common among children with thalassemia major include a yellow or bronze skin color (jaundice), thick bones of the forehead and skull, a flattened nose, and prominent cheekbones. The yellowish skin is due to the increased destruction of red blood cells. As the skull bones grow they thicken in an attempt to increase the supply of red blood cells, which are produced within the bone marrow. Unfortunately, the red blood cells that are produced do not contain normal hemoglobin and are unable to increase the amount of circulating oxygen.

TREATMENT. Depending on the type and severity of thalassemia, treatment can include protection from infection, including the use of prophylactic antibiotics, frequent blood transfusions, and the administration of chelating agents (medications given to bind with the excess iron accumulated from frequent blood transfusions so it can be excreted from the body), removal of the spleen, and/or bone marrow transplantation. If bone marrow transplantation is successful, the need for blood transfusions may be eliminated. Continued health-care supervision is necessary for all individuals with thalassemia. DNA testing is available to identify people who carry the gene.

VITAMIN B12 DEFICIENCY ANEMIA

Vitamin B12, found in meat and dairy products, is another element necessary for RBC production. Although vitamin B12 deficiency anemia is a nutritional disorder, it is rarely caused by a lack of dietary intake of the vitamin except in people who eat a truly vegetarian diet. The most common cause is the malabsorption of vitamin B12, which can result from a variety of medical disorders.

A substance called intrinsic factor that is produced by special cells in the stomach is needed for vitamin B12 to be absorbed by the last segment of the small intestine (the ileum). Lack of intrinsic factor causes a form of vitamin B12 deficiency called pernicious anemia; because it occurs repeatedly in some families, pernicious anemia may have a genetic connection. Pernicious anemia can also be caused by surgically removing all or part of the stomach or by the body's own immune system destroying the cells of the stomach that produce intrinsic factor.

Vitamin B12 deficiency can also be caused by infection, malabsorption syndromes, or parasite infestation involving the ileum, the part of the small intestine where the vitamin is normally absorbed.

SIGNS AND SYMPTOMS. General symptoms of anemia occur (see page 203). In addition, loss of appetite and weight, diarrhea or constipation, abdominal discomfort, a sore and swollen tongue, and a tingling or numbing sensation of the hands and feet may be present. Memory loss, irritability, depression, and a loss of coordination sometimes occur.

TREATMENT. The cause of the vitamin B12 anemia determines the type of treatment. If due to a lack of dietary intake as occurs in true vegetarianism, vitamin B12 supplements can be taken by mouth. When intrinsic factor is absent (pernicious anemia), injections of vitamin B12 are given throughout life. Other treatments may be needed if the anemia is caused by malabsorption syndromes or infections.

IMMUNE SYSTEM DISEASES AND DISORDERS

AUTOIMMUNE THROMBOCYTOPENIC PURPURA (AITP)

Also called idiopathic thrombocytopenic purpura (ITP) and primary thrombocytopenic purpura.

Thrombocytopenia is characterized by a lower-than-normal number of platelets in the blood because of decreased platelet production by the bone marrow or because large numbers of platelets are being destroyed. Diseases such as aplastic anemia, systemic lupus erythematosus, and lymphoma can cause thrombocytopenia, as can certain chemotherapy drugs and other medications, radiation therapy, and viruses. Thrombocytopenia caused by these and other disorders is called secondary thrombocytopenia.

The cause of AITP is unknown, but it is thought to be an abnormal immune system response that causes the body to produce antibodies that attack its own platelets (an autoimmune disorder). AITP occurs most often in women and children. Some forms of thrombocytopenia are associated with genetic disorders and causes.

SIGNS AND SYMPTOMS. Easy bruising; pinpoint hemorrhages on the skin (especially on the legs); nosebleeds; bloody vomit, urine, or stool; heavy menstrual flow; and prolonged bleeding after surgery or trauma can occur as a result of the decreased number of platelets. Bleeding into the brain or severe blood loss from gastrointestinal or internal bleeding can be fatal.

TREATMENT. Steroid medication can be used to suppress the production of platelet-destroying antibodies; other immunosuppressive drugs may also be used. Surgical removal of the spleen may be indicated because platelets are easily destroyed in the spleen, especially when coated with or attached to antibodies. In children, AITP may dissipate without treatment. In recent years, dramatic correction of thrombocytopenia has been achieved by administration of intravenous immunoglobulin (protective protein antibodies). In secondary thrombocytopenia, the underlying cause is corrected when possible. Transfusions of blood or blood components (including platelets) may be needed.

IMMUNE DEFICIENCIES
Also called immunodeficiencies.

Diseases and disorders of the immune system are caused by disturbances in the development of crucial components of the immune system that result in a less-than-competent immune system. One or more of the cellular components (B cells, T cells, phagocytic cells, or components of the complement system) of the immune system apparatus may be affected. Because the immune system components communicate and work together to protect the body, even one abnormality can severely affect immune system function. People with immune deficiencies have increased risk of infections, autoimmune diseases, and cancers. Whenever infections recur, are unusually severe or persistent, or are caused by unusual microorganisms, analysis of the immune system for deficiency or disease is indicated.

Immune deficiency diseases are divided into primary and secondary categories.

PRIMARY IMMUNE DEFICIENCIES
Also called inherited or congenital immune deficiencies.

Primary immune deficiencies are caused by an internal defect or deficiency in one or more immune system components. Although the cause of many of these disorders remains unknown, many primary immune deficiencies are the result of inherited genetic abnormalities. Some primary immune deficiencies are passed down through distinct inheritance patterns such as an autosomal dominant, autosomal recessive, or X-linked pattern; some appear as new, sporadic cases with no previous family history. Some cases of primary immune deficiency appear to be the result of the incomplete or arrested development of one or more immune system components.

Primary immune deficiencies can be further divided into categories according to the component affected. Deficiencies caused by deficient or abnormal B cell function include common variable immunodeficiency (CVI) and X-linked agammaglobulinemia. Deficiencies caused by abnormal T cell function include chronic mucocutaneous candidiasis and DiGeorge anomaly (also called DiGeorge syndrome). Deficiencies of combined B and T cell abnormalities include ataxia telangiectasia, severe combined immunodeficiencies (SCID), and Wiskott-Aldrich syndrome. Deficiencies caused by abnormal or defective phagocytic white blood cell function include Chédiak-Higashi syndrome and chronic granulomatous disease. Deficiencies caused by abnormalities of one or more complement components are designated according to which complement component is dysfunctional or missing: C_1 deficiency, C_2 deficiency, and so on.

There are more than 93 different identifiable primary immune deficiencies. The incidence rates for many of these disorders are unknown; some milder forms are known to occur as frequently as 1 in 500 to 1,000 people, while others occur as infrequently as 1 in 100,000. The primary immunodeficiencies vary in severity and in the age at which they become clinically apparent (show symptoms); some become apparent shortly after birth, and others do not appear until adulthood. As a group, primary immune deficiencies are a significant health problem for both children and adults, occurring more frequently than the leukemias and lymphomas combined.

SECONDARY IMMUNE DEFICIENCIES

Secondary or acquired immune deficiencies are caused by external or outside agents or events that cause a previously healthy immune system to become nonfunctional or incompetent. Certain medications can cause a secondary immune deficiency by suppressing or interfering with the bone marrow's ability to produce blood cells. Chemotherapy drugs and radiation therapy used to treat cancers can cause temporary immune deficiencies by suppressing the bone marrow's production of healthy, functioning blood cells.

Infectious agents can also cause secondary immune deficiencies, such as acquired immunodeficiency syndrome (AIDS), which is associated with the human immunodeficiency virus (HIV). The AIDS virus invades helper/inducer T cells and duplicates itself by using the infected T cell.

Other infections, including measles virus and influenza viruses, can cause a temporary or transient immune deficiency from which the body is able to recuperate. Long-term malnutrition and some cancers can also contribute to or cause immune deficiencies. Sometimes, such as in chronic lymphatic leukemia, Hodgkin disease, or multiple myeloma (all are types of cancer), the secondary immunodeficiency may be so severe it becomes one of the major life-threatening components of the cancer.

SIGNS AND SYMPTOMS. Whereas symptoms vary according to the immune system components affected, general symptoms include susceptibility to infections that occur in unusual organs and are caused by microorganisms that are either unusual or not usually harmful to human beings.

A disorder of B cell function decreases the body's ability to produce protective gamma globulins (proteins called antibodies) against bacteria and some viruses. A disorder of T cell function decreases the body's ability to fight infectious microorganisms, especially viruses and fungi. A disorder of phagocytic cells often results in skin infections. A disorder of the complement system often results in blood infections and meningitis.

Other symptoms associated with immune deficiency disorders include the development of autoimmune and rheumatic-type diseases such as autoimmune hemolytic anemia, autoimmune thrombocytopenic purpura, or rheumatoid arthritis. Gastrointestinal problems, including diarrhea, malabsorption, inflammatory bowel diseases, and even malnutrition, can occur. Red blood cell and platelet counts can be altered in some immune deficiency disorders, causing excessive bleeding and anemia.

TREATMENT. There are treatments but not always cures for immune deficiencies. Depending on the specific type and cause of immune deficiency, treatment may include the infusion of antibodies (for B cell deficiencies) and aggressive, early treatment of all infections. Bone marrow transplantation, thymus transplantation, and even gene therapy are possible treatments for immune deficiencies. Replacement of a genetically abnormal enzyme can correct some specific immune deficiencies.

In gene therapy, a mutant gene is replaced by a normal gene, which becomes part of the body's DNA and is reproduced in subsequent new cells. Gene therapy holds great promise of curing genetic primary immune deficiencies. Several of the primary immune deficiencies have been completely cured by bone marrow transplantation, which is the treatment of choice, especially for the more serious forms of severe combined immunodeficiencies (SCID).

For secondary or acquired immune deficiencies, prevention is the ideal treatment.

Regardless of the type of immune deficiency, early recognition is vital. Without treatment, repeated infection or the development of autoimmune disorders can cause permanent health problems, such as lung damage. Children suspected of having an immune deficiency should not receive live-virus immunizations (oral polio, measles, mumps, and rubella); these can cause critical illness and even death in an immunodeficient child. Routine health care is imperative to maintaining optimal wellness in all people with immune deficiency, regardless of their age or the specific type of deficiency.

LEUKEMIA

Leukemia is the collective name for a group of blood diseases caused by malignant changes in the organs in which blood cells are formed, primarily the bone marrow. This malignant change results in the overproduction of abnormal white blood cells (WBCs). As the abnormal WBCs take over in the bone marrow, the production of normal WBCs, red blood cells (RBCs), and platelets is markedly reduced. Although high numbers of abnormal WBCs circulate within the bloodstream, they are not able to perform the protective and immune functions normally performed by WBCs; hence, the body is left susceptible to infection and injury. The large numbers of abnormal WBCs collect in the bone marrow and other tissues and organs, including the lymph nodes, liver, and spleen. The malignant WBCs may also spread into the central nervous system (brain and spinal cord), kidneys, gastrointestinal tract, and skin, affecting the integrity and function of these organs and tissues. Inhibition of RBC production causes anemia; the decrease in platelet production causes bleeding complications from impaired blood clotting ability; and the decrease in normal WBC production leads to increased infections.

Leukemia occurs more frequently in males than in females, although the ratio varies depending on the type of leukemia. Leukemia is the most common childhood cancer, but the majority of leukemia cases occur in adults.

The exact cause of leukemia is unknown, but both genetic and environmental factors have been implicated. A genetic susceptibility may be inherited. The incidence of leukemia is higher in people with some chromosome disorders such as Down syndrome, Fanconi syndrome, and Klinefelter syndrome.

Environmental factors associated with the development of leukemia include exposure to certain chemical agents such as benzene and some anticancer drugs; exposure to physical agents such as large-dose radiation, whether before or after birth; and specific infectious agents, mainly certain viruses.

SIGNS AND SYMPTOMS. Leukemia symptoms reflect the abnormality and defective function of the blood cells and the congestion and accumulation of excessive WBCs within organs and tissues. Symptoms include susceptibility to infection; fever; easy bruising and bleeding; fatigue; weight loss; pale skin; enlarged lymph nodes, liver, and spleen; bone pain and joint swelling; headache; and shortness of breath, especially with activity.

Leukemia is frequently classified according to the specific line of WBCs that is affected by the leukemic process and whether the onset of the disease was acute (sudden and severe) or chronic (slow and insidious). Cell lines are divided into myelogenous (also called myelocytic) leukemias, which affect the granulocytes (eosinophils, basophils, and neutrophils) or monocytes, and lymphocytic (also called lymphoid) leukemias, which affect the lymphocytes (primarily B cells and T cells). Leukemias are often divided into four major categories: acute myelogenous, chronic myelogenous, acute lymphocytic, and chronic lymphocytic. Many subtypes also exist.

Treatment begins after the specific type of leukemia is diagnosed by means of an examination of a sample of marrow withdrawn from the bone.

ACUTE MYELOGENOUS LEUKEMIA (AML)
Also called acute nonlymphocytic, monocytic, myelogenic, or myelocytic leukemia.

This form of leukemia occurs in all age groups, but the risk may increase with age. AML is characterized by the overproduction of malignant WBCs, primarily granulocytes. AML is often associated with an altered chromosome in bone marrow cells. Symptoms typically appear suddenly or over a few months. Death can occur within six months if treatment is not given.

TREATMENT. Few people achieve cure. Treatment includes chemotherapy; however, the majority of people who experience remission (i.e., appear to be free of the disease) after treatment have a recurrence of AML later. Bone marrow transplantation has been used, which permits intensive radiation and chemotherapy to produce cure or long-term remission.

CHRONIC MYELOGENOUS LEUKEMIA (CML)
Also called chronic myeloid, myelocytic, or granulocytic leukemia.

This leukemia usually affects people 20 to 50 years of age. CML is characterized by the overproduction of malignant granulocytes. About 90% of people with CML have a chromosome rearrangement referred to as the Philadelphia chromosome, in which a small portion of chromosome 22 is dislodged and attached to chromosome 9.

TREATMENT. CML can be treated by oral chemotherapy (anticancer medication taken by mouth) as long as it remains in its chronic, slowly progressing form, but this leukemia eventually transforms into an acute disease similar to AML that is very resistant to treatment. The only chance for cure is bone marrow transplantation which, when used relatively early in the course of the disease, can produce a cure or long-term remission as frequently as 75% of the time.

ACUTE LYMPHOCYTIC LEUKEMIA (ALL)

Also called lymphoblastic leukemia and childhood leukemia.

This form of leukemia primarily affects young children, although it makes up a small percentage of adult cases of leukemia. ALL is characterized by the overproduction of immature lymphocytes (B cells or T cells). Symptoms usually appear rather suddenly.

TREATMENT. The prognosis (expected outcome) used to be poor for children with ALL, with death expected within months from infection or bleeding complications. Today, however, chemotherapy and other treatment regimens, including radiation therapy and long-term, low-dose chemotherapy, achieve complete remission (disappearance of disease symptoms) in 60% to 70% of young children. Some children are completely cured by chemotherapy alone. If ALL recurs after obtaining a good remission, cure can still be achieved with intensive chemotherapy coupled with bone marrow transplantation.

CHRONIC LYMPHOCYTIC LEUKEMIA (CLL)

This form of leukemia is usually seen in older adults aged 40 to 70 , the majority of whom are males over the age of 60. Symptoms may not appear for a long time; thus, this form of leukemia is often discovered during routine physical and laboratory examinations. It is generally less severe than the acute form of lymphocytic leukemia. CLL is characterized by the overproduction of adult (mature) lymphocytes (B cells and T cells).

TREATMENT. This type of leukemia may not require any treatment initially, although each case varies. Red blood cell and platelet levels may be normal. Chemotherapy, steroid medication therapy, and radiation therapy can help people with CLL survive for 5 to 20 years.

LYMPHOMA

Lymphomas are cancers of the lymphatic system that most often originate within the lymph nodes. Lymphoma tumors can also occur, however, in other lymphoid tissues (tissues that have or contain lymphocytes), including the spleen, liver, and gastrointestinal tract. Lymphomas can eventually spread (metastasize) to other nonlymphoid organs if not diagnosed and treated early. The cause of lymphoma is unknown; viral agents, exposure to large-dose radiation, and chemical or physical agents that cause compromised immune system function have been suspected. Lymphomas may be divided into two major categories: Hodgkin and non-Hodgkin lymphomas.

HODGKIN LYMPHOMA

Also called Hodgkin disease.

Males are affected more often than females; the disease is usually seen in people between the ages of 15 and 35 and people over age 50. Hodgkin disease usually begins with cancerous (malignant) changes occurring within a single lymph node or in a single chain or group of lymph nodes. When the enlarged lymph node(s) are biopsied and the tissue is examined under a microscope, large, malignant cells called Reed-Sternberg cells are found. If left untreated, Hodgkin lymphoma eventually spreads to the next set of lymph nodes, the spleen or liver, and beyond.

SIGNS AND SYMPTOMS. A painless, hard, enlarged lymph node (often just one) in the neck, axilla (underarm), or groin area appears and continues to enlarge over time. Fever, weight loss, night sweats, and itchy skin also occur. Enlarged lymph nodes can cause other symptoms if they encroach or press on other structures such as the trachea (windpipe), heart, lungs, liver, stomach, or spleen. If untreated, anemia, susceptibility to infection, and death can occur within a few years.

TREATMENT. Hodgkin lymphoma is one of the most curable adult cancers. Radiation therapy cures as many as 90% of cases if the disease is discovered while only a limited number of lymph nodes are involved. In more advanced disease, treatment may include combined radiation therapy and chemotherapy. Advanced disease that does not respond to therapy is sometimes treated by bone marrow transplantation, using the person's self-donated bone marrow if it is cancer-free; the bone marrow is removed and stored frozen while intensive radiation and chemotherapy are given in an attempt to destroy all the Hodgkin lymphoma cells within the body. Because this intense therapy also destroys bone marrow cells, after therapy the stored healthy bone marrow is returned to the person in the hope that it will resume normal function and production of normal blood cells.

NON-HODGKIN LYMPHOMA

Non-Hodgkin lymphoma is the collective name for all lymphomas that are not Hodgkin lymphomas. Non-Hodgkin lymphomas usually occur in adults over age 40. Non-Hodgkin lymphomas often begin similarly to Hodgkin lymphoma, but may begin in lymphoid tissue other than the lymph nodes, such as in the spleen or liver. Often such lymphomas have spread to other organs before they are discovered.

SIGNS AND SYMPTOMS. Symptoms of non-Hodgkin lymphoma can be very similar to Hodgkin lymphoma and include the painless, hard enlargement of lymph nodes in the neck, axilla (underarm), or groin. Fatigue, fever, weight loss, itching, night sweats, nausea, vomiting, and abdominal pain may also occur.

TREATMENT. Depending on the specific type and degree of spread (metastasis), chemotherapy, steroid medication, and radiation therapy may be used. Bone marrow transplantation may be employed in specific cases and has been used with considerable success in recent years. Although the prognosis (expected outcome) and long-term survival rate have improved tremendously in recent years, each case varies in outcome. Some forms are curable with aggressive treatment.

MULTIPLE MYELOMA

Multiple myeloma is a cancer of plasma cells, which are formed by B cell lymphocytes to produce antibodies. When plasma cells undergo cancerous change, they begin to proliferate within the bone marrow, crowding out other blood cells. The tumor-like overgrowth of plasma cells weakens and destroys bone and releases bone calcium into the bloodstream. The cancerous plasma cells may also invade the spleen, liver, or kidneys; the resulting tumors interfere with organ function. The cancerous plasma cells produce an abnormal protein antibody that can be identified with special blood and urine tests. The cause of multiple myeloma is unknown.

SIGNS AND SYMPTOMS. Spontaneous fractures and constant bone pain occur and can be incapacitating. Weakness, fatigue, and other symptoms of anemia; susceptibility to infection; a tendency to bruise and bleed easily; kidney damage and failure; and elevated blood calcium levels can occur. If the vertebrae of the spine (backbone) fracture, the spinal cord can be damaged, resulting in numbness or permanent loss of body function in varying degrees, depending on the location of the spinal fracture.

TREATMENT. There is usually no cure for multiple myeloma, but chemotherapy and steroid medication can reduce the size of the tumor(s) and relieve the pain and other symptoms. Radiation therapy may also help relieve pain. Treatment may extend life span for many years. Drinking adequate amounts of fluid and staying active help prevent kidney damage and additional bone calcium loss. A few people have apparently been cured by bone marrow transplantation.

POLYCYTHEMIA VERA

Also called primary polycythemia.

Polycythemia vera is a chronic, long-term disorder of unknown cause. It may be a form of blood cancer like leukemia, different only in that red blood cells (RBCs) are affected instead of white blood cells (WBCs). The disorder usually affects adults, males more often than females. In addition to having an elevated number of RBCs, people with polycythemia vera often have elevated numbers of WBCs and platelets.

The increase in blood thickness, in number of platelets, and sometimes in blood volume poses a risk of blood clot formation. Bleeding may be a complication as well, because the platelets may not function as they normally should.

Secondary polycythemia can result when other medical disorders such as heart or lung disease interfere with the distribution of oxygen to body tissues. Lack of oxygen triggers the kidneys to release a hormone (erythropoietin) that stimulates the bone marrow to produce more RBCs in an attempt to get more oxygen to the body's tissues.

SIGNS AND SYMPTOMS. Headache; vision disturbances; dizziness; shortness of breath, especially with physical activity; enlargement of the liver and spleen (hepatosplenomegaly); numbness, burning, or tingling sensations of the hands, feet, arms, or legs; red, ruddy complexion; severe itching; and night sweats can occur. Complications include the formation of blood clots in the legs (thrombophlebitis) or organs, which can contribute to stroke, heart pain (angina), heart attack (myocardial infarction), and kidney damage.

TREATMENT. Phlebotomy, the removal of a predetermined amount of blood, is performed on a regular basis to keep the RBC count within a normal range. An adequate intake of fluids is important for maintaining plasma volume. Blood thinners may be given to reduce the risk of blood clot formation. Treatment with radioactive phosphorus decreases the production of all blood cells but may increase later risk of leukemia. Chemotherapy is sometimes used.

SYSTEMIC LUPUS ERYTHEMATOSUS (SLE)

See page 230.

VON WILLEBRAND DISEASE

One form of this disease is transmitted through an autosomal dominant inheritance pattern, and all forms combined affect 1 in 1,000 individuals. This bleeding disorder is caused by defective von Willebrand factor, a protein that binds with and carries one of the clotting factors (Factor VIII) in the blood. Lack of sufficient clotting factors makes it difficult for bleeding to stop.

SIGNS AND SYMPTOMS. Nosebleeds, bleeding gums, heavy menstrual periods, and easy bruising typically occur.

TREATMENT. Treatment options include supplying the missing or defective protein, suppressing menstruation, and taking drugs that increase the body's production of von Willebrand factor.

SECTION 16
THE BLOOD AND IMMUNE SYSTEMS

Document any defects in the structures of the blood and immune systems, if present, and treatment(s), if known.

Check any of the following diseases and disorders of the blood and immune systems that are or were present.

THE BLOOD

16.1 Aplastic anemia: indicate the age it occurred. Document causes and treatment(s), if known.

16.2 Folic acid deficiency anemia: indicate the age symptoms occurred. Document causes and treatment(s), if known.

16.3 Glucose-6-phosphate dehydrogenase deficiency (G6PD): indicate the age symptoms became apparent. Document treatment(s), if known.

16.4 Hemochromatosis: indicate age symptoms began. Document treatment, if known.

16.5 Hemophilia A: document treatment, if known.

16.6 Hemophilia B: document treatment, if known.

16.7 Hemolytic anemia: indicate age symptoms occurred. Document causes and treatment(s), if known.

16.8 Hereditary spherocytosis: document treatment, if known.

16.9 Iron-deficiency anemia: indicate age symptoms occurred. Document causes and treatment(s), if known.

16.10 Sickle cell anemia: document treatment(s).

16.11 Thalassemia: document the type and treatment(s), if known.

16.12 Vitamin B12 deficiency anemia: indicate the age symptoms occurred. Document causes and treatment(s), if known.

THE IMMUNE SYSTEM

16.13 Autoimmune thrombocytopenic purpura (AITP or ATP): indicate the age at onset. Document the cause and treatments, if known.

16.14 Immune deficiency disorder: document the type of disorder as primary (genetic or present at birth) or secondary (due to an external cause such as infection, medications, etc.). If the exact type of immune deficiency is known, list it here. Indicate the age symptoms of immune deficiency developed and document treatment(s), if known.

16.15 Leukemia: document the specific type of leukemia as acute myelogenous leukemia (AML), chronic myelogenous leukemia (CML), acute lymphocytic leukemia (ALL), chronic lymphocytic leukemia (CLL), if known. Document age at onset and treatment(s), if known.

16.16 Lymphoma: document the type as Hodgkin lymphoma or non-Hodgkin lymphoma. Document age at onset and treatment(s), if known.

16.17 Multiple myeloma: indicate age at onset. Document treatment(s), if known.

16.18 Polycythemia vera: indicate the age it occurred. Document the cause and treatments, if known.

16.19 Von Willebrand disease: document treatment, if known.

16.20 Document other diseases or disorders of the blood and/or immune systems that are or were present, age at onset, and treatment(s), if known.

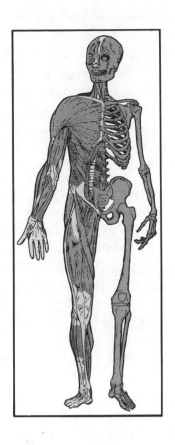

CHAPTER 17

THE MUSCULOSKELETAL SYSTEM

The musculoskeletal system makes up the largest mass of the body, consisting of muscles, bones, joints, tendons, ligaments, and cartilage. These structures account for about 75% of body weight. The musculoskeletal system allows the body to move, gives it shape, and enables people to stand erect. The bony skeleton provides a rigid framework of support for body tissues and organs; protects vital organs such as the brain, spinal cord, heart, and lungs; stores important minerals like calcium and phosphorus; and produces all blood cells (red blood cells, white blood cells, and platelets) within the bone marrow, which is the soft, pulpy substance in the center of the bone.

Muscles attached to bones give movement to the skeleton by contracting and shortening. Special muscles within organs such as the heart and the gastrointestinal tract do not attach to bone; they contract as they perform vital functions such as pumping blood throughout the blood vessels and propelling food throughout the digestive (gastrointestinal) tract. Muscle contraction produces heat, thus helping the body maintain its normal temperature.

STRUCTURES AND FUNCTIONS
THE SKELETON

The human skeleton is made up of 206 bones. Bone is composed of both living and nonliving elements. Bone cells called osteocytes live within the hard, nonliving substance of the bone. Bone grows, and it can actually repair itself as the osteocytes form new bone and break down or reabsorb old bone to make room for the new. This process of new bone formation and old bone reabsorption continues throughout life, although the rate of new bone growth slows with age. Growth in size is usually completed by late adolescence to early adulthood. Bones usually become weaker in late adulthood because the absorption rate of old bone usually exceeds the formation rate of new bone.

Blood vessels and nerves course throughout bone tissue. Blood vessels deliver oxygen and nutrients to the bone cells, and nerves provide a communication pathway to the brain, which is the mechanism through which bone pain is perceived.

The nonliving substance of bone produced by the osteocytes is laid down in layers, giving bone its strength and hardness. Calcium is the primary mineral stored within this nonliving substance; other minerals include phosphorus, magnesium, and fluoride. These stored minerals can be released from the bone into the bloodstream as needed. For example, the calcium level in the blood must be within a specific range for the body to stay in chemical balance; when blood calcium levels fall below that range, calcium is released from

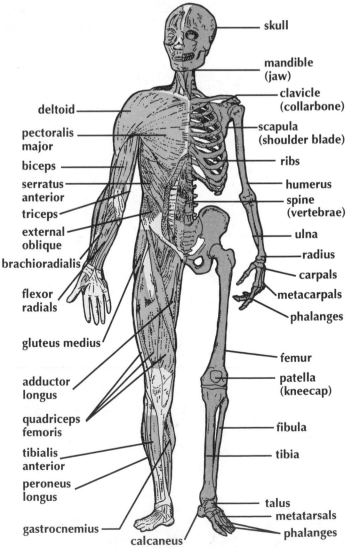

Figure 17.1. Some of the muscles and bones of the body

bone to bring the level up. Hormones produced by various glands regulate the movement of calcium from bone to blood and back, as well as the degree to which calcium is absorbed from the digestive tract and reabsorbed from the urine by the kidneys. These hormones include parathyroid hormone, calcitonin, growth hormone, glucocorticoid hormones, and sex hormones. Vitamin D also plays a large role in maintaining optimal blood calcium levels so that bone tissue remains strong. Because vitamin D can be synthesized in the body when the skin is exposed daily to adequate amounts of sunlight, and because vitamin D increases the amount of calcium retrieved by both the digestive tract and the kidneys, this vitamin is also considered to be a hormone.

Bone is covered by a thick, tough, fibrous layer of tissue called the periosteum. The periosteum contains blood vessels and nerves; many muscles and their tendons are attached to the periosteum. Cartilage, which is located at the ends of bones that come together to form a joint, is not covered by periosteum. Under the periosteum lies compact bone, the hardest layer, which contains large numbers of bone-forming cells (osteocytes). The inner layer of bone, called spongy bone or cancellus bone, is less dense and has a lace-like or sponge-like appearance. The central or inner cavity of bone, called the medullary cavity, contains bone marrow, the soft pulpy substance that produces blood cells (see figure 17.2).

Bones are grouped according to shape: the arm and leg bones are long bones; the ankle and wrist bones are short bones; the skull, breastbone (sternum), and ribs are flat bones; and the vertebrae of the spine (backbone) are irregular bones.

CARTILAGE

Cartilage is a tough, fibrous substance that is strong yet flexible. Cartilage is located at various sites, including in the ear and nose, between the ribs

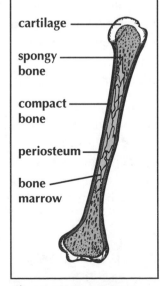

Figure 17.2. Anatomy (structure) of bone

cartilage
spongy bone
compact bone
periosteum
bone marrow

and the breastbone (sternum), at the end of the long bones of the arms and legs, and between the vertebrae of the spine (backbone). Cartilage at the end of the long bones is called articular or hyaline cartilage; it provides for growth of bone length by transforming into bone as the cartilage cells, called chondrocytes, form new cartilage. Cartilage also protects the bones from wear and tear by forming a cushion between bones when they join together to form joints.

LIGAMENTS

Ligaments are strong bands of tough, fibrous tissue that help hold the skeletal bones together and provide stability to bone joints. Ligaments also support and hold in place internal organs such as the stomach, liver, kidneys, spleen, and uterus.

JOINTS AND ARTICULATIONS

The structure formed where two or more bones come together is called a joint or articulation. Some joints are stiff; others allow movement. The degree of movement is determined in part by the shape of the bones and the type of tissue within the joint.

Joints can be classified into three major types: fibrous, cartilaginous, and synovial. Fibrous joints, also called synarthroses, are immovable joints in which the bones are joined by tough fibrous tissue. Bones of the skull are joined by fibrous joints.

Cartilaginous joints, also called amphiarthroses, are slightly movable joints in which the bones are joined by cartilage tissue. Bones of the pelvis and also the ribs and the breastbone (sternum) are joined by cartilaginous joints.

Synovial joints, also called diarthroses, move freely and are limited only by the shape of the bones and the attached ligaments, muscles, and tendons. Most of the joints in the human body, including the shoulder, elbow, knee, and hip, are synovial joints. The ends of the bones that come together to form a synovial joint are lined with cartilage, and the joint is surrounded by a membranous sac called the joint capsule. The capsule is lined with a special membrane (synovial membrane) that produces a special fluid (synovial fluid) that fills the capsule. Synovial fluid lubricates the joint and acts as a shock absorber during weight-bearing activities like walking, jogging, and running (see figure 17.3).

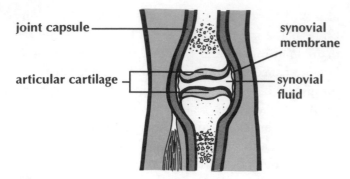

Figure 17.3. Structure of a joint

joint capsule

articular cartilage

synovial membrane

synovial fluid

Subtypes of synovial joints are designated by the type and degree of movement they allow. Subtypes include ball-and-socket joints like the shoulder and hip; hinge joints like the elbow, finger, toe, and knee; pivot joints like the portion of the elbow joint that allows the hand to be rotated palm-up and palm-down; gliding joints like those in the wrist and between the vertebrae of the spine (backbone); saddle joints like the base of the thumb; and condyloid joints like those in the wrist and the base of the index finger.

MUSCLES

Muscles consist of living cells called muscle fibers, which vary in size and shape. Muscle fibers contract to shorten their length to cause body or organ movement. Muscle fibers require calcium and energy to contract. Some muscle cells store calcium within themselves; some muscle cells absorb calcium from surrounding body fluid. Glucose (blood sugar) and glycogen (a complex form of glucose) are the primary sources of energy used by muscle cells, although they can also use fats and proteins if necessary. Many muscle cells store glycogen for future use.

Muscle fibers get oxygen and nourishment from blood that circulates in and around the muscles. Oxygen is used by muscle cells to change glucose and glycogen into energy. However, if the muscle cells' need for energy outdistances the available supply of oxygen, as for example during prolonged exercise, energy can be produced by means that do not require oxygen.

The three major types of muscle tissue are skeletal muscle, smooth muscle, and cardiac muscle.

SKELETAL MUSCLE. Skeletal muscle, also called striated (striped) muscle, gives the skeletal system movement. There are more than 600 skeletal muscles in the body. These are attached to bones, other muscles, and skin; their movement is voluntarily controlled. That is, the movement of skeletal muscle is consciously determined and regulated.

Skeletal muscle fibers are grouped into bundles, and bundles are grouped together to form the mass of the muscle. The muscle is covered by a layer of tough, slick tissue (fascia) that can extend beyond the mass of the muscle to form a tendon. Skeletal muscle may be directly attached to the outer covering of the bone (periosteum), or the muscle may attach to the periosteum by a tendon. Often, the origin or beginning point of the muscle, which is generally located toward the center of the body, is attached directly to the periosteum of the bone, whereas the insertion or end of the muscle attaches via its tendon(s) at a point away from the body, across a joint and onto another bone. Often, opposing muscles attach to opposite sides of bones. This arrangement enables movement in two directions. As one muscle or muscle group contracts, the opposing muscle or muscle group relaxes, and the bones to which the muscles are attached move closer together. The joint is the pivot point. An example of opposing muscles is the triceps and biceps of the upper arm, which bend the elbow (see figure 17.4). There is always a slight amount of contraction in skeletal muscles, which maintains the body's posture and position.

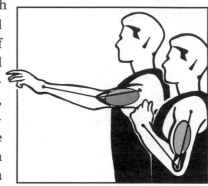

Figure 17.4. Opposing muscles of the upper arm, which bend the elbow

VISCERAL MUSCLE. Visceral muscle, also called smooth or involuntary muscle, is the type of muscle found in the hollow organs and structures of the body: the gastrointestinal system (esophagus, stomach, small and large intestines), blood vessels, uterus, and even the pupil of the eye. Visceral muscle is not consciously controlled; it is controlled by the autonomic (automatic) branch of the nervous system.

CARDIAC MUSCLE. Cardiac muscle is found only in the heart. It has built-in pacemaker cells that give it the ability to stimulate itself to contract without conscious thought or effort. Cardiac muscle beats at a rhythmic pace throughout life without tiring, unless it is damaged. The nervous system can cause the heart rate to quicken or slow in times of excitement and stress or when bearing down and straining, but the base rate of contraction is determined by the pacemaker cells within the cardiac muscle itself.

BURSAE. Bursae are small sacs made of tough, fibrous tissue filled with fluid (synovial fluid). They form small cushions at joints, such as the elbow, shoulder, hip, and knee. Bursae can be located between bone and tendon, skin and bone, muscle and muscle, tendon and ligament, etc. Bursae help reduce friction between moving structures at a joint and allow the structures to glide over one another.

STRUCTURAL BIRTH DEFECTS
CLUBFOOT

Also called talipes equinovarus.

Tho incidence is approximately 1 to 3 in 1,000; it is more common in males than in females. Clubfoot is a term used for various deformities of the foot that encompass abnormal positionings of the ankle and foot.

SIGNS AND SYMPTOMS. In the most common deformity, referred to as talipes equinovarus, the foot is turned inward with the toes extended downward in varying degrees of severity. Although in some types of clubfoot the ankle remains fairly flexible, the classic form involves the bones of the ankle and foot, making the joint stiff and rigid. In the classic defect, manual manipulation to straighten the foot cannot be performed. Overcrowding in the uterus late in pregnancy may cause flexible deformities, which are correctable without surgery; an insult or interruption during embryonic development may result in stiff deformities.

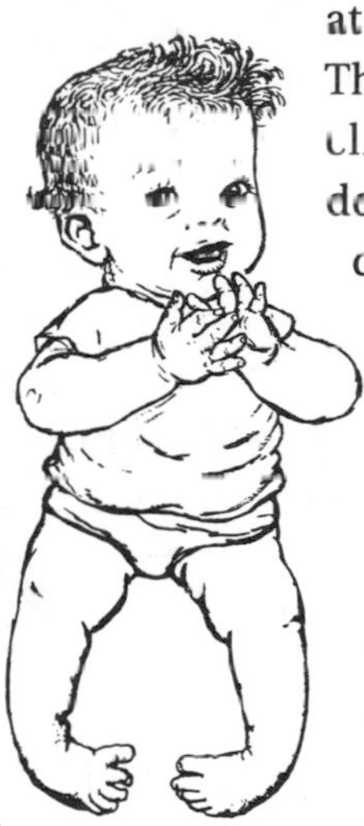

Figure 17.5. Infant with bilateral clubfoot

TREATMENT. Soon after birth, when the bones are fairly pliable and rapidly growing, the foot is manually straightened as much as possible. A cast is applied and replaced every few days initially, then every few weeks, progressively correcting the foot's position. Braces and other splinting devices may also be used. Some deformities are corrected more easily than others; those that do not respond to these methods may require surgical correction.

CONGENITAL HIP DISLOCATION

Incidence is approximately 1 in 500 to 1,000 live births; it is more common in females than in males. The hip joint is a ball-and-socket joint, where the head of the thigh bone (the femur) fits into the socket (the acetabulum) that is located on the sides of the pelvic bones. Congenital dislocation of the hip may involve either of these structures.

SIGNS AND SYMPTOMS. In some instances, the thigh bone is only partially out of the socket; in others, the bone is totally out of the socket (dislocated). In some cases the hip socket is underdeveloped (hip dysplasia). Hip dislocation is usually detected shortly after birth.

TREATMENT. The dislocation is easier to correct sooner than later. Splinting devices such as the Pavlik harness keep the head of the thigh bone directed into the socket at all times. Casting and/or surgery may be necessary. The defect becomes more difficult to correct as the child ages, with permanent damage and early deterioration of the bone occurring if treatment is delayed too long.

DISEASES AND DISORDERS
ACHONDROPLASIA

Sometimes known as short limb dwarfism.

The incidence of achondroplasia is approximately 1 in 10,000 live births and is seen in all races and in both sexes. It is transmitted through an autosomal dominant inheritance pattern. About 80% of all cases are the result of new mutation that occurred in the egg or sperm, so there is seldom any family history. Increased age of the father may contribute to its occurrence.

SIGNS AND SYMPTOMS. Abnormal bone growth, particularly in the long bones of the arms and legs, results in short limbs. A person with achondroplasia may have a large-appearing head with a prominent forehead and jaw, bowed legs, and short, broad hands and feet. The torso (trunk) is usually of normal size. Many people with achondroplasia have swayback of the lower spine (lordosis) or other abnormal spinal curvatures. Sometimes the vertebrae (backbones) are weak in structure, which can result in spinal cord compression; this can cause a wide variety of complications, from pain and/or numbness in the legs to a cessation of breathing, which can result in death.

Most people with achondroplasia have normal intelligence. Children may be slow to achieve physical developmental milestones such as sitting, standing, and walking only because of their loose joints and the disproportion of their limbs to their bodies.

TREATMENT. Procedures to break and lengthen bones can be performed, but these procedures can take many months and are painful. Infants and children with achondroplasia should be monitored closely for bone abnormalities so that serious complications can be avoided. Some bone abnormalities, like severely bowed legs, can be surgically corrected.

ANKYLOSING SPONDYLITIS

Also called rheumatoid spondylitis and Marie-Strümpel disease.

Ankylosing spondylitis is considered rheumatoid arthritis of the spine. It is an inflammatory disorder that begins in the sacroiliac joint, the region of the lower back where the spinal column and the pelvis (hip bones) meet. Initially, the ligaments, tendons, cartilage, and joint capsules of the spinal column bones (vertebrae) become irritated, red, and swollen; eventually they are converted into bone tissue resulting in a stiff, rigid spine that becomes increasingly painful and difficult to bend. In some cases ankylosing spondylitis may involve other synovial joints, including the shoulder, hip, and knee; sometimes the entire body is affected. If the ribs are involved, chest movement is severely restricted, making it very difficult to breathe deeply and expand the lungs. Other complications include inflammation of the iris of the eye (iritis) and disturbance of the heart's rhythm. Ankylosing spondylitis slowly worsens over the years.

The precise cause of this disorder is unknown, but it is thought to occur in people who have a genetic susceptibility and have also been exposed to an environmental trigger; for example, a virus. Approximately 9 in 10 people who have ankylosing spondylitis have a specific tissue type or tissue marker on their body cells, which supports the idea of a genetic connection. Ankylosing spondylitis occurs in males more than females, with symptoms usually beginning anytime from the late teens to 40 years of age.

SIGNS AND SYMPTOMS. Symptoms caused by ankylosing spondylitis range from mild to severe and can affect the entire body. Back pain and early morning back stiffness are characteristic symptoms, although the pain may come and go in severity. As the disorder progresses, the person begins to lean forward in an effort to reduce the back pain; eventually the spinal column hardens irreversibly in this forward, slumped position. Other involved joints can become painful, stiff, and eventually nonfunctional as the joint tissues turn to bone. Generalized or systemic symptoms that sometimes occur include low-grade fever, fatigue, weight loss, and arthritis-like discomfort in other joints.

TREATMENT. Ankylosing spondylitis cannot be halted or cured, but medication can be used to reduce the pain and inflammation. Frequent physical therapy and exercise of the affected joints help retain as much proper body alignment and joint function as possible. Joint surgery is sometimes indicated.

BURSITIS

Bursitis is the inflammation of one or more bursae. The inflammation is usually related to excessive use of the joint involved. Bursae of the shoulder are frequently affected, although bursitis can develop within bursae of the knees, elbows, hips, big toes, or other joints. Bursitis may or may not accompany tendonitis (inflammation of one or more tendons).

SIGNS AND SYMPTOMS. Bursitis causes deep pain and swelling in the joint in which the bursa is located. Symptoms usually disappear in a few weeks.

TREATMENT. Medication can be used to reduce inflammation. Injections of steroid medication to the affected area are sometimes used.

DEGENERATIVE JOINT DISEASE (DJD)

Also known as osteoarthritis, osteoarthrosis, and "wear-and-tear" arthritis.

DJD is probably the most common arthritic disorder. Unlike other forms of arthritis, DJD is not an inflammatory disorder with redness, warmth, or swelling; it is a mechanical wearing down of the joints. DJD causes the cartilage at the ends of the synovial joint bones to yellow, weaken, pit, and eventually deteriorate. Without their protective cartilage cushion, the bones of the joint begin to grind against one another, changing their shape and weakening the joint. Painful bone spurs often develop within the joint, adding to the discomfort. The involved joint(s) wear down over a period of several years so slowly that DJD is often accidentally discovered on x-ray before symptoms have appeared. As the disease progresses, joint pain and loss of function occur. DJD often affects only one joint, but it can affect more. The hands and the weight-bearing joints, including the spinal column, hips, and knees, are most commonly affected (see figure 17.6).

The cause of DJD remains unknown. The cartilage may be abnormal in structure or composition, or may be digested by enzymes present in the joint fluid. Some researchers believe the immune system may be involved, and there could be genetic susceptibility.

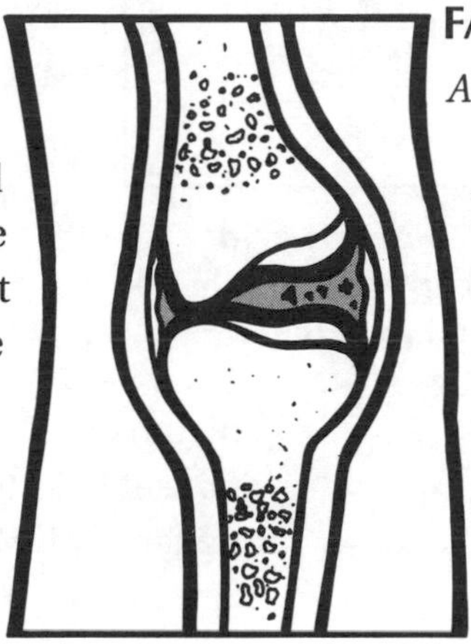

DJD has primary and secondary forms. Primary DJD is frequently more severe, with swelling, warmth, and redness similar to other forms of arthritis, and it tends to have a higher familial or genetic tendency.

Figure 17.6
DJD: degeneration of articular cartilage and deformity of joint

Secondary DJD is most often associated with joint trauma, overuse, infection, etc. Obesity increases the risk of DJD because of increased stress and pressure on the joints, especially the weight-bearing joints. People in occupations that require heavy use of the joints—such as jack-hammer operators, construction workers, and pianists—and people who participate in athletics that increase wear and tear on joints, are at increased risk. Women are affected by DJD more frequently than men. DJD is usually seen after age 40, and incidence increases with age.

SIGNS AND SYMPTOMS. Symptoms of DJD are frequently mild, but can include joint pain and loss of function, often in only one joint. Pain frequently increases with joint use and is worse at the end of the day. In rare cases, DJD may be crippling. Bony lumps sometimes develop in the end or middle joints of the fingers; this occurs more often in women than in men.

TREATMENT. Medication can be used to relieve inflammation and pain. Inflammation of an affected joint, thought to be caused by small fragments (possibly bone) floating in the synovial fluid, is sometimes treated with joint aspiration, a procedure in which synovial fluid is drawn off the joint through a small hollow needle and replaced with a small amount of cortisone (a steroid medication). Although cortisone reduces inflammation, it can be used only a limited number of times. Surgery, such as total hip joint replacement, is sometimes indicated. Weight reduction (if necessary) and exercises to improve posture and strengthen muscles may help slow the progression of DJD.

FAMILIAL HYPOPHOSPHATEMIC RICKETS
Also called vitamin D–resistant rickets.

The incidence is approximately 1 in 25,000 live births. This disorder is usually more severe in males than females and follows an X-linked dominant inheritance pattern.

SIGNS AND SYMPTOMS. The mutant gene inherited with this disorder causes an abnormality in special structures (receptors) within the kidney that convert and absorb active vitamin D. The resulting lack of active vitamin D causes soft bones, curving of the legs (bow legs), and short stature, although growth in infancy is usually normal.

TREATMENT. Vitamin D–resistant rickets is so named because it is unresponsive to normal doses of vitamin D therapy. Treatment requires high doses of vitamin D and additional dietary phosphorous.

GOUT
Also known as gouty arthritis and crystal-induced arthritis.

Gout is an arthritic disorder that occurs roughly 90% of the time in men over age 40. It is thought to occur when the body either produces too much uric acid or has a decreased ability to clear uric acid from the blood through the kidneys. Primary gout may be an inherited disorder. The mode of transmission is suspected to be an X-linked inheritance pattern; thus, mainly males are affected and females are carriers who are usually unaffected. Secondary gout is caused by another medical disorder, such as leukemia or cancer of the blood-forming organs (bone marrow, liver, spleen); it can also be caused by certain medications, including aspirin and certain diuretics (drugs used to increase urine output).

In gout, uric acid crystalizes into particles in the fluid of a synovial joint, causing sudden and severe inflammation, pain, swelling, redness, and warmth.

Without treatment, this acute gout attack or flare-up lasts 3 to 10 days or more, after which the joint returns to normal.

Chronic gout, however, is manifested by frequent flare-ups and can lead to permanent joint damage. Excess uric acid can also form into kidney stones, or deposits in joint cartilage and other tissues, including the skin, as small nodules. Called *tophi*, these nodules are usually found in people who have had gout for 10 years or more.

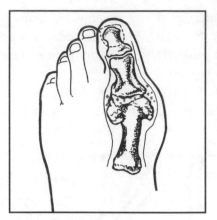

Figure 17.7. Gout: uric acid crystals build up and cause bone destruction and joint deformity

SIGNS AND SYMPTOMS. Acute gout usually occurs suddenly and affects only a single joint, often the big toe, but it can occur in other joints such as the ankle or knee. Symptoms, aside from intense joint pain, include redness, swelling, and warmth in the joint area. Fever, fatigue, and headache may also be present.

TREATMENT. Gout is an incurable long-term disorder that can be successfully managed with appropriate treatment. Medication can be used to decrease the pain and inflammation during acute attacks and to reduce the amount of uric acid in the body. Resting the affected joint during flare-ups is helpful.

In the past, a diet low in purine (a compound related to uric acid) was thought to decrease the amount of uric acid in the body, but this diet is controversial. It is now known that the body itself produces a certain amount of uric acid with or without a low-purine diet. Alcohol, aspirin, diuretics, and excess stress (physical and emotional) can precipitate gout flare-ups and should be avoided when possible. Maintaining a healthy body weight and avoiding fasting or fad diets is important, because quick weight losses can trigger gout flare-ups. An adequate daily intake of fluids is important to help prevent uric acid kidney stone formation. People with gout should be tested routinely for kidney damage that could be caused by uric acid deposits within kidney tissues.

MUSCULAR DYSTROPHY (MD)

MD is the collective name for a group of chronic hereditary diseases marked by the progressive (wors-ening) wasting of muscles and the degeneration and deterioration of skeletal muscle strength. All types of MD are genetic disorders; the pattern of inheritance varies. The most prevalent forms of muscular dystrophy are myotonic, Duchenne, Becker, limb-girdle, facioscapulohumeral, congenital, oculopharyngeal, and distal.

MYOTONIC MUSCULAR DYSTROPHY

Also known as myotonia atrophica and Steinert disease.

Myotonic MD is the most common type of adult MD, with an incidence of 1 in 10,000 live births; it is transmitted through an autosomal dominant inheritance pattern. The age of onset is 20 to 40 years, and it occurs in both males and females. Myotonic MD usually progresses slowly, sometimes over a period of 50 or 60 years. Affected women are at risk for life-threatening complications during labor and delivery.

SIGNS AND SYMPTOMS. A characteristic symptom of myotonic MD is a delayed relaxation of muscles after they are contracted (used). Progressive weakness of all body muscles frequently begins in the face, neck, hands, and feet, and is followed by eyelid droop (ptosis), facial weakness, and poorly articulated speech. Muscle degeneration (wasting) occurs slowly, and often does not restrict the performance of daily tasks.

A rare form of myotonic MD called congenital myotonic MD occurs almost exclusively in the infants of women affected with myotonic dystrophy. Symptoms at birth include profound muscle weakness evidenced by difficulty in breathing, sucking, and swallowing. These infants initially require special care but often improve. Varying degrees of mental retardation and delayed motor skills may become apparent in late infancy or early childhood.

DUCHENNE MUSCULAR DYSTROPHY (DMD)

Also known as pseudohypertrophic muscular dystrophy.

DMD is, unfortunately, the most common and severe form of childhood MD. Its incidence is approximately 1 in 5,000 live male births. Two thirds of all reported DMD cases are thought to be inherited through an X-linked inheritance pattern; the remainder are thought to be the result of a new mutation on the X chromosome in the egg. A new mutation on the X chromosome of a sperm results in a carrier female who is at risk of transmitting DMD to her son.

In DMD a protein called dystrophin is missing from muscle tissues, causing muscles to shrink, weaken, and waste away (atrophy). In the early stages of DMD, fat deposited into the weakening muscles gives the false appearance of the child's having excellent muscular development. The first muscles affected are those of the pelvis, upper arms, and upper legs.

SIGNS AND SYMPTOMS. Infants with DMD appear healthy at birth and throughout their first year, but between the ages of one and three the signs of muscle weakening and wasting appear. Sitting and walking may be delayed; the child begins to move about clumsily, falls frequently, develops a waddling gait, complains of fatigue and leg pain, and has difficulty keeping up with other children, especially in activities like skipping and running. As the child ages, the muscle degeneration (wasting) continues; by age 12, many children with DMD require the use of a wheelchair. As DMD progresses, the child may lose all voluntary muscle control; eventually even the heart and breathing muscles are affected. Most boys with DMD die between the ages of 15 and 25, usually from heart failure or infection.

BECKER MUSCULAR DYSTROPHY

This form of MD is transmitted through an X-linked inheritance pattern; thus, it occurs primarily in males, usually those between 2 and 16 years of age. However, onset can occur as late as age 25. Incidence is 1 in 30,000 live male births. Becker MD is caused by milder mutations in the same gene that causes Duchenne MD. In Duchenne MD the muscle protein dystrophin is absent. In Becker MD, the mutant gene causes a decrease in the amount of dystrophin or abnormalities in its structure. Daughters born to fathers who have Becker MD will be carriers of the mutant gene and can pass it on to their sons.

SIGNS AND SYMPTOMS. The symptoms of Becker MD are similar to those of Duchenne MD but are generally less severe and progress more slowly. The first muscles affected are those of the pelvis, upper arms, and upper legs. People with Becker MD typically have a longer life expectancy than those with Duchenne MD.

LIMB-GIRDLE MUSCULAR DYSTROPHY

Limb-girdle MD occurs in both males and females and is transmitted through an autosomal recessive inheritance pattern. The onset of limb-girdle MD commonly occurs in late childhood to early adulthood. It rarely appears in older adults.

SIGNS AND SYMPTOMS. A slow, progressive weakness begins in the muscles of the shoulders, hips, and pelvis and those muscles that encircle the waist. For many years following the first onset of symptoms, walking is usually possible; however, in some cases, muscle weakness progresses quickly, necessitating the use of walking aids. Heart and lung function may become involved late in the disease. Limb-girdle MD can shorten life span.

FACIOSCAPULOHUMERAL MUSCULAR DYSTROPHY (FMD)
Also called Landouzy-Dejerine muscular dystrophy.

FMD occurs in both males and females and is transmitted through an autosomal dominant inheritance pattern. Symptoms usually appear between the teenage and early adult years.

SIGNS AND SYMPTOMS. The first muscles affected are those of the face, shoulders, and upper arms. Early signs include difficulty closing the eyes, a forward sloping of the shoulders, and difficulty raising the arms above the head. The progression of FMD is slow, and may span several decades, with long periods of stability alternating with bursts of rapid muscle deterioration and extreme muscle weakness. Although FMD is sometimes mild, in its most severe form it causes disability and decreased life span.

CONGENITAL MUSCULAR DYSTROPHY

Congenital MD is a very rare muscular dystrophy that is present at birth and occurs in both males and females. It is transmitted through an autosomal recessive inheritance pattern.

SIGNS AND SYMPTOMS. Generalized muscle weakness is sometimes accompanied by joint deformities caused by muscle shortening. Congenital MD progresses slowly or may stay unchanged; the severity of symptoms can vary greatly. Life span may be shortened.

OCULOPHARYNGEAL MUSCULAR DYSTROPHY

Oculopharyngeal MD occurs in both males and females, with symptoms beginning anytime between the ages of 40 and 70. It is transmitted through an autosomal dominant inheritance pattern.

SIGNS AND SYMPTOMS. Drooping eyelids, usually the first indicator of oculopharyngeal MD, is followed by other signs of eye and facial muscle weakness. This slowly progressing disease can also affect the muscles of the throat, leading to difficulty in swallowing, which increases the risk and occurrence of choking episodes and repeated lung infections such as pneumonia. Difficulty eating and maintaining adequate nutrition can become major problems. Eventually the muscles of the shoulders and pelvis may weaken. Life span can be affected.

DISTAL MUSCULAR DYSTROPHY

This relatively mild, slowly progressing form of MD occurs in both males and females and is transmitted through an autosomal dominant inheritance pattern. Symptoms usually begin between ages 40 and 60.

SIGNS AND SYMPTOMS. The earliest symptom is weakness of the hand muscles, which causes clumsiness and difficulty with fine hand coordination. As distal MD progresses it affects the muscles of the forearms and lower legs. The life span of affected people is usually not altered.

EMERY-DREIFUSS MUSCULAR DYSTROPHY

Emery-Dreifuss is a rare form of MD that affects primarily males and is transmitted through an X-linked inheritance pattern. It progresses slowly, with symptoms beginning from childhood to the early teen years.

SIGNS AND SYMPTOMS. Muscles of the shoulders, upper arms, and lower legs become weak and wasted (atrophied). Joints of the elbows, knees, and ankles may become distorted and disfigured from muscle shortening. People with Emery-Dreifuss MD sometimes have abnormal heart rhythm.

TREATMENT. There is no cure for the muscular dystrophies. Continuous care from a team of health-care providers, which includes physical, occupational, and respiratory therapists, helps people with MD maintain optimal muscle function and independence, and helps prevent complications for as long as possible. Special limb or body braces, wheelchairs, hydraulic lifts, bathroom aids, and speech and communication aids may be needed.

OSTEOGENESIS IMPERFECTA (OI)

OI occurs in several forms. Their combined incidence is approximately 1 in 10,000 to 20,000 live births. Clinically, there are more than four types of osteogenesis imperfecta. Types I and IV follow an autosomal dominant inheritance pattern and are the most common; types II and III may be either dominant or recessive and are the most severe. However, the vast majority of lethal type II are autosomal dominant and are the result of mosaicism (some body cells have normal genes and some cells have the mutant gene for OI) or a new gene mutation that occurred in the egg or sperm. A defect in the formation of collagen, one of the proteins that give the body's connective tissues elasticity, results in brittle bones that fracture and break easily.

SIGNS AND SYMPTOMS. People with OI characteristically have fragile, brittle bones with loose joints and often abnormal curvatures of the spine. Impaired hearing, abnormal tooth formation or crowding, and a blueness of the white part of the eye (the sclera) may also be present.

TREATMENT. There is no cure for the collagen formation defect; treatment focuses on prevention of fractures and other complications.

OSTEOMYELITIS

Osteomyelitis is an inflamation and infection of the bone that is usually caused by bacterial microorganisms that enter bone tissue through a penetrating wound or injury, such as a gunshot or stab wound, a nail that is stepped on, or a bone fracture that pokes through the skin. Bone tissue can also be infected by bacteria that have traveled through the bloodstream from another site of infection in the body. Having bone surgery, diabetes mellitus, or rheumatoid arthritis, or being elderly or malnourished can make bone tissue susceptible to infection.

When bacteria enter bone tissue, infection begins and spreads throughout the central cavity that holds the bone marrow, as well as to the hard bone layers. Bone and surrounding tissues become inflamed and swollen. Blood clots can form within the tiny blood vessels that serve the bone. As a result, bone tissue can die from lack of oxygen and nourishment.

SIGNS AND SYMPTOMS. Pain, swelling, and warmth over the infected bone can be extreme and worsen when the bone or joint is moved. Generalized symptoms include fever and fatigue.

TREATMENT. Osteomyelitis is treated with antibiotics, and hospitalization may be required. The bone or joint is usually immobilized and rested. Infected or dead bone tissue sometimes requires surgical removal. Osteomyelitis can recur, and sometimes it becomes chronic.

OSTEOPOROSIS

Osteoporosis is probably the most common bone disorder. It affects women more than men; it usually occurs after age 45 and increases with age. X-rays of as many as 9 in 10 women over the age of 75 reveal signs of osteoporosis.

Osteoporosis is a decrease in bone mass caused by the loss of calcium from both spongy and hard bone. This loss of calcium makes bones porous and spongy in appearance as well as brittle, fragile, and weak in structure. Bones with osteoporosis are more vulnerable to fractures. Although all bones can be affected, the vertebrae (backbone), hip (pelvis), wrist, and bones of the forearms are most often affected.

Although the exact cause of osteoporosis is unknown, both genetic and environmental factors seem to be involved. A major risk factor of osteoporosis is not achieving maximum peak bone mass as an adult. Peak bone mass, which is attained at about age 30 to 35, is the point at which bone is at its strongest and highest density. Until that time, the buildup of new bone and the breakdown of old bone is about equal. After age 35, bone breakdown exceeds the rate of new bone formation, and bone mass begins to decline. As a result, the process of osteoporosis begins and continues as part of the normal aging process. Peak bone mass is affected by genetics, nutrition (especially with respect to lifelong intake of calcium and vitamin D), exercise, tobacco and alcohol use, and medical disorders that interfere with bone formation or with the body's ability to absorb and use calcium and vitamin D.

The female hormone estrogen, produced by the ovaries until menopause, appears to play a role in maintaining calcium within the bone, and thus maintaining bone mass. After natural menopause or menopause induced by the removal of both ovaries, the amount of estrogen in a woman's body is markedly reduced. This reduction appears to increase the loss of bone calcium, and osteoporosis becomes more severe. Men generally achieve a higher peak bone mass than women and do not have the sudden hormonal alterations that women have. Perhaps that is why the majority of cases of osteoporosis—and the most severe cases—occur in women. Among women who have low peak bone mass to begin with, osteoporosis becomes significant faster.

Other risk factors associated with osteoporosis include family history; a body that is small and thin-framed; a sedentary lifestyle that does not include adequate or regular weight-bearing exercises like walking, jogging, or playing tennis; tobacco use; long-term alcohol use; long-term low intake of dietary calcium and vitamin D; medical disorders such as malabsorption syndromes; endocrine disorders such as hyperthyroidism and hyperparathyroidism; kidney or liver disorders; long-term use of medications such as heparin (an anticoagulant or blood thinner), steroids, and certain anticonvulsants and antibiotics; and prolonged periods of immobility.

SIGNS AND SYMPTOMS. Symptoms of osteoporosis include low back pain, hip pain, and a susceptibility to bone fractures, especially of the hips, wrist, and vertebrae (usually in the form of compression). In severe osteoporosis, fractures can occur spontaneously without associated trauma or injury. As the bones of the spine compress, height decreases and the upper back slumps forward.

TREATMENT. Although osteoporosis has no cure, treatment can slow its progress. When calcium levels in the blood drop, bones release calcium into the blood. An adequate daily intake of calcium maintains adequate levels of calcium in the blood so that none is lost from bone. Obesity puts unnecessary stress on osteoporitic bones; maintaining a healthy body weight eliminates that stress. Routine weight-bearing exercise helps keep calcium in the bones. Estrogen hormone replacement therapy is sometimes used after menopause to slow the process of osteoporosis.

Because the loss of bone mass cannot be reversed and treatment can only slow its progression, prevention is the most effective way to fight osteoporosis. Children should learn the importance of a diet that includes adequate calcium and vitamin D and the importance of routine physical activity and exercise.

PAGET DISEASE OF BONE

Also known as osteitis deformans.

Paget disease of bone occurs in males more than females. It usually affects people over age 40, although it occurs rarely in younger people.

Paget disease of bone is initially characterized by an increase in the activity rate of cells that break down old bone. This process stimulates cells that form new bone to increase their activity as well, and they begin overproducing new bone. This hurriedly formed new bone is laid down in an irregular, abnormal pattern that makes the bone structurally weak, despite increased thickness and high mineral (including calcium) content. Affected bones become more susceptible to fractures, which can occur with little or no injury to the bone.

Paget disease of bone may affect many bones or only a local area of bone. The bones most often affected are the skull, vertebrae (backbone), long bones (including the thigh and lower leg bones), and the pelvis. Paget disease of bone usually progresses slowly. Many people have few or no evident symptoms and are diagnosed after the disease is discovered during a routine health examination.

SIGNS AND SYMPTOMS. Deep pain and warmth can occur in affected bones, some of which develop arthritic changes. The skull bones can become noticeably enlarged, which makes the face look small even though the facial bones are not usually affected. Thickening of the skull can compress nerves within the skull, resulting in hearing loss. Dizziness, headache, and intermittent ringing in the ears may also occur. In severe cases the flow of cerebral spinal fluid in and around the brain becomes obstructed, resulting in hydrocephalus ("water on the brain"). When the spine is affected it stiffens and becomes rigid and bent forward. The rib cage (ribs and breastbone) may also stiffen. When the pelvis and legs are affected the legs become bowed, sometimes severely. Resulting gait disturbances such as limping and waddling can interfere with walking.

TREATMENT. Medications can be used to reduce the pain and inflammation and depress the abnormal activity of the bone cells. People with Paget disease of bone who have no symptoms are usually not treated, but they should be evaluated routinely.

RHEUMATOID ARTHRITIS (RA)

RA is the most debilitating form of arthritis. It affects women more severely and more often than it does men. RA usually occurs between 20 and 60 years of age, although it can occur at any age. RA is a chronic (long-term), progressive disease causing inflammation and destruction of synovial joints. RA usually affects the same joints on both sides of the body; for example, both hands, shoulders, hips, or knees. It affects other tissues of the body as well.

RA begins with the inflammation of the synovium, the special lining of the joint capsule that surrounds the joint. This inflammation causes the synovium to redden and thicken, as well as excess synovial fluid to accumulate within the joint. Abnormal tissue that forms within the joint destroys the cartilage on the ends of the bones inside the capsule. This eventually erodes bone tissue, muscles, tendons, and ligaments, which results in joint destruction and instability. Fibrous scar tissue that forms within the damaged joint ultimately becomes bone tissue, consolidating or fusing the joint and causing complete loss of joint function. The bones may lose stored calcium, causing a loss of hardness and susceptibility to bone fracture. The inflammation that occurs with RA can involve other structures and organs, including the blood vessels, heart, lungs, and eyes. Inflammation of arteries that lead to internal organs can reduce the amount of blood and oxygen to those organs and interfere with their function and/or cause permanent damage.

The cause of RA is unknown but is suspected to be an immune system disorder in which antibodies (protective proteins produced by special blood cells of the immune system) attack the joint tissue. Many people with RA, but not all, have an abnormal antibody called rheumatoid factor in their blood and within the joint fluid. It is not known exactly where rheumatoid factor is produced, but it may be produced by special cells within the synovium (the joint lining). Approximately two-thirds of people with RA have a specific tissue type or tissue marker on their body cells, indicating an inherited genetic susceptibility to RA. Some researchers feel RA may be caused by an infectious agent such as a virus or bacterium or an infectious agent combined with a genetic susceptibility. RA occurs in some syndromes, including Sjogren syndrome and Felty syndrome.

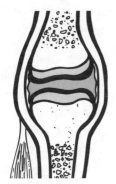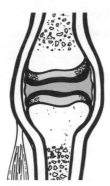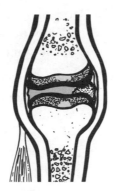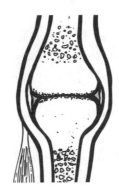

Figure 17.8. Rheumatoid arthritis: the progression of cartilage and bone destruction seen in RA, which results in joint destruction and loss of function

SIGNS AND SYMPTOMS. The symptoms of RA may begin suddenly or develop gradually. They frequently start with the hands but may eventually affect all of the synovial joints. Redness, warmth, swelling, discomfort and pain occur in affected joints, along with joint stiffness that is usually worse in the morning. Early symptoms of RA sometimes come and go in periodic flare-ups. Joint deformity, loss of function, and loss of muscle mass occur from joint disuse late in the disease. Body-wide or systemic symptoms include fatigue, loss of appetite and weight, low-grade fever, sweats, and rheumatoid nodules (round, nontender, movable lumps) that form beneath the skin in areas such as the wrist, along the forearm, elbow, knee, and under the toes. Rheumatoid nodules can come and go.

TREATMENT. There is no cure for RA. A balance of rest and exercise is an important part of the treatment for RA. Because it is a systemic, body-wide disease, people often feel ill and tire early in the day. Exercise is important for maintaining as much strength and joint flexibility as possible. The body must be properly aligned at all times, even when at rest. A well-balanced diet is also important. Applying hot and cold compresses can help relieve discomfort and swelling. Medications such as aspirin, nonsteroidal anti-inflammatory drugs, gold salt injections, some anticancer medications, and steroid medications (usually for short-term use only) can be used to reduce inflammation, swelling, and pain.

When begun early, treatment may lead to remission of symptoms, which could last several years. Surgery is sometimes performed to restore joint function. It is important that people not use treatments or therapies that have not been proved appropriate and safe in the treatment of RA. Many false cures are on the market. A health-care provider should always be consulted before an unproven treatment is tried. A physician who specializes in rheumatoid disorders can provide the best treatment.

SCOLIOSIS

Scoliosis is an abnormal lateral (to the side) curvature of the spine that takes the spinal column (backbone) out of its normal alignment. Scoliosis can progress until the abnormal curvature and rotation of the spine are so severe that heart and lung function are affected. Scoliosis can sometimes be caused by structural defects of the spine or poor posture, but the majority of cases are idiopathic, meaning the cause is unknown. However, it is believed that most cases of idiopathic scoliosis are genetically determined either through an autosomal dominant inheritance pattern or from multifactorial causes. Other causes of scoliosis include neuromuscular disorders that weaken muscles, paralysis of spinal muscles, or bone-weakening disorders such as rickets. Scoliosis in infants most often affects males; scoliosis in children and adolescents most often affects females.

SIGNS AND SYMPTOMS. Scoliosis can cause one shoulder to be higher than the other, one arm to hang closer to the body than the other, one shoulder blade to be more prominent than the other, and clothes to hang unevenly off the shoulders and hips. The abnormal lateral curvature of the spine may be visible or may be felt on physical examination. An x-ray can determine its severity.

TREATMENT. Braces may be recommended for children and adolescents to straighten the spine as the bones mature and harden. These braces are usually worn 23 hours a day and require frequent adjustments as the spine grows and begins to straighten. Exercises to maintain muscle strength while a brace is worn are an important part of treatment. Severe scoliosis may require surgery. Treatment in severe scoliosis should begin as soon as possible; scoliosis that does not require immediate treatment should be reevaluated yearly. School screening programs have helped identify many children who need further evaluation for scoliosis.

SYSTEMIC LUPUS ERYTHEMATOSUS (SLE)

Also known as lupus.

SLE is a disorder of the collagen-containing connective tissue of the body. Collagen is a tough, fibrous protein found in bones, joints, cartilage, ligaments, tendons, and the linings and tissues of many organs, including the kidneys, heart, lungs, gastrointestinal tract, arteries, skin, and nervous system (including the brain). SLE can be a body-wide disease. It is considered to be a serious rheumatoid disease associated with inflammation and damage of collagen tissues. SLE can occur at almost any age; it usually becomes apparent in people under age 40 and affects women in 9 out of 10 cases.

Although the exact cause of SLE remains unknown, it is thought that some factor or event causes the immune system to produce faulty or abnormal antibodies that attack the body's own tissues. Family history is a significant risk factor; some families have higher incidences of SLE than the general population. Some researchers suspect a genetic predisposition to the development of SLE that does not materialize until triggered by an external environmental factor such as a virus or medication.

Often, the first symptoms mimic those of rheumatoid arthritis. However, SLE usually does not cause the crippling or deformity in affected joints that long-term rheumatoid arthritis can.

Damage to internal organs can result as the abnormal antibodies attach to specific protein elements in the blood and accumulate within organ tissue. This type of tissue/organ damage is most clearly evident within the kidneys and can result in kidney failure.

SIGNS AND SYMPTOMS. SLE symptoms tend to come and go. Some people experience permanent remission (an absence of symptoms of the disease). Symptoms —which can be mild or severe—depend on which tissues and organs are affected. Symptoms can include arthritis-like pain, redness, and synovial joint swelling that comes and goes; a mask-like red, raised, scaly rash that appears on the bridge of the nose and extends to both cheeks, or appears on other areas of the body; purple bruise-like areas that appear on the fingers, toes, elbows, and forearms; kidney failure; anemia due to decreased numbers of red blood cells, sometimes accompanied by a decreased number of blood platelets; chest pain; nervous system symptoms that include headache, memory loss, behavior changes, and depression; nausea, vomiting, diarrhea, and abdominal pain; generalized symptoms such as excessive and unexplained fatigue, muscle weakness, weight loss, and low-grade fever; and an intolerance to sunlight. In some people, symptoms of SLE are aggravated or occur with certain triggers such as exposure to sunlight, physical or emotional stress, infections, extreme fatigue, and certain medications and chemicals.

TREATMENT. SLE is a chronic, long-term, recurrent disorder for which there is no cure. Treatment is aimed at preventing organ damage and reducing the degree of inflammation within collagen tissues. Medications are used to depress the immune system in order to decrease pain and inflammation and reduce the amount of abnormal antibodies. Adequate rest, good nutrition, moderate exercise, and avoidance of triggers that worsen SLE symptoms are important aspects of disease management. People with SLE should have routine health examinations.

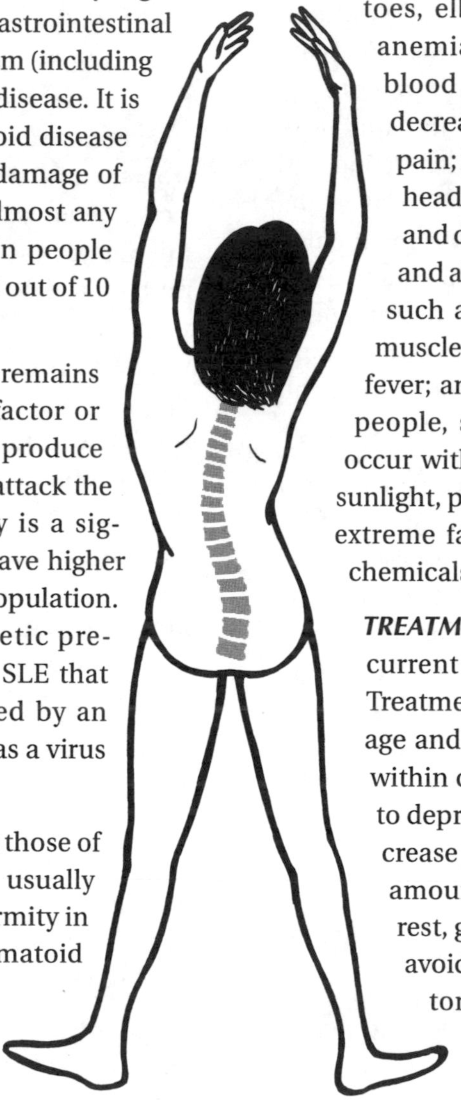

Figure 17.9. Scoliosis: abnormal lateral curvature and rotation of the spine

SECTION 17
THE MUSCULOSKELETAL SYSTEM

Check any of the following structural defects of the musculoskeletal system that were present at birth.

17.1 Clubfoot: indicate whether the right or left ankle was affected. Document treatment(s), if known.

17.2 Congenital hip dislocation: indicate whether the right or left hip was affected. Document the treatment(s), if known.

17.3 Document any other structural defects of the musculoskeletal system, if present, and treatment(s), if known.

Check any of the following diseases and disorders of the musculoskeletal system that are or were present.

17.4 Achondroplasia: document treatment(s), if known.

17.5 Ankylosing spondylitis: indicate age when symptoms began. Document treatment(s), if known.

17.6 Bursitis: indicate age(s) bursitis occurred. Document which joint area(s) were affected and treatment(s), if known.

17.7 Degenerative joint disease (DJD): indicate age when DJD was diagnosed. Document which joints were affected and treatment(s), if known.

17.8 Familial hypophosphatemic rickets: document treatment(s), if known.

17.9 Gout: indicate age when gout first occurred. Document which joint(s) were affected and treatment(s), if known.

17.10 Muscular dystrophy: document the specific type: myotonic muscular dystrophy, Duchenne muscular dystrophy, Becker muscular dystrophy, limb-girdle muscular dystrophy, fascioscapulohumeral muscular dystrophy, congenital muscular dystrophy, oculopharyngeal muscular dystrophy, distal muscular dystrophy, Emery-Dreifuss muscular dystrophy, or other. Indicate age when symptoms began and treatment(s), if known.

17.11 Osteogenesis imperfecta (OI): document the specific type, if known, and treatment(s), if known.

17.12 Osteomyelitis: indicate which bone(s) or joint(s) were affected and age when osteomyelitis occurred. Document the cause and treatment(s), if known.

17.13 Osteoporosis: indicate age when osteoporosis was discovered. Document treatment(s), if known.

17.14 Paget disease of bone: indicate age when it was discovered. Document treatment, if known.

17.15 Rheumatoid arthritis (RA): indicate age when RA was diagnosed. Indicate which joints were affected and document treatment(s), if known.

17.16 Scoliosis: indicate age when scoliosis was discovered. Document treatment(s), if known. Document other abnormal curvatures of the spine, such as lordosis or kyphosis, if present.

17.17 Systemic lupus erythematosus (SLE): indicate age when symptoms began. Document treatment(s), if known.

17.18 Document other diseases or disorders of the musculoskeletal system that are or were present, the age at onset, and treatment(s) received, if known.

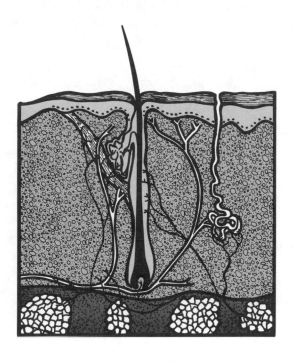

CHAPTER 18

THE INTEGUMENTARY SYSTEM

The integumentary system is the skin, hair, and nails. The skin is considered to be the largest organ of the body. The skin has been said to be a mirror that reflects a person's overall state of health, perhaps because many diseases and disorders that affect internal organs and systems cause changes or symptoms in the skin.

STRUCTURES AND FUNCTIONS

The skin has many functions. It is a protective armor, a tough but pliable barrier that shields the internal systems from the environment and its harmful agents. The skin is a water-resistant barrier that holds in water and other fluids; thus, it plays a very important role in maintaining fluid and chemical balances within the body. Normally, a small amount of water is lost through the skin; however, large breaks in the skin from injuries, such as serious burns, can allow massive amounts of water to be lost, causing critical, life-threatening water and chemical imbalances.

Blood vessels located in the skin help regulate body temperature by dilating and constricting. Dilation increases heat loss through the skin; constriction prevents it. Exposing the skin to sunlight or other sources of ultraviolet light allows the body to synthesize vitamin D, an element important for the normal growth and strength of bones. Last, but not least, the skin is rich with nerve endings and sensory receptors that allow the individual to identify different levels of temperature, pressure, pain, and touch.

Skin has three layers: the epidermis, dermis, and subcutaneous layers (see figure 18.1).

THE EPIDERMIS

The epidermis is the outermost layer of skin; it consists mainly of keratin, a strong protein. Cells within the epidermis continuously divide to produce new cells. As the older cells die, the newer cells push them to the outside of the layer where they are shed. Through this continuous replacement of cells, the epidermis completely replaces itself every three to four weeks. Melanocytes, the special cells that produce the pigment melanin, are located within the epidermis. Melanin gives skin, hair, and eyes their color and protects the skin from ultraviolet light damage. The amount of melanin produced by the melanocytes is influenced by genetic factors, hormones, and the environment.

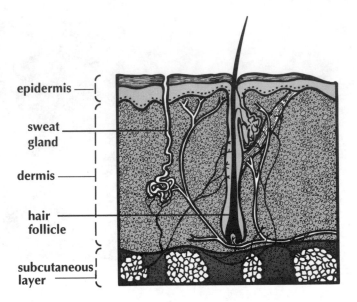

Figure 18.1. Structures and layers of the skin

THE DERMIS

The middle skin layer is the dermis. This "elastic" layer of skin contains sensory and nerve endings, blood vessels, and lymphatic vessels. Hair shafts and sweat and oil (sebaceous) glands are rooted in the dermis and open through the epidermis to the outside of the body.

THE SUBCUTANEOUS LAYER

The innermost layer of the skin is the subcutaneous layer; it consists of fat globules (adipose tissue) that hold the epidermis and dermis layers firmly to the body. This fatty layer also helps pad the body from injury and helps insulate against heat loss.

DISEASES AND DISORDERS

ACNE VULGARIS

Acne vulgaris appears most often during adolescence, although it can occur at other times throughout life. Genetic susceptibility seems apparent, and acne vulgaris may be multifactorial in cause.

Acne vulgaris affects the sebaceous (oil) glands attached to the hair follicles within the dermis. These glands produce oils that lubricate the hair shafts. When the glands become blocked, they form comedones, commonly known as whiteheads or blackheads. The dermis becomes inflamed, possibly because oil from the glands and other irritants leak into the dermis. In severe cases, scarring can result.

SIGNS AND SYMPTOMS. The inflammation and irritation within the dermis layer create swollen bumps, cysts, and/or pus-filled nodules. Acne appears most often on the face, neck, back, and chest, but can involve other skin areas as well.

TREATMENT. Oral medication and medicated creams and ointments are prescribed to treat acne. Helpful personal hygiene practices include keeping hair and skin clean, and avoiding oil-based creams, lotions, and makeups, as well as tightly fitting hats and collars. Scrubbing the face too hard can actually worsen the inflammation that is already present. Maintaining a balanced and nutritional diet, getting enough sleep, and reducing stress may also be helpful in reducing acne symptoms.

Note: Some acne medications, including iso-tretinoin, can cause severe birth defects if taken during pregnancy and should be taken only under the supervision of a health-care provider. Medications should never be shared with anyone.

ALBINISM

The incidence is approximately 1 in 17,000 live births; it is seen in all racial and ethnic groups. Almost all cases follow an autosomal recessive pattern, although there are autosomal dominant and X-linked types as well. There are, in fact, many, many forms of albinism.

Albinism is characterized by a reduction or absence of color (pigment) in the skin, hair, and/or eyes. Melanin is the substance that normally gives these tissues their color. Specific enzymes must be produced by specific genes for the body to produce melanin. Tyrosinase, one of the enzymes needed to produce melanin, is absent in many people with albinism. The gene that produces tyrosinase can be abnormal in various ways, which may explain the different degrees of color absence seen in people with albinism. Some people with albinism do produce tyrosinase, and researchers speculate that another

enzyme important in melanin production must be genetically mutant in these people. Some forms of albinism cause decreased color in the skin, hair, and eyes; some forms affect primarily the eyes.

SIGNS AND SYMPTOMS. In hair and skin, color can be reduced or absent. In the eyes, albinism can affect the retinas, the nerve pathways from the retinas to the brain, and the iris, causing visual problems including nearsightedness, farsightedness, and astigmatism, as well as sensitivity to light. Jerking eye movements, known as nystagmus, or crossed eyes, known as strabismus, can also occur.

TREATMENT. There is no way to replace melanin or to prevent the visual problems caused by albinism. Sunscreens rated 20 or higher and sunglasses and/or tinted lenses can help prevent damage from the sun's harmful ultraviolet rays, a job that melanin usually performs. Vision can be improved with corrective eyeglasses or contact lenses. Surgery can sometimes correct eye muscle abnormalities that cause strabismus. Developmental abnormalities of the retina or eye nerves cannot usually be repaired.

ATOPIC DERMATITIS

Also known as eczema and allergic dermatitis.

Atopic dermatitis is a genetically influenced inflammatory disorder of the skin. People with atopic dermatitis are thought to have inherited a low threshold to skin allergens (things that cause allergic reactions like itching and redness). Affected people frequently have or develop other allergic disorders such as asthma and hay fever at some point in their lives. Atopic dermatitis is seen most often in infants and children.

SIGNS AND SYMPTOMS. With atopic dermatitis the skin is extremely sensitive, itchy, and dry. Eczema-type lesions appear as small bumps, blisters, and/or scaly patches on the skin. Allergens that trigger atopic dermatitis include fabrics such as wool, nylon, or fur, harsh detergents, perfumes, some foods, changes in weather temperature and/or humidity, and possibly stress.

Complications of atopic dermatitis include secondary infection of the lesions, usually caused by microorganisms (germs) entering through breaks in the skin that were caused by intense scratching.

TREATMENT. Prevention by avoiding triggering agents is the best treatment for atopic dermatitis. People are instructed to use only mild detergents, wear cotton clothing, and avoid perfumed lotions and soaps and extreme changes in temperature. Medication and/or special ointments and creams may be prescribed to relieve symptoms.

CANCERS OF THE SKIN

As a group, cancers of the skin are the most common form of cancer in the United States, and their incidence has been increasing. It has been speculated that this increase is related to the thinning of the ozone layer that encircles the earth; the thinner the ozone layer, the more of the sun's skin-damaging ultraviolet rays reach the earth. Another cause could be the growing number of people who spend more recreational and/or retirement time engaging in sun-soaked activities. In general, skin cancers occur most frequently in people who are fair-skinned, who live close to the equator, and who are elderly.

A major risk factor for skin cancer is long-term exposure to the sun's ultraviolet rays. Skin damage from sun exposure builds over the years; by the time most people are in their twenties, they have already received enough sun exposure to increase their risk of developing skin cancer in their later years. People who experienced one or more severe sunburns as children have a higher incidence of skin cancer than those who did not. People who work outdoors, or who are exposed to irritating chemicals like pesticides, coal tar, pitch, arsenic, creosote, and radium are at higher risk of developing skin cancers. Artificial sources of ultraviolet light, including tanning beds or booths and some types of radiation/light therapies, increase risk as well. A genetic predisposition is apparent in a significant number of cases.

Types of skin cancer include basal cell carcinoma, squamous cell carcinoma, and malignant melanoma, all of which involve the epidermis layer of the skin.

BASAL CELL CARCINOMA (BCC)

This most common skin cancer usually occurs on sun-exposed areas of the skin. Although this type of skin cancer rarely spreads to other areas of the body, it can erode a large amount of surrounding tissue, including muscle and bone.

SIGNS AND SYMPTOMS. Lesions of BCC appear as waxy, transparent growths with ulcerated centers, or as shiny yellow or gray plaques.

TREATMENT. Treatment can include surgical removal, freezing, burning, or laser therapies; radiation therapy; various types of chemotherapy (including topical application); or a combination of these.

SQUAMOUS CELL CARCINOMA (SCC)

This skin cancer can occur on almost any area of the skin. It easily spreads to other parts of the body.

SIGNS AND SYMPTOMS. Lesions of SCC are red, raised, scaly patches that may bleed if irritated or traumatized.

TREATMENT. Treatment can include surgical removal, freezing, burning, or laser therapies; radiation therapy; various types of chemotherapy (including topical application); or a combination of these.

MALIGNANT MELANOMA

This most severe of the skin cancers is a cancerous growth of the pigment (melanin) producing cells, the melanocytes. Melanomas usually develop on the trunk, legs, or feet, but can develop in other skin areas as well, including within the eye or along the nailbeds. Malignant melanoma invades the deeper layers of skin and can readily spread (metastasize) to other areas of the body. Melanoma is fatal if not diagnosed and treated early. Malignant melanoma can either develop within a preexisting mole or birthmark or appear as a new skin lesion.

SIGNS AND SYMPTOMS. These lesions are usually uneven (asymmetric) in shape, with ragged, irregular edges; a lesion can have several colors, including brown, pink, gray, white, and tan. Melanomas become bigger with time and often bleed when traumatized.

TREATMENT. Surgical removal of the lesion is highly successful when performed early. Other treatments, including chemotherapy or radiation therapy, may be used to treat cancer spread (metastasis).

CELLULITIS

Cellulitis is a widespread inflammation and bacterial infection that affects all layers of the skin and sometimes extends into deeper areas around muscles and organs. Types of cellulitis occur within the tissues around the eye, on the floor of the mouth, around the uterus, or on the arms or legs.

SIGNS AND SYMPTOMS. The affected tissue becomes swollen, red, hot to the touch, and painful.

TREATMENT. Antibiotics are given by mouth or intravenously; hospitalization may be required.

ICHTHYOSIS

Several types of ichthyosis exist: ichthyosis vulgaris, the most common type, is an autosomal dominant disorder; lamellar ichthyosis is an autosomal recessive disorder; and ichthyosis linearis circumflexa is an autosomal recessive disorder. X-linked ichthyosis (see page 238) occurs only in males and is manifested by large, thick brown scales on the skin.

SIGNS AND SYMPTOMS. All types of ichthyosis involve abnormalities of skin texture that result in dryness and scaliness. The severity varies with the type.

TREATMENT. Topical creams and lotions containing agents that reduce the thickness of the skin can be used. Agents that irritate the skin, such as harsh soaps, should be avoided.

IMPETIGO CONTAGIOSA

Impetigo is a bacterial infection of the skin most often seen in children. It sometimes develops in preexisting insect bites, areas of skin infected with poison ivy, or skin affected by eczema when the skin has been broken by scratching.

SIGNS AND SYMPTOMS. Impetigo lesions first appear as red spots; then small blisters form, break open, and scab over. Lesions usually appear on areas of skin that are exposed to the environment, such as the face, arms, legs, and scalp.

TREATMENT. Impetigo is treated with antibiotics and antiseptic skin cleansers.

NEUROFIBROMATOSIS

See page 101.

PSORIASIS VULGARIS

Psoriasis is a recurring, chronic condition involving the epidermis, the outside layer of skin. The most common type is psoriasis vulgaris. Psoriasis is typically seen in people 10 to 50 years of age and is more common among Whites than Blacks. The exact cause is unknown, but psoriasis does occur at higher incidences in some families. Environmental factors that aggravate psoriasis include infection, hormonal changes that occur during adolescence, and certain medications. Stress may also aggravate psoriasis.

Normally, cells of the epidermis die and are replaced with new cells in three to four weeks; with psoriasis the process takes three to four days. This overactivity of cell growth causes psoriatic lesions.

SIGNS AND SYMPTOMS. Psoriasis vulgaris lesions are distinct, round, irritated areas with silvery scales. They usually develop on the scalp, elbows, knees, chest, or back, but can occur anywhere on the skin. The lesions may or may not itch and can be aggravated by cold weather, illness, stress, and some medications.

Complications of psoriasis include infected lesions and exfoliative psoriasis, a condition in which the entire skin surface is covered with lesions. A few people have psoriatic arthritis, a potentially crippling form of arthritis associated with psoriasis vulgaris.

TREATMENT. No cure exists for psoriasis, but treatments can decrease the severity of the lesions. Such treatments, which are numerous and have varying degrees of success, include topical steroid skin ointments and tar preparations, and exposure to ultraviolet light in combination with creams or oral medications. In cases resistant to other treatments, low-dose oral (by mouth) chemotherapy may be used.

SCABIES

Scabies is the infestation of the skin by the scabies mite *Sarcoptes scabiei;* scabies is most often seen in children. When the female mite gets on the skin, she finds snug areas, such as between the fingers or toes, under the arms, or in the groin, where she burrows into the outer skin layer and lays her eggs.

SIGNS AND SYMPTOMS. Approximately 30 days or more after infestation, redness and intense itching begin at the sites where the mite(s) have burrowed into the skin.

TREATMENT. One treatment of medication that is applied to the skin usually kills the mite(s). Scabies is spread from person to person, so often the entire family must be treated.

TINEA INFECTIONS
Also called ringworm.

Tinea infections are fungal infections of the skin caused by a variety of fungal organisms. There are no worms involved in ringworm infections. Ringworm infections are most often seen in children and can occur along the groin, feet, hair, or other areas of the skin. The infection spreads outward in a circular pattern creating rings, often with normal tissue in the center. Types of ringworm infection are named according to the area of the body they infect. Following is a list of those types and their symptoms.

TINEA CORPORIS

Ringworm infection of the epidermis that causes scaly, inflamed, ring-like lesions.

TINEA PEDIS

Commonly known as athlete's foot infection.

This infection causes itching, burning, and small blisters and cracks in the skin between the toes and on the soles of the feet. It is not as easily spread from person to person as once believed. Wearing shoes that allow airflow to the feet and cotton socks can help prevent this infection, as can keeping feet clean and dry.

TINEA CRURIS

Commonly known as jock itch.

These lesions are similar to those seen in tinea corporis, but they occur in the groin area and/or scrotum, causing itching.

TINEA CAPITIS

This ringworm infection causes the hair to break off at the scalp, leaving a circular bald spot where lesions occur. The infection usually begins within the root of a hair shaft and extends about one inch in diameter to the surrounding area of scalp. Lesions are often scaly and/or scabbed. Hair usually returns after the lesions fade, generally within three months.

TREATMENT. Tinea infections are treated with antifungal medications taken by mouth and/or applied to the skin.

TUBEROUS SCLEROSIS

See page 104.

WARTS

Also known as verrucae.

Warts are raised, skin-colored bumps, callous-like in appearance, caused by a viral infection. One or many warts may occur at a time, usually located on the hands, fingers, or face, but they can occur anywhere. The different types of warts are named according to the area of the skin in which they are located.

PLANTAR WARTS

Occurring on the soles of the feet, these warts are just about the only type that causes pain and discomfort.

GENITAL WARTS

This type is a sexually transmitted disease (STD), which appears as soft, cauliflower-like growths along the anogenital tissues. Genital warts are caused by a virus that is easily spread from person to person through direct contact.

TREATMENT. Warts often disappear on their own, but they can also be removed with surgical, burning, or freezing techniques, as well as with topical agents that dissolve the warts by destroying the causative virus.

X-LINKED ICHTHYOSIS

The incidence is approximately 1 in 6,000 live male births and is an X-linked disorder. Ichthyosis causes thick, dry, rough, scaly skin. In 90% of the cases, X-linked ichthyosis is related to a deficiency of the enzyme steroid sulfatase.

SIGNS AND SYMPTOMS. Infants may be born with thick, brown, scaly skin; ichthyosis can also develop later in infancy. Scaling is typically noted on the neck, abdomen, back, extremities, and buttocks. Another common finding is clouding of the corneas.

TREATMENT. Topical agents (creams or lotions) that contain aspirin (ASA), lactic acid, urea, or propylene glycol are used to loosen the outermost layer of skin (epidermis) and thus reduce its thickness.

XERODERMA PIGMENTOSUM

The incidence is approximately 1 in 50,000 to 500,000 live births. People with xeroderma pigmentosum have a defect in the enzymes necessary for cellular repair from ultraviolet light or irradiation damage. It primarily affects the eyes and skin.

SIGNS AND SYMPTOMS. People with xeroderma pigmentosum are extremely sensitive to light, including sunlight. Exposure to the sun causes excessive freckling and skin lesions that worsen with further exposure. Cancers of the skin, including basal cell and squamous cell carcinomas and malignant melanomas, occur early in life. Opacities and/or tumors of the eye may also develop. Death may occur before age 20 because of associated cancer(s).

TREATMENT. There is no cure for xeroderma pigmentosum. Avoiding exposure to the sun and receiving regular health-care evaluations with cancer screenings may minimize complications.

SECTION 18
THE INTEGUMENTARY SYSTEM

18.1 Acne vulgaris: indicate age(s) that acne vulgaris occurred. Document treatment(s), if known.

18.2 Albinism: document the specific form of albinism, if known.

18.3 Atopic dermatitis: indicate age that symptoms occurred. Document treatment(s), if known.

18.4 Cancer of the skin: document whether the cancer was basal cell carcinoma, squamous cell carcinoma, or malignant melanoma. Document the location of the cancer. Indicate age(s) that the cancer(s) occurred. Document treatment(s), if known.

18.5 Cellulitis: document the location where the cellulitis occurred. Document age when it occurred and treatment(s), if known.

18.6 Ichthyosis: document the specific form of ichthyosis, if known.

18.7 Impetigo contagiosa: indicate age(s) the infection occurred. Document treatment(s), if known.

18.8 Psoriasis vulgaris: indicate age that symptoms began. Document treatment(s), if known.

18.9 Xeroderma pigmentosum: document treatments, if known.

18.10 Document any other diseases or disorders of the integumentary system that are or were present, the age at onset, and treatment(s), if known.

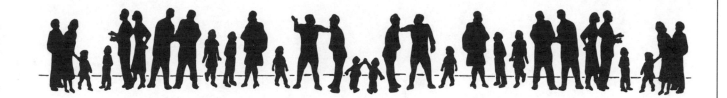

UNIT III
YOUR HEALTH PEDIGREE

This unit guides you in drawing your family pedigree and adding health information about yourself and your blood relatives. The resulting family health pedigree can be shared with your health-care provider to help him or her manage your health care in the best way possible.

As you record the health histories of family members, put a question mark in the appropriate box on the form if you think someone had a particular disease or disorder *but have no way to confirm this* (for example, if the person is deceased and you are unable to obtain health records). Also write a note on that person's form stating why you think he or she had that disease or disorder and the source of your information.

Having a family history of a disease does not always mean that you are at a higher risk for developing the same disease. Some diseases have various causes.

For example, some cases of hypothyroidism can be attributed to genetic causes, while other cases can be attributed to an environmental cause, such as the surgical removal of the thyroid gland. (Surgery is an environmental cause because it is an *external* event that results in the disease.) Still other cases of hypothyroidism are *idiopathic*, which means that the cause is unknown.

To *interpret* your health history, see your health-care provider. He or she can often infer from your complete family health history and pedigree whether or not a genetic component exists in the occurrence of specific diseases among family members. Without assistance from a health professional, there is a chance you may misinterpret your health pedigree, causing unnecessary worry or failure to receive appropriate preventive health care.

HOW TO CREATE YOUR HEALTH PEDIGREE

If you have been filling out your personal copy of the *GENETIC CONNECTIONS™ HEALTH HISTORY FORM* as you moved from one chapter to another in this book, you are ready to proceed in gathering the health histories of key members of your family and constructing your health pedigree.

This section takes you through one step at a time to help you:

1. Fill out the *LINEAR PEDIGREE WORKSHEET.*
2. Graph your pedigree.
3. Collect health information on blood relatives.
4. Transform your family pedigree into a family health pedigree.
5. Share your family health pedigree with your health-care providers.
6. Keep family medical files.
7. Keep yourself up to date on health issues.

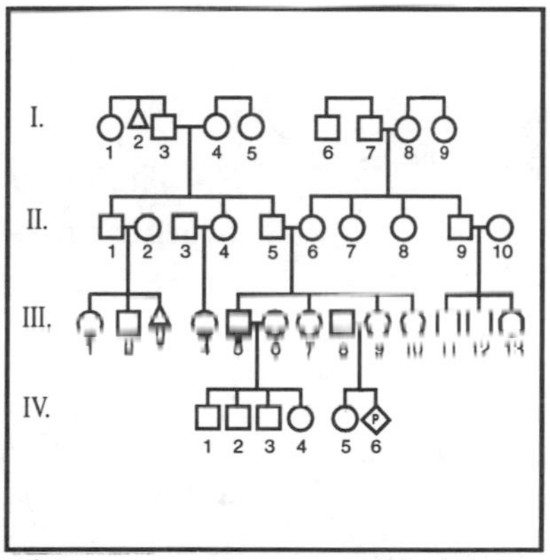

Figure A-1. Example of family pedigree. See also page 251

STEP 1: FILL OUT THE WORKSHEET

Remove the *LINEAR PEDIGREE WORKSHEET* from Appendix B. Fill in the names of all family members from your grandparents' generation to your own by carefully following directions **a** through **d** below.

Unlike genealogy pedigrees, which trace surnames from one generation to the next, a health pedigree is concerned with following gene-related illnesses. Therefore, it is sufficient to begin with your grandparents' generation and work forward to your own. Although you may include earlier, older generations, the earlier the generation, the fewer genes you have in common.

The most important thing is to begin somewhere, even if you limit your pedigree to just your own generation. The information you gather can be a valuable resource to pass on to your children and subsequent generations.

a. Begin at the top of Column I, which is located along the right side of the worksheet. List the full names of your **paternal grandfather's siblings**. Your paternal grandfather is your father's father; his siblings are your great aunts and great uncles. List them by birth order; that is, in the order in which they were born, beginning with the oldest.

It is important to include all pregnancy losses, such as miscarriages and terminations, as well as stillbirths and infant deaths. List the infant's name, if one was given. Also list the year the loss occurred, the type of loss, and the infant's sex, if known.

Notice that one box on the worksheet is specifically labeled so you can fill in the name of your **paternal grandfather**. Next is a box specifically labeled for the name of your **paternal grandmother** (your father's mother). Continue by listing your **paternal grandmother's siblings** according to birth order.

On the lower half of Column I, list the full names of your **maternal grandfather's siblings**, also according to birth order. These are the siblings of your mother's father.

Next list the names of your **maternal grandfather** and **maternal grandmother** (your mother's parents) in the boxes specifically labeled for them, and then list your **maternal grandmother's siblings** by birth order.

When you complete Column I, trace the marriage and descent lines that lead to Column II and double check that in each case the right partners are joined.

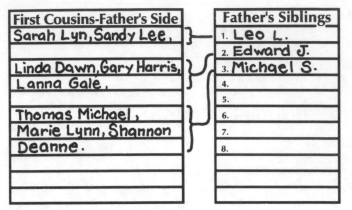

Figure A-2.

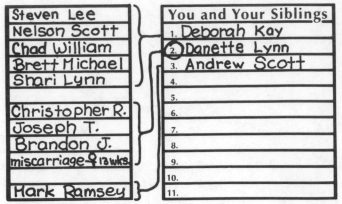

Figure A-3.

b. In Column II of the worksheet (to the left of Column I) list your father's siblings—your aunts and uncles on your father's side of the family, also known as your **paternal aunts and uncles**. List them by birth order. Remember to list all pregnancy losses, stillbirths, and infant deaths.

Put your father's name in the box specifically labeled for your **father**; put your mother's name in the box specifically labeled for your **mother.**

Then list your mother's siblings—your aunts and uncles on your mother's side of the family, also known as your **maternal aunts and uncles**. List them by birth order.

If you wish, you can list the names of the **spouses** of your aunts and uncles so they will be represented on your family pedigree, but you will not collect health history data about them because they are not your blood relatives. Simply write their names in the appropriate column next to the aunt or uncle to whom they are or were married.

When you have completed your list of family members in Column II, double check that your father and mother are listed in the appropriate boxes and are connected to the correct set of parents.

c. In Column III of the worksheet (to the left of Column II) list your **first cousins** on your **father's** side. Begin with the names of the children—in birth order—of the aunt or uncle who is listed first in Column II. List them from left to right.

Between Columns II and III, draw a bracket that connects the cousins who are siblings to their parents, as illustrated in **figure A-2**. Repeat the process for the rest of your paternal aunts and uncles listed in Column II.

Next, write **your** name and those of **your siblings** —by birth order—in the box that is joined to your parents. Notice that this box is located between the listing of your paternal and maternal cousins.

The spouses of your sisters and brothers (i.e., your **brothers-in-law and sisters-in-law**) can be listed on the right half of your sibling box, although you will not collect health data on them because they are not blood relatives. If you are married list the name of **your spouse** beside your name. Highlight your name and that of your spouse, if applicable, with a check mark, asterisk, or marking pen, as this is *your* linear pedigree.

Then list your **first cousins** on your **mother's** side of the family to complete Column III. Bracket siblings (also as illustrated in figure A-2) and connect them to their parents as you did for your paternal first cousins.

d. If you or any of your siblings have children, list their names in Column IV. Group **your children** and **your nieces and nephews** by family. Begin by listing the children of your oldest sibling according to birth order; bracket them and adjoin them to their parents. See **figure A-3**.

Again, include all pregnancy losses, stillbirths, and infant deaths.

STEP 2: GRAPH THE PEDIGREE

With your *LINEAR PEDIGREE WORKSHEET* completed, you are ready to graph the frame of your family pedigree. Tools you will need include paper, template (included with this book), lead pencil (preferably mechanical), and a soft pencil eraser.

As you are guided through the following process, study the sample illustrations to clarify each step. Your first pedigree will be practice; use a sheet of your own lined or graph paper, or one of the 11" x 17" sheets of graph paper provided in the back of this book. Starting with a practice sheet allows you to get a feel for what you are doing, and helps you determine the spacing that is needed so you can fit your entire pedigree on a single sheet of paper.

ABOUT PEDIGREES

Although the pedigree you are in the process of constructing will show some genealogical data, its main purpose is to illustrate medical and health data, which is why it is referred to as a *health* pedigree. A pedigree can show complex family structure, including offspring by adoption and offspring conceived using special fertility procedures such as artificial insemination with donor sperm and/or donor ovum and surrogate mothership.

Symbols are used to designate specific information on pedigrees. **Figure A-4** shows a symbol key. Study it to become familiar with those symbols that apply to your family. Some general rules pertain to pedigree graphing. For example:

- Males are designated by squares and are usually graphed on the left side when couples are represented; females are represented by circles.

- The paternal, or father's side of the family, is represented on the left side of a pedigree.

- Marriages are designated by a marriage line that runs horizontally from one spouse to the other.

- Divorce or separation is designated by a break in the marriage line.

- Children of the same parents are grouped by a sibling line and are connected to their parents by a vertical descendant (or descent) line.

- Individuals of the same generation are graphed along the same generation line.

Historically, pedigree symbols have not been standardized; two health professionals might use different symbols to mean the same thing. This increases the possibility of misinterpretation of the pedigree by other health professionals. Recognizing this as a major problem, the National Society of Genetic Counselors (NSGC) formed a Pedigree Standardization Task Force to officially research the problem and establish recommendations for standardization. Figure A-4

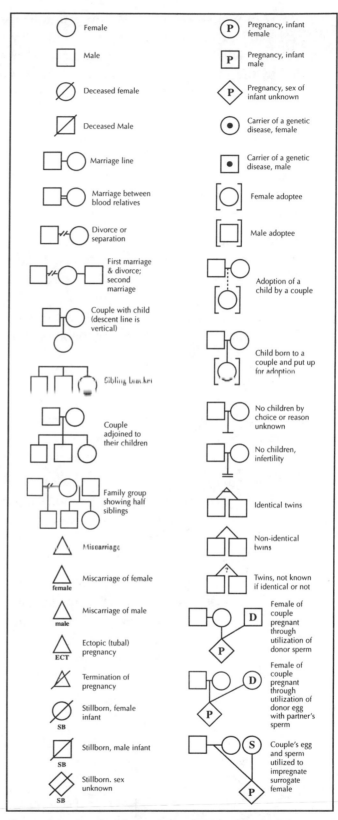

Figure A-4. Symbol key adapted from the NSGC Pedigree Standardization Task Force: "Recommendations for Standardized Human Pedigree Nomenclature," R. L. Bennett, et al., *American Journal of Human Genetics*, 56:3 (March 1995), University of Chicago Press (used with permission)

displays a sample of those symbols chosen by the Task Force for standardizing human pedigree graphing. This is not a complete representation of symbols recommended by the Task Force, but it does include those that most families need to complete their health pedigrees.

If you do not find all the symbols you need for your family health pedigree, you may request a copy from your local library of "Recommendations for Standardized Human Pedigree Nomenclature," *American Journal of Human Genetics* (March 1995).

a. Begin to graph your pedigree by counting the generations you are including so you can get an idea of how "tall" your pedigree has to be. For example, if your worksheet includes your grandparents, your parents, and your children, nieces, and nephews—in addition to yourself—you need four generation lines on your pedigree.

Generation lines run horizontally across the paper and are labeled with roman numerals. **Generation I** is the earliest or oldest generation that you are including, so it is placed at the top of the pedigree. Each subsequent generation is numbered in sequence.

You may want to turn your paper so it is wider than it is long. In pencil, number the generation lines along the left edge, allowing ample space between generations. All members of the same generation are drawn along the same generation line. See **figure A-5**.

b. Look at the *LINEAR PEDIGREE WORKSHEET* you just completed to see which generation is the largest—and therefore needs the most room on your paper. Divide your graph paper so that you can represent everyone in the largest generation side by side along

the appropriate generation line. You will use the template provided in this book to help you lightly draw, in pencil, the appropriate symbols from figure A-4 that represent each individual in that largest generation.

Beginning with the largest generation, assign the leftmost position on your paper to the first name listed for that generation on your *LINEAR PEDIGREE WORKSHEET*. The names will thereby remain in birth order. Continue representing each person as you move down the list of names, working from left to right on the graph paper.

Note: When graphing couples, remember to keep males on the left side and females on the right. For example, when graphing a maternal aunt and her husband, draw his symbol first and then your aunt's, even though her name is listed first on the *LINEAR PEDIGREE WORKSHEET* and his name is listed second in the "spouse" column.

Allow ample space between symbols. Important health information will later be documented below each person. See **figure A-6**.

If you did not finish graphing your own generation, do so now in the same manner as just described in the preceding paragraphs. You (and your spouse) and your siblings should be positioned between your first cousins on your father's side (to the left) and your first cousins on your mother's side (to the right).

Bracket siblings together with sibling lines and connect the representation of each sibling to that line. Draw marriage lines between spouses as needed without connecting the spouses of siblings to the sibling bracket. See **figure A-7**.

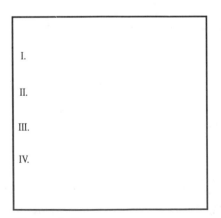

Figure A-5.

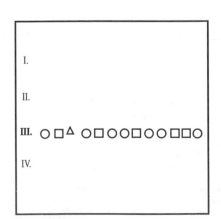

Figure A-6.

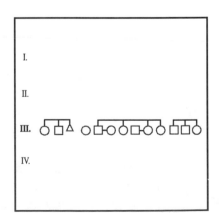

Figure A- 7.

c. Above your own generation is the line for **your parents' generation**. Working from left to right, graph the individuals of this generation as they are listed in Column II of your *LINEAR PEDIGREE WORKSHEET.*

Try to center your aunts and uncles above the symbols for their children (your first cousins), and your parents above the symbols for you and your siblings. Centering parents above their children will help keep your pedigree properly aligned and easier to interpret.

Bracket your parents' siblings with sibling lines and connect each sibling to that line. Draw marriage lines between spouses, as needed. Finally, connect all sibling groups in your generation to their parents with descent lines. See **figure A-8**.

d. Above your parents, graph your grandparents' generation line. Again allow ample spacing between generation lines. On the left half of your paper, graph from left to right a representation of your **paternal grandfather** and his siblings, then your **paternal grandmother** and her siblings, keeping the same order as on Column I of your worksheet.

Again bracket siblings with sibling lines, connecting the representation of each sibling to that line. Draw a marriage line between your paternal grandparents, making sure this grouping is drawn on your father's side of the pedigree—the left.

On the right side of your paper, draw from left to right your **maternal grandfather** and his siblings, then your **maternal grandmother** and her siblings, keeping the same order as listed in Column I of your worksheet.

Bracket siblings, draw a marriage line between your maternal grandparents, and make sure these groupings are drawn on your mother's side of the pedigree at the right of your paper.

Use descent lines to connect your mother's and father's sibling groups to their parents. See **figure A-9**.

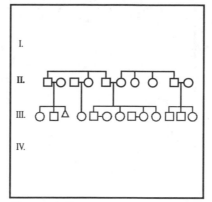

Figure A-8.

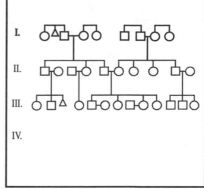

Figure A-9.

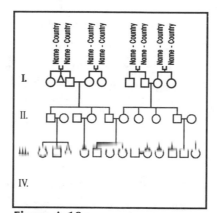

Figure A-10.

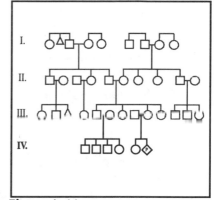

Figure A-11.

Note: If you wish to write in the names of your **great grandparents** (your grandparent's parents) and their countries of origin, follow the example demonstrated in **figure A-10**. You will not, however, be instructed to collect health history data on them.

e. If you have **children** and **nieces and nephews**, use the bottom or youngest generation line to add them, working from left to right as they are listed in Column IV of your worksheet.

Bracket siblings together with sibling lines and connect each sibling to the line. Connect sibling groups to their parents with descent lines.

In case you do not have adequate space to graph members of this generation directly under their corresponding parents, you can draw diagonal descent lines. See **figure A-11**.

f. If you are married, your **spouse** should complete a **HEALTH HISTORY FORM**, fill out a separate copy of the **LINEAR PEDIGREE WORKSHEET**, and follow steps 1 and 2 to create his or her own family pedigree.

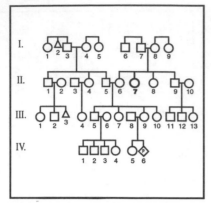

Figure A-12.

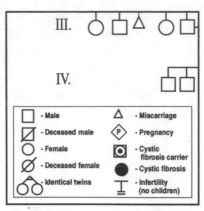

Figure A-13.

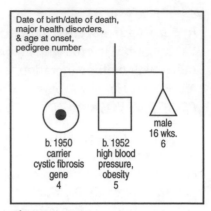

Figure A-14.

Your children are represented on the separate pedigrees that you and your spouse each construct.

g. Once you have completed your practice pedigree, trace it onto a clean sheet of graph paper, making whatever minor adjustments in spacing are needed to better align your pedigree.

When your pedigree is redrawn, make sure roman numerals are assigned to each generation line. Then assign arabic numerals (1, 2, 3, etc.) to each individual along each generation line, working from left to right. This gives each person a two-part pedigree number by which you can identify him or her. For example, the individual highlighted in **figure A-12** has the pedigree number II-7. Later you will write each person's pedigree number in the top right-hand corner of his or her individual *HEALTH HISTORY FORM*.

In a lower corner of your pedigree, create a key or legend identifying the symbols you used in constructing your pedigree, as illustrated in **figure A-13**. This will ensure the correct interpretation of your pedigree by health-care professionals.

STEP 3: COLLECT HEALTH INFORMATION ON BLOOD RELATIVES

For all blood relatives that you listed on your *LINEAR PEDIGREE WORKSHEET*, complete a *GENETIC CONNECTIONS™ HEALTH HISTORY FORM*. It may be easiest to start with the members of your immediate family and then branch out to more distant relatives. For those family members whose health care you participate in or are in charge of, such as your spouse, children, and parents, complete as much of the health history data as possible. For them, the *HEALTH HISTORY FORM* should be used as an ongoing health record for your personal health files.

For more distant relatives (those outside your immediate family unit), your priority is to document the occurrence of disorders known to run in your family, as well as major chronic illnesses such as heart disease and cancer, disorders that could be genetic in cause, and the other illnesses and events, such as accidents, that have had a major effect on their lives or their health status.

You may wish to gather this health information yourself, or to send each relative a copy of the *GENETIC CONNECTIONS™ HEALTH HISTORY FORM* to complete and return to you. This may be somewhat difficult for others to do, however, if they do not recognize the medical terms used on the form and do not have access to this book for reference.

The most pertinent information to collect on blood relatives is indicated on the *HEALTH HISTORY FORM* with asterisks. You need not collect answers to questions not marked with an asterisk.

Individual family members are the most accurate source for their own health histories. Nevertheless, some family members may refuse to disclose health information to you, and that is their prerogative. Often, if you explain why you are collecting the data and its importance to your health and your children's, cooperation may be gained. Assure the hesitant family member that the information is to be shared only with your health-care providers and immediate (adult) family members, and that it will be kept confidential.

To understand why the confidentiality of health information is so important, you may find it helpful to reread the article in Unit I written by genetic ethicist Carol Isaacson Barash, Ph.D. The article begins on page 6.

If a blood relative is deceased, obtain what information you can from living relatives who were closest to that person. Always document the source of information if it does not come from the individuals themselves. For deceased relatives, it may be necessary to gather information from more than one source. Death certificates may state the cause of death (although some states delete this information to protect the privacy of the deceased and their living relatives). But death certificates usually do not give much information about the health status of the deceased. For example, a death certificate that lists congestive heart failure as the cause of death may not tell you about the underlying health disorder that caused the congestive heart failure.

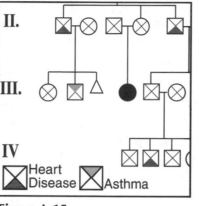

Figure A-15.

Copies of death certificates can be obtained from the Bureau of Vital Statistics in the capital city of the state in which the death occurred. See Appendix E for a description of other potential sources of health information on deceased family members.

STEP 4: TRANSFORM YOUR FAMILY PEDIGREE INTO A FAMILY HEALTH PEDIGREE

As the **HEALTH HISTORY FORM** for each member of your family is completed, you can begin transferring pertinent data onto the family pedigree. This transforms it into a *family health pedigree*. Date of birth, date or age and cause of death, genetic diseases, major chronic illnesses, age at onset of a disease—all this information should be documented, whenever applicable. Note the placement of such data and the placement of pedigree numbers in **figure A-14**.

Because abbreviations for medical disorders save space, use them. But it is important to use standard, medically accepted abbreviations when listing health disorders and diseases. You can use the abbreviations that are used in this book, or clearly print the entire name of the illness or disorder. Add to the pedigree key the abbreviations you are using.

Some people use color on their pedigrees to designate specific diseases that appear repeatedly within families. Color can be powerful in calling attention to diseases and disorders that appear repeatedly on your family health pedigree, but color is not essential for creating a good health pedigree.

One effective way of using color is to lightly mark an X on each circle and square on your pedigree, dividing each into four quadrants or uniform pie slices. Indicate a specific disease by using a unique color within one quadrant—selecting the same quadrant for each family member in whom that disease has occurred. For example, you may choose to show heart disease with the color red within the upper right quadrant. If you use color, be sure to draw a color key or legend on your pedigree chart below the symbol key that designates what disease each color represents to avoid misinterpretation by health care professionals. See **figure A-15**.

STEP 5: SHARE YOUR FAMILY HEALTH PEDIGREE WITH YOUR HEALTH-CARE PROVIDERS

The basic purpose of compiling your family health history and pedigree is to share the information with your health-care provider. This will give him or her more information about your health strengths and risks than could possibly be derived from medical testing. With the information contained in your family health pedigree, your health-care provider can construct a plan of care that specifically meets your needs. This may mean that you will be advised to change some of your eating habits, lose weight, exercise regularly, see your health-care provider every six months instead of once a year, begin screenings earlier, and perhaps see a specialist for certain health disorders you are at risk of developing. Your family health pedigree will assist your health-care provider in practicing preventive medicine, which can help delay, lessen the severity of, or prevent a disease to which you are genetically predisposed.

For example, let's say you have a strong family history of early heart disease. Knowing this, your health-care provider can instruct you on preventive measures, such as the importance of limiting fat in your diet, maintaining a healthy body weight, participating in aerobic exercise routinely, and avoiding tobacco use. Your health-care provider might also begin to monitor you for beginning signs and symptoms of heart disease and test you earlier and more frequently than someone who has no family history of heart disease. Your health-care provider might even prescribe medications. Such preventive measures might actually help you escape the heart attack you perhaps were genetically destined to have.

If you do not have a health-care provider, get one. These professionals are your link to optimal health. If you are not comfortable with the health-care provider you have, seek a new one. If you ever have doubts about a response your health-care provider gives you, seek a second opinion, or a third. Remember, you are the consumer, and the product you are buying is health care.

STEP 6: KEEP FAMILY MEDICAL FILES

In completing steps 1 through 5 described so far, you have already begun step 6—keeping accurate, current health files for yourself and your immediate family. Your family's health history forms are records that should be handled with as much care as tax, insurance, and automobile records.

If you or a member of your immediate family— such as a child—needs to see a doctor or receive emergency medical care, the health form can be taken along so that accurate health history information can be relayed to attending doctors and nurses. This helps ensure that prompt, safe, and effective care is received.

It is important to keep your compiled health records and family health pedigree updated as births, deaths, and illnesses or other health-related events occur. You may want to store other important documents in your health files, such as copies of personal medical records, medical test reports, physical examination reports, hospital admission and discharge summary records, birth certificates, copies of dental records, fingerprint cards of your children, death certificates, family photographs, and so on.

Be sure to label the family photographs that you include in your health files with the date and the subject's name and corresponding pedigree number. Having a photograph of each family member can sometimes be helpful because photographs can reveal interesting or prevalent familial traits that were not brought out on the health history forms.

Safeguard your health records. One of the most important legacies you can pass on to your children is a copy of your compiled family health history and pedigree. Plastic sheet protectors work well to prevent pencil smearing and to protect the health forms and pedigrees and other health records from air and moisture damage.

See the order blank at the back of this book for ordering custom storage units for your health records.

You may consider storing copies of your health files in a location other than your home—for example, in a safe-deposit box—in case your personal files at home are destroyed.

STEP 7: KEEP YOURSELF UP TO DATE ON HEALTH ISSUES

By using this book you have taken a giant step toward becoming an educated participant in your good health. But this is only a start. It is up to you to continue learning about health and disease and your personal risks.

There are many ways to keep up to date on health issues and concerns. You can gather information from local and national health and resource organizations, public health departments, local and national newspapers and magazines—and from your health-care providers.

Almost every day you can read or hear about new health discoveries and events. You can learn a great deal by simply paying attention to the world around you.

See Appendix F for a partial listing of health and support organizations that provide information.

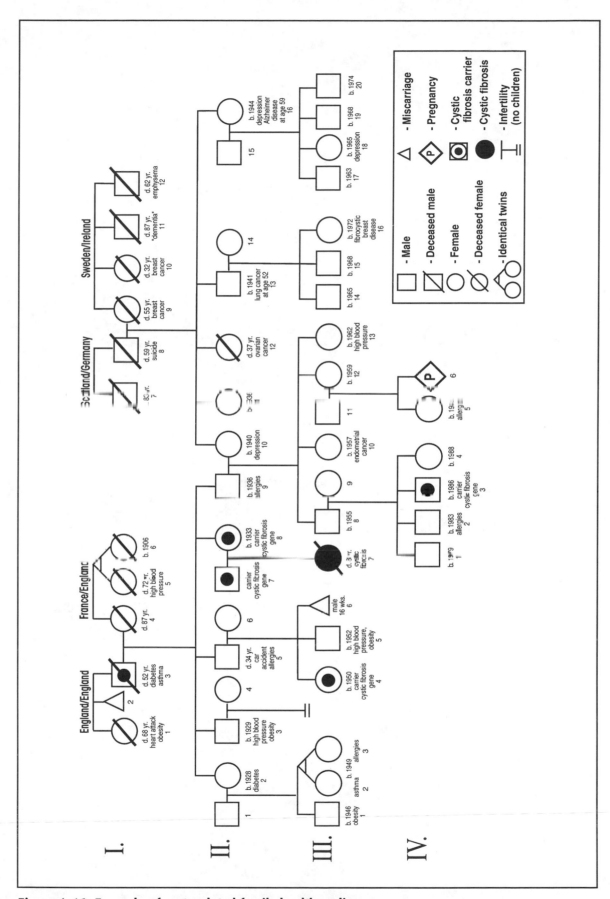

Figure A-16. Example of a completed family health pedigree

GENETIC CONNECTIONS™
Health History Form

Pedigree No. _____

Section 1 - Genetic Inheritance

*1.1 Name: _____ Maiden: _____
  (first)   (middle)   (confirmation)   (last)
☐A; ☐DS; ☐DO

*1.2 Mother's name: _____ Father's name: _____

  Biologic parents (if different than listed above): _____

*1.3 Date of birth: _____ ; Place of birth: _____

*1.4 Immigration: To: _____ ; Date: _____ ; Mode of transportation: _____

*1.5 Name of spouse: _____ ; Marriage date: _____ ; County, state: _____

  Date widowed: _____ ; Date of divorce: _____

  Children: 1. _____ ; ☐AI; ☐AO;☐DS; ☐DO   5. _____ ☐AI; ☐AO;☐DS; ☐DO

  2. _____ ; ☐AI; ☐AO;☐DS; ☐DO   6. _____ ☐AI; ☐AO;☐DS; ☐DO

  3. _____ ; ☐AI; ☐AO;☐DS; ☐DO   7. _____ ☐AI; ☐AO;☐DS; ☐DO

  4. _____ ; ☐AI; ☐AO;☐DS; ☐DO   8. _____ ☐AI; ☐AO;☐DS; ☐DO

  Previous spouse: _____ ; Marriage date: _____ ; County, state: _____

  Date widowed: _____ ; Date of divorce: _____

  Children: 1. _____ ; ☐AI; ☐AO;☐DS; ☐DO   5. _____ ☐AI; ☐AO;☐DS; ☐DO

  2. _____ ; ☐AI; ☐AO;☐DS; ☐DO   6. _____ ☐AI; ☐AO;☐DS; ☐DO

  3. _____ ; ☐AI; ☐AO;☐DS; ☐DO   7. _____ ☐AI; ☐AO;☐DS; ☐DO

  4. _____ ; ☐AI; ☐AO;☐DS; ☐DO   8. _____ ☐AI; ☐AO;☐DS; ☐DO

  Previous spouse: _____ ; Marriage date: _____ ; County, state: _____

  Date widowed: _____ ; Date of divorce: _____

  Children: 1. _____ ; ☐AI; ☐AO;☐DS; ☐DO   5. _____ ☐AI; ☐AO;☐DS; ☐DO

  2. _____ ; ☐AI; ☐AO;☐DS; ☐DO   6. _____ ☐AI; ☐AO;☐DS; ☐DO

  3. _____ ; ☐AI; ☐AO;☐DS; ☐DO   7. _____ ☐AI; ☐AO;☐DS; ☐DO

  4. _____ ; ☐AI; ☐AO;☐DS; ☐DO   8. _____ ☐AI; ☐AO;☐DS; ☐DO

*1.6 Places of residence: _____ ; From: _____ ; To: _____
  (address)   (city/state)   (county)

  _____ ; From: _____ ; To: _____

  _____ ; From: _____ ; To: _____

  _____ ; From: _____ ; To: _____

*1.7 Education history: _____

  _____

  _____

*1.8 Occupation/trade history: _____ ; From: _____ ; To: _____ ; Hazards: _____

  _____ ; From: _____ ; To: _____ ; Hazards: _____
  (include health hazards
  exposed to)   _____ ; From: _____ ; To: _____ ; Hazards: _____

  _____ ; From: _____ ; To: _____ ; Hazards: _____

*1.9 Military service: Station: _____ ; Dates: _____ ; Branch of Service _____

  Station: _____ ; Dates: _____ ; Branch of Service _____

  Station: _____ ; Dates: _____ ; Branch of Service _____

*1.10 Political and religious affiliations: _____

*1.11 Special/unique achievements: _____

  _____

*1.12 Avocations/hobbies: _____

*1.13 Date of death: _____ ; Place of death: _____ ; Age: _____ ; Cause: _____

FORM NO.0795-1 © SONTERS PUBLISHING, INC.

Section 2 - Prenatal History

2.1 Prenatal exposure to chemical substances:

☐ Prescription medication: Drug name: _____ ; ☐ 1st trimester; ☐ 2nd trimester; ☐ 3rd trimester

☐ Tobacco; If cigarettes, number of packs per day mother smoked: _____ ; ☐ 1st trimester; ☐ 2nd trimester; ☐ 3rd trimester

☐ Alcohol; Describe mother's use as ☐ seldom; ☐ occasional; ☐ daily ☐ 1st trimester; ☐ 2nd trimester; ☐ 3rd trimester

☐ Illicit drug use; type(s): _____ ; ☐ 1st trimester; ☐ 2nd trimester; ☐ 3rd trimester

2.2 Prenatal exposure to infections:

Type: _____ ; ☐ 1st trimester; ☐ 2nd trimester; ☐ 3rd trimester

Type: _____ ; ☐ 1st trimester; ☐ 2nd trimester; ☐ 3rd trimester

2.3 Maternal medical conditions/complications:

☐ Chronic hypertension; ☐ PIH; ☐ Diabetes mellitus; ☐ Gestational diabetes; ☐ Rh incompatibility; ☐ Other: _____

2.4 Maternal bleeding complications:

☐ Threatened miscarriage; ☐ Incompetent cervix; ☐ Placenta previa; ☐ Abruptio placentae; ☐ Other: _____

2.5 Maternal premature rupture of membranes: ☐ Yes; ☐ No

2.6 Other complications of labor and/or delivery: _____

_____

_____

Section 3 - Birth History

3.1 Birth: ☐ Vaginal; ☐ Cesarean section

*3.2 ☐ Term infant; ☐ Preterm infant; ☐ Post-term infant; Approximate gestational age: _____

3.3 Birth weight: _____ ; 3.4 Birth length _____

3.5 Blood type: ☐ A; ☐ B; ☐ AB; ☐ O; Rh: ☐ Positive; ☐ Negative

3.6 Blood transfusion history:

Date: _____ ; ☐ Whole blood; ☐ Fresh frozen plasma; ☐ Platelets; ☐ Clotting agent; ☐ Other: _____

Date: _____ ; ☐ Whole blood; ☐ Fresh frozen plasma; ☐ Platelets; ☐ Clotting agent; ☐ Other: _____

Date: _____ ; ☐ Whole blood; ☐ Fresh frozen plasma; ☐ Platelets; ☐ Clotting agent; ☐ Other: _____

Date: _____ ; ☐ Whole blood; ☐ Fresh frozen plasma; ☐ Platelets; ☐ Clotting agent; ☐ Other: _____

*3.7 Chromosome abnormality: ☐ Cri du chat; ☐ Down syndrome; ☐ Edwards syndrome; ☐ Patau syndrome; ☐ Fragile X syndrome;

☐ Klinefelter syndrome; ☐ Turner syndrome; ☐ Other: _____

*3.8 Complications after birth:

☐ Apnea; ☐ Hyaline membrane disease; ☐ Bronchopulmonary dysplasia; ☐ Meconium aspiration syndrome; ☐ Retinopathy of prematurity;

☐ Necrotizing enterocolitis; ☐ Jaundice; ☐ Infection/sepsis; ☐ Other: _____

_____

_____

Section 4 - Physical Attributes

*4.1 Maximum adult height: _____ ; *4.2 Average adult weight: _____

*4.3 Skin tone: ☐ Fair; ☐ Medium; ☐ Dark; ☐ Other: _____

*4.4 Eye color: ☐ Blue; ☐ Brown; ☐ Gray; ☐ Green; ☐ Hazel; ☐ Other: _____

*4.5 Hair color: ☐ Blond; ☐ Brunette; ☐ Auburn; ☐ Red; ☐ Black; ☐ Other: _____ ; Approximate age graying began: _____

*4.6 Hair loss ("balding") began at age: _____

Other: _____

_____

Section 5 - Health Practices

*5.1 Healthy eating pratices followed: ☐ Yes; ☐ No; Special diets: _____

5.2 Dates and results of blood cholesterol screenings: _____

_____

*5.3 Participate in regular exercise: ☐ Yes; ☐ No

*5.4 Alcohol use: ☐ Occasional; ☐ Frequent; ☐ Daily; ☐ Other: _____ ; Age use began: ____ ; Age when use ended (if applicable): ____

*5.5 Tobacco use: ☐ Cigarettes – packs smoked per day ____ ; ☐ Chewing tobacco; ☐ Snuff; Age when use began: _____

Age when use ended (if applicable): _____

Health Practices continued

*5.6   Hours per day of second-hand smoke exposure: _____ ; Years of exposure: _____

*5.7   Substance abuse/chemical dependence: ☐ Yes; ☐ No;   Specific substance: _____
       Age chemical use began: _____ ; Age use ended: _____

*5.8   Sleep disorders: ☐ Insomnia; ☐ Narcolepsy; ☐ Sleep apnea syndrome; ☐ Sleep walking (adult); ☐ Sleep-eating; ☐ Other: _____

*5.9   Accident history: _____
       _____
       Resulting mental/physical limitations: _____

*5.10 Childhood communicable disease history:

	Age	Immunization	Resulting physical/mental limitations
☐ Chickenpox	_____	_____	_____
☐ Diphtheria	_____	_____	_____
☐ Haemophilus influenza type B	_____	_____	_____
☐ Hepatitis A	_____	_____	_____
☐ Hepatitis B	_____	_____	_____
☐ Measles	_____	_____	_____
☐ Mumps	_____	_____	_____
☐ Pertussis	_____	_____	_____
☐ Poliomyelitis	_____	_____	_____
☐ Rubella	_____	_____	_____
☐ Tetanus	_____	_____	_____
☐ Other: _____	_____	_____	

*5.11 Receive routine medical examinations: ☐ Yes; ☐ No; Name, address and phone number of primary care physician: _____
       _____

*5.12 Receive routine dental care: ☐ Yes; ☐ No; ☐ Periodontal disease; ☐ Dentures; ☐ Partial plates; ☐ Bridges; ☐ Dental implants
       ☐ Other: _____

*5.13 Allergies: _____
       _____

*5.14 Learning disability: _____

*5.15 Surgical history: _____
       _____
       _____
       _____
       _____

*5.16 General anesthesia complications: ☐ Psuedocholinesterase deficiency; ☐ Malignant hyperthermia; ☐ Other: _____

5.17   Medications : _____
       _____
       _____
       _____

Section 6 - The Eyes and Ears

EYES:

*6.1   ☐ Cataracts: ☐ Right eye; ☐ Left eye; Documentation: _____
       ☐ Intraocular lens implant: ☐ Right eye; ☐ Left eye

6.2   ☐ Conjunctivitis: ☐ Right eye; ☐ Left eye; Documentation: _____

*6.3   ☐ Glaucoma: ☐ Right eye; ☐ Left eye; ☐ Documentation: _____

*6.4   ☐ Loss of sight : ☐ Right eye; ☐ Left eye; ☐ Documentation: _____

*6.5   ☐ Refractive errors: ☐ Hyperopia; ☐ Myopia; ☐ Astigmatism; Documentation: _____

*6.6   ☐ Retinal detachment: ☐ Right eye; ☐ Left eye; Documentation: _____

*6.7   ☐ Retinal degenerative disorder: ☐ Right eye; ☐ Left eye; Documentation: _____

*6.8   ☐ Retinoblastoma: ☐ Right eye; ☐ Left eye; Documentation: _____

*6.9   ☐ Strabismus : ☐ Right eye; ☐ Left eye; Documentation: _____
       ☐ Other eye disorders: _____
       _____
       _____

FORM NO.0795-1 © SONTERS PUBLISHING, INC.

The Eyes and Ears continued

EARS:

*6.10 ☐ Hearing loss : ☐ Right ear; ☐ Left ear; Documentation: _____

*6.11 ☐ Meniere disease: ☐ Right ear; ☐ Left ear; Documentation: _____

 6.12 ☐ Otitis media: ☐ Right ear; ☐ Left ear; Documentation: _____

*6.13 ☐ Otosclerosis : ☐ Right ear; ☐ Left ear; Documentation: _____

*6.14 ☐ Other ear disorders: _____
_____
_____

Section 7 - Nervous System

*7.1 ☐ Encephalocele; Documentation: _____

*7.2 ☐ Spina bifida occulta; ☐ Spina bifida cystica; Type: _____ ; Documentation: _____
_____

*7.3 ☐ Other nervous system structural defects: _____
_____

*7.4 ☐ Alzheimer disease; Documentation: _____

*7.5 ☐ Amyotrophic lateral sclerosis; Documentation: _____

*7.6 ☐ Cerebral palsy; Type :_____ ; Documentation: _____

*7.7 ☐ Encephalitis; Type :_____ ; Documentation: _____

*7.8 ☐ Epilepsy; Type :_____ ; Documentation: _____

*7.9 ☐ Familial dysautonomia; Documentation: _____

*7.10 ☐ Febrile seizures; Documentation: _____

*7.11 ☐ Galactosemia; Documentation: _____

*7.12 ☐ Guillain-Barré syndrome; Documentation: _____

*7.13 ☐ Huntington disease; Documentation: _____

*7.14 ☐ Hydrocephalus; Documentation: _____

*7.15 ☐ Infantile autism; Documentation: _____

*7.16 ☐ Meningitis; Type :_____ ; Documentation: _____

*7.17 ☐ Menkes syndrome; Documentation: _____

*7.18 ☐ Migraine headaches; Documentation: _____

*7.19 ☐ Multiple sclerosis; Documentation: _____

*7.20 ☐ Myasthenia gravis; Documentation: _____

*7.21 ☐ Neurofibromatosis; ☐ Type 1; ☐ Other: _____
Documentation: _____

*7.22 ☐ Parkinson disease; Documentation: _____

*7.23 ☐ Phenylketonuria; Documentation: _____

 7.24 ☐ Rabies; Treatment: ☐ Yes; ☐ No

*7.25 ☐ Reye syndrome; Documentation: _____

*7.26 ☐ Tay-Sachs disease; Documentation: _____

*7.27 ☐ Tourette syndrome; Documentation: _____

*7.28 ☐ Tuberous sclerosis; Documentation: _____

*7.29 ☐ Tumor of the brain; ☐ Tumor of the spinal cord; Documentation: _____
_____

*7.30 ☐ Other nervous system disorders: _____
_____
_____

Section 8 - Mental Illness

*8.1 ☐ Anxiety disorder; Type:_____ ; Documentation: _____

*8.2 ☐ Eating disorder; Type:_____ ; Documentation: _____
_____

Section 8 - Mental Illness continued

*8.3 ☐ Mood disorder; Type: _____ ; Documentation: _____
_____

*8.4 ☐ Schizophrenia; Type: _____ ; Documentation: _____
_____

*8.5 ☐ Other mental illnesses: _____
_____
_____

Section 9 - The Cardiovascular System

*9.1 ☐ Congenital heart defects; Type: _____ ; Documentation: _____
_____

*9.2 ☐ Other cardiovascular system structural defects: _____
_____

*9.3 ☐ Aneurysm; Documentation: _____

*9.4 ☐ Atherosclerosis; Documentation: _____

*9.5 ☐ Cerebral vascular accident; Documentation: _____

*9.6 ☐ Congestive heart failure; Documentation: _____

*9.7 ☐ Coronary artery disease; Documentation: _____

*9.8 ☐ Abnormal heart rate; Documentation: _____

*9.9 ☐ Endocarditis; Documentation: _____

*9.10 ☐ Familial hypercholesterolemia; Type: _____ ; Documentation: _____

*9.11 ☐ High blood pressure; Documentation: _____

*9.12 ☐ Marfan syndrome; Documentation: _____

*9.13 ☐ Myocardial infarction; Documentation: _____

*9.14 ☐ Myocarditis; Documentation: _____

*9.15 ☐ Pericarditis; Documentation: _____

*9.16 ☐ Peripheral vascular disease; Documentation: _____

*9.17 ☐ Rheumatic heart disease; Documentation: _____

*9.18 ☐ Other heart valve disorders; Documentation: _____

*9.19 ☐ Other cardiovascular system disorders: _____
_____
_____

Section 10 - The Respiratory System

*10.1 ☐ Choanal atresia; Documentation: _____

*10.2 ☐ Other respiratory system structural defects: _____
_____

10.3 ☐ Acute bronchitis; Documentation: _____

*10.4 ☐ Asthma; Documentation: _____

10.5 ☐ Bronchiolitis; Documentation: _____

*10.6 ☐ Cancer of the throat/vocal cords; Documentation: _____
_____

*10.7 ☐ Cancer of the lungs; Documentation: _____
_____

*10.8 ☐ Chronic obstructive pulmonary disease; Documentation: _____
_____

10.9 ☐ Croup; Documentation: _____

*10.10 ☐ Cystic fibrosis; Documentation: _____

*10.11 ☐ Emphysema; Documentation: _____

FORM NO.0795-1 © SONTERS PUBLISHING, INC.

The Respiratory System continued

10.12 ☐ Epiglottitis; Documentation: _____

10.13 ☐ Pharyngitis; Documentation: _____

10.14 ☐ Pleurisy; Documentation: _____

*10.15 ☐ Lung disease – pneumoconiosis; Type: _____ ; Documentation: _____

_____

10.16 ☐ Pneumonia; Documentation: _____

10.17 ☐ Tonsillitis; Documentation: _____

10.18 Dates and results of tuberculosis skin testing: _____

   * ☐ Tuberculosis infection; Documentation: _____

*10.19 ☐ Other respiratory system disorders: _____

_____

_____

Section 11- The Gastrointestinal System

*11.1   ☐ Cleft lip; ☐ Cleft palate; Documentation: _____

*11.2   ☐ Diaphragmatic hernia; Documentation: _____

*11.3   ☐ Esophageal atresia; ☐ Tracheoesophageal fistula; Documentation: _____

_____

*11.4   ☐ Gastroschisis; Documentation: _____

*11.5   ☐ Hirschsprung disease; Documentation: _____

*11.6   ☐ Imperforate anus; Documentation: _____

*11.7   ☐ Omphalocele; Documentation: _____

*11.8   ☐ Pyloric stenosis; Documentation: _____

*11.9   ☐ Other gastrointestinal system structural defects: _____

_____

11.10 ☐ Appendicitis; Documentation: _____

*11.11 ☐ Celiac disease; Documentation: _____

*11.12 ☐ Gallstones; Documentation: _____

*11.13 ☐ Cirrhosis of the liver; Documentation: _____

*11.14 ☐ Colorectal cancers; Documentation: _____

_____

11.15 ☐ Diverticulosis; ☐ Diverticulitis; Documentation: _____

*11.16 ☐ Esophageal cancer; Documentation: _____

_____

*11.17 ☐ Gastric cancer; Documentation: _____

_____

11.18 ☐ Gastritis; ☐ Acute; Documentation: _____

            ☐ Chronic; Documentation: _____

11.19 ☐ Hemorrhoids; Documentation: _____

*11.20 ☐ Hepatitis; Type: _____ ; Documentation: _____

*11.21 ☐ Hiatal hernia; Type _____ ; Documentation: _____

*11.22 ☐ Intestinal polyposis; Documentation: _____

*11.23 ☐ Liver cancer; Documentation: _____

_____

*11.24 ☐ Oral cancers; Type: _____ ; Documentation: _____

_____

*11.25 ☐ Pancreatic cancer; Documentation: _____

_____

*11.26 ☐ Pancreatitis; ☐ Acute; Documentation: _____

            ☐ Chronic; Documentation: _____

*11.27 ☐ Peptic ulcer disease; Type _____ ; Documentation: _____

11.28 ☐ Peritonitis; Documentation: _____

The Gastrointestinal System continued

*11.29 ☐ Regional enteritis; Documentation: _____

*11.30 ☐ Ulcerative colitis; Documentation: _____

*11.31 ☐ Other gastrointestinal disorders: _____

_____

_____

Section 12 - The Urinary System

*12.1 ☐ Epispadias; Documentation: _____

*12.2 ☐ Extrophy of the bladder; Documentation: _____

*12.3 ☐ Hypospadias; Documentation: _____

*12.4 ☐ Kidney (renal) agenesis; Documentation: _____

*12.5 ☐ Kidney (renal) hypoplasia; Documentation: _____

*12.6 ☐ Other urinary system structural defects: _____

_____

*12.7 ☐ Adult polycystic kidney disease; Documentation: _____

*12.8 ☐ Alport syndrome; Documentation: _____

*12.9 ☐ Bladder cancer; Documentation: _____

_____

*12.10 ☐ Congenital nephrosis; Documentation: _____

*12.11 ☐ Cystinuria; Documentation: _____

12.12 ☐ Cystitis; Documentation: _____

*12.13 ☐ Glomerulonephritis; Documentation: _____

*12.14 ☐ Infantile polycystic kidney disease; Documentation: _____

*12.15 ☐ Kidney (renal) cancer; Documentation: _____

_____

*12.16 ☐ Nephrogenic diabetes insipidus; Documentation: _____

12.17 ☐ Nephrosis; Documentation: _____

12.18 ☐ Pyelonephritis; Documentation: _____

*12.19 ☐ Urolithiasis; Type _____ ; Documentation: _____

*12.20 ☐ Wilms tumor; Documentation: _____

*12.21 ☐ Other urinary system disorders: _____

_____

_____

Section 13 - The Male Reproductive System

*13.1 ☐ Cryptorchidism; Documentation: _____

*13.2 ☐ Other male reproductive system structural defects _____

_____

13.3 ☐ Benign prostatic hyperplasia; Documentation: _____

*13.4 ☐ Cancer of the prostate; Documentation: _____

_____

13.5 Dates and results of Prostatic Specific Antigen (PSA) testing: _____

_____

*13.6 ☐ Cancer of the testis; Documentation: _____

_____

13.7 ☐ Epididymitis; Documentation: _____

13.8 ☐ Orchitis; Documentation: _____

13.9 ☐ Prostatitis; Documentation: _____

*13.10 ☐ Other male reproductive system disorders: _____

_____

_____

FORM NO.0795-1 © SONTERS PUBLISHING, INC.

14.1 ☐ Age at menarche: _____ ;   14.2 ☐ Age at menopause; Documentation: _____

*14.3 ☐ Female reproductive system structural defects: _____
_____

*14.4 ☐ Breast cancer; Documentation: _____
_____

*14.5 ☐ Cervical cancer; Documentation: _____
_____

*14.6 ☐ Endometrial cancer; Documentation: _____
_____

*14.7 ☐ Endometriosis; Documentation: _____

14.8 ☐ Fibrocystic breast disease; Documentation: _____

*14.9 ☐ Ovarian cancer; Documentation: _____
_____

14.10 ☐ Pelvic inflammatory disease; Documentation: _____

*14.11 ☐ Other female reproductive system disorders: _____
_____

Obstetric History

	A	B	C	D	E	F	G	H	I	J	K
1.											
2.											
3.											
4.											
5.											
6.											
7.											
8.											
9.											
10.											
11.											
12.											

KEY FOR OBSTETRIC HISTORY GRAPH

Column A: Age/year the pregnancy occurred.
Column B: Infant(s) delivered term (or post-term).
Column C: Infant(s) delivered preterm.
Column D: Miscarriage/termination of pregnancy.
Column E: Number of infants pregnancy produced.
Column F: Number of live infants delivered.

Column G: Vaginal (V) vs cesarean section (C/S) birth.
Column H: Sex of infant(s): Male (M), Female (F).
Column I: Infant birth weight(s).
Column J: Health condition of infant at birth.
Column K: Maternal medical conditions or bleeding disorders occurring during the pregnancy; complications occurring during labor and delivery.

Section 15 - The Endocrine System

*15.1 ☐ Structural defects of endocrine system glands: _____
_____

*15.2 ☐ Addison disease; Documentation: _____

*15.3 ☐ Congenital adrenal hyperplasia; Documentation: _____

*15.4 ☐ Cushing syndrome; Documentation: _____

Section 15 - The Endocrine System continued

*15.5 ☐ Diabetes insipidus; Documentation: _____

*15.6 ☐ Diabetes mellitus; Type: _____ ; Documentation: _____

*15.7 ☐ Gigantism; ☐ Acromegaly; Documentation: _____

*15.8 ☐ Goiter; Documentation: _____

*15.9 ☐ Hyperparathyroidism; Documentation: _____

*15.10 ☐ Hyperthyroidism; ☐ Graves disease; Documentation: _____

*15.11 ☐ Hypoparathyroidism; Documentation: _____

*15.12 ☐ Hypothyroidism; Documentation: _____

*15.13 ☐ Pheochromocytoma; Documentation: _____

*15.14 ☐ Thyroid cancer; Documentation: _____

_____

*15.15 ☐ Thyroiditis; ☐ Hashimoto thyroiditis; Documentation: _____

*15.16 ☐ Other endocrine system disorders: _____

_____

_____

Section 16 - The Blood and Immune Systems

*16.1 ☐ Blood and immune system structural defects: _____

_____

*16.2 ☐ Aplastic anemia; Documentation: _____

16.3 ☐ Folic acid deficiency anemia; Documentation: _____

*16.4 ☐ Glucose-6-phosphate dehydrogenase deficiency; Documentation: _____

*16.5 ☐ Hemochromatosis; Documentation: _____

*16.6 ☐ Hemophilia A; Documentation: _____

*16.7 ☐ Hemophilia B; Documentation: _____

*16.8 ☐ Hemolytic anemia; Documentation: _____

*16.9 ☐ Hereditary spherocytosis; Documentation: _____

16.10 ☐ Iron deficiency anemia; Documentation: _____

*16.11 ☐ Sickle cell anemia; Documentation: _____

*16.12 ☐ Thalassemia; Type: _____ ; Documentation: _____

16.13 ☐ Vitamin B_{12} deficiency anemia; Documentation: _____

*16.14 ☐ Autoimmune thrombocytopenic purpura; Documentation: _____

*16.15 ☐ Immune deficiency disorder; Type: _____ ; Documentation: _____

*16.16 ☐ Leukemia; Type: _____ ; Documentation: _____

_____

_____

*16.17 ☐ Lymphoma; Type: _____ ; Documentation: _____

_____

*16.18 ☐ Multiple myeloma; Documentation: _____

_____

*16.19 ☐ Polycythemia vera; Documentation: _____

*16.20 ☐ Von Willebrand disease; Documentation: _____

*16.21 ☐ Other blood and immune system disorders: _____

_____

_____

FORM NO.0795-1 © SONTERS PUBLISHING, INC.

Section 17 - The Musculoskeletal System

*17.1 ☐ Clubfoot; Documentation: _____

*17.2 ☐ Congenitial hip dislocation; Documentation: _____

*17.3 ☐ Other musculoskeletal structural defects: _____

_____

*17.4 ☐ Achondroplasia; Documentation: _____

*17.5 ☐ Ankylosing spondylitis; Documentation: _____

17.6 ☐ Bursitis; Documentation: _____

*17.7 ☐ Degenerative joint disease; Documentation: _____

*17.8 ☐ Familial hypophosphatemic rickets; Documentation: _____

*17.9 ☐ Gout; Documentation: _____

*17.10 ☐ Muscular dystrophy; Type: _____ ; Documentation: _____

_____

*17.11 ☐ Osteogenesis imperfecta; Type: _____ ; Documentation: _____

17.12 ☐ Osteomyelitis; Documentation: _____

*17.13 ☐ Osteoporosis; Documentation: _____

*17.14 ☐ Paget disease of bone; Documentation: _____

*17.15 ☐ Rheumatoid arthritis; Documentation: _____

*17.16 ☐ Scoliosis; Documentation: _____

*17.17 ☐ Systemic lupus erythematosis; Documentation: _____

*17.18 ☐ Other musculoskeletal disorders: _____

_____

_____

Section 18 - The Integumentary System

18.1 ☐ Acne vulgaris; Documentation: _____

*18.2 ☐ Albinism; Type; _____ ; Documentation: _____

*18.3 ☐ Atopic dermatitis; Documentation: _____

*18.4 ☐ Cancer of the skin; Type _____ ; Documentation: _____

_____

18.5 ☐ Cellulitis; Documentation: _____

*18.6 ☐ Ichthyosis; Type: _____ ; Documentation: _____

18.7 ☐ Impetigo contagiosa; Documentation: _____

*18.8 ☐ Psoriasis vulgaris; Documentation: _____

*18.9 ☐ Xeroderma pigmentosum; Documentation: _____

*18.10 ☐ Other integumentary system disorders: _____

_____

_____

APPENDIX B — LINEAR PEDIGREE WORKSHEET

COLUMN IV
Children, Nieces, Nephews

COLUMN III
First Cousins – Father's Side

You and Your Siblings

Spouses

First Cousins – Mother's Side

1.
2.
3.
4.
5.
6.
7.
8.
9.
10.
11.
12.

COLUMN II

Father's Siblings

Spouses

Father

Mother

Mother's Siblings

Spouses

1.
2.
3.
4.
5.
6.
7.
8.
9.
10.
11.
12.
13.
14.
15.
16.
17.
18.
19.
20.
21.
22.
23.

COLUMN I

Paternal Grandfather's Siblings

Paternal Grandfather

Paternal Grandmother

Paternal Grandmother's Siblings

Maternal Grandfather's Siblings

Maternal Grandfather

Maternal Grandmother

Maternal Grandmother's Siblings

1.
2.
3.
4.
5.
6.
7.
8.
9.
10.
11.
12.
13.
14.
15.
16.
17.
18.
19.
20.

FORM NO. 0795-2 © SONTER'S PUBLISHING, INC.

YOUR RIGHTS TO ACCESS
YOUR MEDICAL RECORDS

Penny S. Smith, B.S.N., J.D.

Information that is most pertinent to your health care is to be found in medical and hospital records. A medical record contains patient information such as name, address, sex, occupation, family relationships, lifestyle, insurance and payment information, and medical data.

Medical records are confidential. Access to these records is limited by federal and state law to the patient, the health-care providers who are treating the patient, certain medical researchers and hospital administrative staff, and anyone legally authorized by the patient to see the records.

At times, however, accessing even your own medical record can be difficult.

Although medical records belong to the health-care provider, in most jurisdictions patients must be allowed to see and to copy their medical records if they request it. However, laws differ by area, so it is important to learn about the medical record laws in your health-care provider's locality.

Release of medical records to employers and insurance companies (and other third parties) is allowed only with the written consent of the patient. Only the information relevant to the patient's condition or treatment is given, unless specific permission to do otherwise is granted in writing.

Some health-care providers resist showing patients their medical records because they are afraid that medical data, terminology, and abbreviations may be misinterpreted and cause the patient unnecessary alarm. If you experience this kind of resistance, offer to review your records together with your health-care provider so there can be no misunderstandings. If access is still denied, health-care regulation agencies such as the American Medical Association or the State Board of Healing Arts can direct you in your next move. If all else fails, usually an attorney can resolve the matter quickly.

Confidentiality continues to be a concern with regard to a patient who is deceased. For example, ordinarily you do not have access to the medical records of your deceased family members. Research indicates that when there is a question about a deceased family member's having carried a genetic disorder, third parties who have a legitimate interest in gaining medical information may be granted access to the deceased family member's medical record. Third parties in this situation have been defined to include family members who might unknowingly also carry the genetic disorder. Whether or not an interest is legitimate may be determined by the seriousness of the genetic disorder and the probability of its occurrence in the individual family member requesting access to the record.

The advice of an attorney can help you in determining your rights under those circumstances.

IF YOU ARE AN ADOPTEE

It can be very difficult for individuals who are adopted to gather a complete family health history if they do not know, or have access to, their biological parents. Adoption records are often closed and difficult to access. Hawaii is the only state in the United States that has an open record policy; a few states offer the original birth certificate through the Department of Human Services.

More and more states are developing adoption registries by which adopted persons and birth parents alike can register personal information in the hope that their birth relative has, or will, do the same. If the registry identifies a match between birth relatives who are searching for each other, the individuals are contacted. There are also private, national, and international adoption registries set up to help adoptees and birth parents find each other.

Many adoptees do not know where to begin the search for their birth parents, and vice versa. They struggle with trying to decide whether or not to search, attempting to weigh potential benefits against potential drawbacks. One good place to start for information to help in making such a decision is the National Adoption Information Clearinghouse in Rockville, Maryland. The clearinghouse offers a comprehensive booklet entitled "Searching for Birth Relatives," which discusses major issues facing all parties from all sides and lists valuable resources and support organizations.

For a copy, write to: National Adoption Clearinghouse, 11426 Rockville Pike, Suite 410, Rockville, MD 20852. Or call 301-231-6512. Your first copy is free.

HOW TO LEARN ABOUT DECEASED FAMILY MEMBERS

If you have difficulty obtaining health information on deceased family members who need to be included in your family health history and pedigree, you may want to search specific records that could give you some health data. Listed here are some of the documents and records you can gather, together with tips on how to obtain them. Not all of them contain health data.

VITAL STATISTICS RECORDS

These records include death, birth, marriage, and divorce records. Birth and death records can be obtained by contacting the Bureau of Vital Statistics in the capital city of the state in which the birth or death occurred. The Bureau of Vital Statistics also maintains marriage and divorce records; however, these records are of less value from a health perspective than from a genealogical perspective.

BIRTH CERTIFICATES contain the individual's name; place of birth; time and date of birth; weight and length at birth; full name of each parent, including the mother's birth name; age of each parent; and the name of the health-care provider attending the birth. Although a birth certificate is considered a confidential record, it may be released to immediate family members or to legal guardians or representatives upon request. Rules can vary from one state to another.

DEATH CERTIFICATES can include information about the deceased such the name; place of death; time, date, and year of death; cause of death; place of birth; names of parents and surviving spouse; occupation and military service; and the names of the informant of the death, the health-care provider or coroner who pronounced the death, and the funeral home and burial cemetery or crematory. Death certificates are confidential, but may be released to family members on written request. Rules can vary from state to state.

When an American citizen dies abroad, a certificate of death in a foreign country—called a Report of Death of an American Citizen—is filed. To obtain information about receiving a copy of this report contact:

Department of Correspondence
U.S. Department of State
202-647-0518

MILITARY RECORDS

Military health records contain valuable health information that can be accessed by immediate family members of deceased veterans. Living members in active duty and those who have retired or been discharged can also obtain valuable health information from their own military health records. To access the records of veterans from World War I (1914) and after, write to:

National Records Center
9700 Page Boulevard
St. Louis, MO 63132

To request a form that will expedite your request, telephone the number that corresponds to the appropriate branch of service:

Army: 314-538-4261   Air Force: 314-538-4243
Navy, Marine Corps, and Coast Guard: 314-538-4141

It is important to list as much information about the veteran as you can, including full name, date of enlistment, Social Security Number, military service number, and the last unit of assignment. (If you want access to the health files of a family member who died in service, also ask for a copy of the certificate of death, called the Report of Casualty.) It is best if you mail your request return receipt, certified, or registered. For additional assistance, contact your local Veterans Affairs Office or the appropriate branch of the Armed Services through the:

Secretary of Defense, 703-545-6700

OBITUARIES

An often-overlooked source of information is the deceased's obituary notice, which can usually be found in newspaper archives. Years ago, an obituary might have stated the cause of death and any diseases the individual had. Although current obituaries do not usually offer this information, they might suggest that a memorial be made in the deceased's name to a health organization.

Sometimes the type of organization is a clue to the deceased's health status and/or cause of death.

FAMILY JOURNALS AND OLD LETTERS

Old family journals and letters sometimes contain health information about family members who are now deceased, although the information can be difficult to verify. Ask living relatives if this type of family documentation exists and who is likely to have it.

Genealogists are experts in investigating ancestral records. For books written to help the reader become a genealogical sleuth, visit your local library. You will find many excellent resources. Also, contact your state or local genealogical society for information and assistance on how and where to begin a record search. The National Genealogical Society (703-525-0050) can direct you to your state's association.

RESOURCES

Volunteer organizations provide services and activities, including sharing general information, making referrals, and offering support while assisting with special needs. Such organizations publish a variety of excellent educational materials for use by the general public, health professionals, educators, and administrators.

Here is a list of some of the national volunteer organizations and other resources that deal with genetic issues. The reference section of your public library contains information about other volunteer organizations that you can contact for information and support. Volunteer when possible.

PART 1

ALLIANCE OF GENETIC SUPPORT GROUPS
35 Wisconsin Circle, Suite 440
Chevy Chase, MD 20815-7015   800-336-GENE

ALZHEIMER'S ASSOCIATION; ALZHEIMER'S DISEASE
AND RELATED DISORDERS ASSOCIATION, INC.
919 North Michigan Avenue, #1000
Chicago, IL 60611-1676   800-272-3900

AMERICAN CANCER SOCIETY, INC.
1599 Clifton Road NE
Atlanta, GA 30329-4251   800-227-2345

AMERICAN DIABETES ASSOCIATION, INC.
1660 Duke Street
Alexandria, VA 22314   800-232-3472

AMERICAN DIGESTIVE DISEASE SOCIETY
7720 Wisconsin Avenue, Suite 217
Bethesda, MD 20814   301-652-9293

AMERICAN HEART ASSOCIATION
7272 Greenville Avenue
Dallas, TX 75231   800-242-1793

AMERICAN LUNG ASSOCIATION
1740 Broadway
New York, NY 10019   800-LUNG-USA

AMERICAN PARKINSON DISEASE ASSOCIATION (THE)
60 Bay Street, Suite 401
Staten Island, NY 10301   800-223-2732

AMERICAN SELF-HELP CLEARINGHOUSE
Saint Clares Riverside Medical Center
25 Pocono Road
Denville, NJ 07834-2995   201-625-7101

AMERICAN SPEECH-LANGUAGE-HEARING ASSOCIATION
10801 Rockville Pike
Rockville, MD 20852   800-638-8255

ARTHRITIS FOUNDATION
AMERICAN JUVENILE ARTHRITIS ORGANIZATION
1314 Spring Street NW
Atlanta, GA 30309   800-283-7800

ASSOCIATION OF BIRTH DEFECT CHILDREN, INC.
827 Erma Avenue   800-313-2232
Orlando, FL 32803   407-245-7035

ASTHMA AND ALLERGY FOUNDATION OF AMERICA
1125 15th Street NW, Suite 502
Washington, DC 20005   800-7-ASTHMA

COALITION FOR HERITABLE DISORDERS
OF CONNECTIVE TISSUE
382 Main Street
Port Washington, NY 11050   800-862-7326

CYSTIC FIBROSIS FOUNDATION
6931 Arlington Road
Bethesda, MD 20814   800-FIGHT-CF

DEPRESSION AND RELATED AFFECTIVE
DISORDERS ASSOCIATION (DRADA)
Meyer 3-181, 600 North Wolfe Street
Baltimore, MD 21287-7381   410-955-4647

EPILEPSY FOUNDATION OF AMERICA
4351 Garden City Drive   800-332-1000
Landover, MD 20785   301-459-3700

FOUNDATION FIGHTING BLINDNESS (THE);
NATIONAL RETINITIS PIGMENTOSA FOUNDATION, INC.
1401 Mt. Royal Avenue, 4th Floor
Baltimore, MD 21217   800-683-5555

IMMUNE DEFICIENCY FOUNDATION
25 West Chesapeake Avenue, Suite 206
Towson, MD 21204   800-296-4433

LEUKEMIA SOCIETY OF AMERICA
600 Third Avenue
New York, NY 10016   800-955-4572

MARCH OF DIMES BIRTH DEFECTS FOUNDATION
125 Mamaroneck Avenue
White Plains, NY 10605   800-367-6630

MEDIC ALERT FOUNDATION
2323 Colorado Avenue
Turlock, CA 95380   800-344-3226

MOTHERS UNITED FOR MORAL SUPPORT (MUMS)
150 Custer Court
Green Bay, WI 54301   414-336-5333

MUSCULAR DYSTROPHY ASSOCIATION
3300 East Sunrise Drive
Tucson, AZ 85718-3208   800-572-1717

NATIONAL ALLIANCE FOR THE MENTALLY ILL (NAMI)
200 North Glebe Road, Suite 1015
Arlington, VA 22203-3754   800-950-6264

NATIONAL DIGESTIVE DISEASE
  INFORMATION CLEARINGHOUSE
2 Information Way
Bethesda, MD 20892-3570   301-654-3810

NATIONAL DOWN SYNDROME CONGRESS
1605 Chantilly, Suite 250
Atlanta, GA 30324   800-232-6372

NATIONAL DOWN SYNDROME SOCIETY
666 Broadway, Suite 810
New York, NY 10012   800-221-4602

NATIONAL EASTER SEAL SOCIETY
300 West Monroe Street, Suite 1800
Chicago, IL 60606-4802   800-221-6827

NATIONAL INFORMATION CENTER FOR CHILDREN
  AND YOUTH WITH DISABILITIES
P.O. Box 1492
Washington, DC 20013   800-695-0285

NATIONAL INSTITUTES OF HEALTH
9000 Rockville Pike
Bethesda, MD 20892   301-496-4000

NATIONAL KIDNEY FOUNDATION
30 East 33rd Street
New York, NY 10016   800-622-9010

NATIONAL MATERNAL AND CHILD HEALTH
  CLEARINGHOUSE
8201 Greensboro Drive, Suite 600
McLean, VA 22102   703-821-8955

NATIONAL ORGANIZATION FOR RARE DISORDERS
  (NORD)
P.O. Box 8923
New Fairfield, CT 06812   800-999-6673

SICKLE CELL DISEASE ASSOCIATION OF AMERICA
200 Corporate Pointe, Suite 495
Culver City, CA 90230-7633   800-421-8453

SIDS ALLIANCE
1314 Bedford Avenue, Suite 210
Baltimore, MD 21208   800-221-SIDS

SPINA BIFIDA ASSOCIATION OF AMERICA
4590 MacArthur Blvd., Suite 250
Washington, DC 20007   800-621-3141

The DIRECTORY OF NATIONAL GENETIC VOLUNTARY ORGANIZATIONS AND RELATED RESOURCES is compiled by the Alliance of Genetic Support Groups for the purpose of linking medical and educational professionals, service providers, and those affected by genetic conditions with appropriate support organizations and resources.

For information on the Directory, please contact the Alliance of Genetic Support Groups, 35 Wisconsin Circle, Suite 440, Chevy Chase, MD 20815; 800-336-GENE.

Alliance
of Genetic Support Groups
A Coalition of Voluntary Organizations and Professionals

PART 2

RESOURCES ABOUT GENETIC CONFIDENTIALITY

ALLIANCE OF GENETIC SUPPORT GROUPS
35 Wisconsin Circle, Suite 440
Chevy Chase, MD 20815   800-336-GENE
A coalition of voluntary organizations and professionals
that serves as an umbrella organization for national and
local genetic disease support groups, as a consumer
advocate, and as an information source

COUNCIL FOR RESPONSIBLE GENETICS
5 Upland Road, Suite 3
Cambridge, MA 02140   617-868-0870
A public interest organization of scientists and
nonscientists devoted to promoting public awareness of
new genetic technologies, the social and environmental
problems arising from these technologies, and the need
for public access to understandable information; and a
consumer advocate and information source

NATIONAL SOCIETY OF GENETIC COUNSELORS, INC.
233 Canterbury Drive
Wallingford, PA 19086

DISABILITY RIGHTS CENTER
Washington, DC   202-337-4119

**LAWYERS COMMITTEE FOR CIVIL RIGHTS
UNDER THE LAW**   202-371-1212

NATIONAL EMPLOYMENT & LAW PROJECT 212-870-2121

NATIONAL HOUSING LAW PROJECT   415-548-9400

THE BOSTON WOMEN'S HEALTH BOOK COLLECTIVE
240A Elm Street
Somerville, MA 02144   617-625-0277
A consumer advocate and information source

CENTER FOR PUBLIC INTEREST LAW
University of San Diego School of Law
San Diego, CA   619-260-4806

THE COUNCIL OF STATE GOVERNMENTS
3560 Iron Works Pike, P.O. Box 11910
Lexington, KY 40578-1910   602-231-1939

VOICE—VICTIMS OF INSURANCE COMPANY ERRORS
                                         310-372-7439
A grassroots nonprofit group furthering consumer
education and participation in insurance reform

**COUNCIL OF REGIONAL NETWORKS FOR GENETIC
SERVICES (CORN)**
Atlanta, GA   404-727-1475

Regional groups

**GENETICS NETWORK OF NEW YORK STATE, PUERTO
RICO AND THE VIRGIN ISLANDS (GENES)**
Albany, NY   518-486-2215

GREAT LAKES REGIONAL GENETICS GROUP (GLaRGG)
Madison, WI   608-265-2907

GREAT PLAINS GENETICS SERVICE NETWORK (GPGSN)
Iowa City, IA   319-356-4860

**MID-ATLANTIC REGIONAL HUMAN GENETICS
NETWORK (MARHGN)**
Philadelphia, PA   215-985-6760

**MOUNTAIN STATES REGIONAL GENETIC SERVICES
NETWORK (MSRGSN)**
Denver, CO   303-692-2423

NEW ENGLAND REGIONAL GENETICS GROUP (NERGG)
Mt. Desert, ME   207-288-2704

PACIFIC NORTHWEST REGIONAL GENETICS GROUP
(PacNORGG) Eugene, OR   503-346-2610

PACIFIC SOUTHWEST REGIONAL GENETICS NETWORK
(PSRGN) Berkeley, CA   510-540-2852

SOUTHEASTERN REGIONAL GENETICS GROUP
(SERGG) Atlanta, GA   404-727-5844

TEXAS GENETICS NETWORK (TEXGENE)
Austin, TX   512-458-7700

STATE COMMISSIONS AGAINST DISCRIMINATION

STATE DIVISIONS OF CONSUMER AFFAIRS

STATE DISABILITY LAW CENTERS

STATE DISABILITY RIGHTS CENTERS

STATE INSURANCE COMMISSIONERS

**STATE LEGISLATURES, SCIENCE, TECHNOLOGY AND
POLICY COMMISSIONS**

BIBLIOGRAPHY

PART 1 — SOURCES USED IN THIS BOOK

Abel, E. L., & Sokol, R. J. "Fetal alcohol syndrome is now leading cause of mental retardation." *Lancet* ii:1222 (1986).

Alcohol, Drug Abuse, & Mental Health Administration. "Fetal alcohol syndrome." *Alcohol Alert* #13 (PH 297) (July 1991). Bethesda: National Institute on Alcohol Abuse & Alcoholism.

Alper, J. S., & Natowicz, M. R. "Genetic testing & insurance." *British Medicine Journal* Vol. 307 (Dec. 1993).

Alter, M., & Margolis, H. "Sexually transmitted diseases: The emergence of hepatitis B as a sexually transmitted disease." *Medical Clinics of North America* Vol. 74 #6. (Nov. 1990).

American Academy of Pediatrics & American College of Obstetricians & Gynecologists. *Guidelines for Perinatal Care*. 3d ed. Washington, DC: 1992.

American Cancer Society. *Cancer Facts & Figures 1992*. Pub. #5008.

____. *Cancer Facts & Figures*. 1986.

____. *Cancer Facts for Men*. Pub. #2008, 1990.

____. *Cancer Facts for Women*. Pub. #2007, 1990.

____. *Taking Control: 10 Steps to a Healthier Life & Reduced Cancer Risk*. Pub. #2019.05, 1985.

American College of Obstetricians & Gynecologists. *ACOG Guide to Preconception Care*. Washington, DC: 1990.

____. *Exercise During Pregnancy & the Postnatal Period*. Washington, DC: 1985.

____. *Standards for Obstetric-Gynecologic Services*. 7th ed. Washington, DC: 1989.

American Heart Asso. (Missouri affiliate). *Conference on Women & Heart Disease: Summary of Proceedings, May 18, 1991*. Columbia, MO: 1991.

American Heart Asso.. *Abnormalities of Heart Rhythm: A Guide for Parents*. Pub. #50-058-A CP, 1983.

____. *About High Blood Pressure: Control, Risk, Lifestyle, Weight*. Pub. #50-052-D CP, 1989.

____. *About Your Heart & Exercise*. Pub. #51-1017 CP, 1989.

____. *Cholesterol & Your Heart: Lower Blood Cholesterol Level*. Pub. #50-1018 CP, 1989.

____. *Coronary Risk Factor Statement for the American Public*. Pub. #50-072-A CP, 1991.

____. *Exercise & Your Heart*. Pub. #51-1018 CP, 1989.

____. *Facts About Congestive Heart Failure*. Pub. 51-1003 CP, 1987.

____. *Fact Sheet on Heart Attack, Stroke & Risk Factors*. Pub. #51-1033 COM, 1991.

____. *Heart Attack*. Pub. #51-1012 CP (1989).

____. *If Your Child Has a Congenital Heart Defect: A Guide for Parents*. Pub. #50-1109 CP, 1991.

____. *The Marfan Syndrome*. Pub. #71-1020 CP, 1991.

____. *1992 Heart & Stroke Facts*. Pub. #55-0386 COM, 1991.

____. *Silent Epidemic: The Truth About Women & Heart Disease*. Pub. #64-9571 CP, 1989.

____. *Understanding Angina*. Pub. #50-1031 CP, 1991.

Amyotrophic Lateral Sclerosis Asso.. *Link* (Spring 1993). Woodland Hills, CA.

____. *ALS & the ALS Asso.*. (March 1992). Woodland Hills, CA.

Angier, N. "Scientists discover the gene in a nervous system disease." *New York Times* (July 13, 1990).

Bennett, R. L., Steinhaus, K. A., Uhrich, S. B., & O'Sullivan, C. K. "Recommendations for standardized human pedigree nomenclature." *American J. of Human Genetics* 56:3 (March 1995). University of Chicago Press.

Bergsma, D. *Birth Defects Compendium*. 2d ed. New York: AR Liss: 1979.

Bernhardt, B. A. "The Marfan syndrome: A booklet for teachers." Port Washington, NY: National Marfan Foundation, 1992.

Billings, P., & Hubbard, R. "Fragile X testing: Who benefits? School-sponsored genetic screening program raises specter of discrimination." *geneWATCH* 9 (Jan. 1994).

Bishop, J. "Scientists find first clues on how genes could cause nerve tumors." *Wall Street Journal* (Aug. 10, 1990).

Bobak, I. M., & Jensen, M. D. *Essentials of Maternity Nursing*. 3d ed. St. Louis: Mosby-Year Book, 1991.

Brunner, L. S., & Suddarth, D. S. *Textbook of Medical Surgical Nursing*. 6th ed. Philadelphia: Lippincott, 1988.

Buyse, M. L. *Birth Defects Encyclopedia*. London: Blackwell, 1990.

Carlin, M. E. *Cri-Du-Chat Syndrome*. Miami, FL: Division of Genetics, University of Miami, n.d.

Casey, C. T. "Fragile X syndrome: Improving understanding & diagnosis." *J. American Medical Asso.* Vol. 271 (Feb. 1994).

Castiglia, P. T., & Harbin, R. E. *Child Health Care Process & Practice*. Philadelphia: Lippincott, 1992.

Clayman, C. B. *American Medical Asso.: Genes & Inheritance*. New York: Reader's Digest Asso., 1993.

Cleft Palate Foundation. *Cleft Lip & Cleft Palate: The First Four Years*. Pittsburgh, PA: 1989.

Council of State Governments. *Advances in Genetic Information: A Guide for State Policy Makers. Environmental Issues, Insurance, Criminal Justice, Health Care, Genetic Testing, Civil Liberties*. Lexington, KY: 1993.

Darrow, W. W., & Valdiserri, R. O. *New Directions for Health Promotion to Prevent HIV Infection & Other STDs*. Atlanta, GA: Centers for Disease Control, n.d.

Dippel, N., & Becknal, B. "Bulimia." *J. of Psychosocial Nursing* 25(9):12-17 (1987).

Doenges, M., Townsend, M., & Moorhouse, M. *Psychiatric Nursing Care Plans*. Philadelphia: F. A. Davis, 1989.

Dudek, S. G. *Nutrition Handbook for Nursing Practice*. 2d ed. Philadelphia: Lippincott, 1993.

Emery, A. E. H., & Rimoin, D. L. *Principles & Practice of Medical Genetics*. Edinburgh: Churchill Livingstone, 1983.

Furrow, B., Johnson, S., Jost, T., & Schwartz, R. *Health Law*. N.p.: West Publishing, n.d.

Garver, K. L., & Marchese, S. G. *Genetic Counseling for Clinicians*. Chicago: Year Book Medical Publishers, 1986.

Gorlin, R. J., Cohen, M. M., & Levin, S. J. *Syndromes of the Head & Neck*. 3d ed. New York: Oxford University Press, 1990.

Gormley, M. V. *Family Diseases: Are You at Risk?* Baltimore: Genealogical Publishing, 1989.

Groer, M. W., & Shekleton, M. E. *Basic Pathophysiology: A Holistic Approach*. 3d ed. St. Louis: Mosby-Year Book, 1989.

Hennessey, J. C. *The Inheritance of RP & Allied Retinal Degenerative Diseases*. Baltimore: RP Foundation, 1991.

Hoekelman, R. A. *Primary Pediatric Care*. 2d ed. St. Louis: Mosby-Year Book, 1992.

Hook, E. B. "Rates of chromosome abnormalities at different maternal ages." *Obstet Gynecol* 58:282-85 (1981).

Huntington's Disease Society of America. *The Marker* Vol. 5 #3 (Fall/Winter 1992).

____. *The Marker* Vol. 6 #2 (Summer 1993).

Ignatavicius, D., & Bayne, M. V. *Medical Surgical Nursing: A Nursing Process Approach*. Philadelphia: W. B. Saunders, 1991.

The Immune Deficiency Foundation. *Primary Immune Deficiency Diseases: An Overview*. Columbia, MD: 1988.

Institute of Medicine, National Academy of Sciences. *Assessing Genetic Risks: Implications for Health & Social Policy*. Washington, D.C.: National Academy Press, 1994.

Jauchem, J. "Advances in treatment of the Marfan syndrome." *Research Resources Reporter* Vol. 10 #8 (Aug. 1986) DHHS Publication.

Johnson, B. *Adaption & Growth: Psychiatric Mental Health Nursing*. St. Louis: Lippincott, 1993.

Johnson, G. E., Hannah, K. J., & Zerr, S. R. *Pharmacology & the Nursing Process*. 3d ed. Toronto: W. B. Saunders, 1992.

Juvenile Diabetes Foundation International. "Diabetes & your heart." (series/#13). New York: n.d.

____. "Diet, exercise & diabetes." (series/#12).

____. "What you should know about diabetes." (series/#3).

Kapp, M. B. "Don't ask, don't tell? Ethical & legal implications of advances in genetic testing technology." *Legal Medicine* (1994).

Kozier, B., Erb, G., & Olivieri, R. *Fundamentals of Nursing: Concepts, Process & Practice*. 4th ed. Redwood City, CA: Addison-Wesley, 1991.

Larson, D. E., et al. *Mayo Clinic Family Health Book*. New York: William Morrow, 1990.

Lauer, Barness, et al. *National Cholesterol Education Program Expert Panel on Blood Cholesterol Levels in Children & Adolescents*. American Heart Asso. Pub. #71-0008 CP, 1991.

LeBieu, S. *Our Immune System*. Columbia, MD: Immune Deficiency Foundation: 1990.

Lehne, R. A., et al. *Pharmacology for Nursing Care*. Philadelphia: W. B. Saunders, 1990.

Long, B. C., Phipps, W. J., & Cassmeyer, V. L. *Medical-Surgical Nursing: A Nursing Process Approach*. 3d ed. St. Louis: Mosby-Year Book, 1993.

McEwen, J. E., & Reily, P. R. "State legislative efforts to regulate use & potential misuse of genetic information." *American J. of Human Genetics* Vol. 51 #3 (Sept. 1992).

McFarland, G., & Thomas, M. *Psychiatric Mental Health Nursing: Application of the Nursing Process*. St. Louis: Lippincott, 1992.

McKenry, L. M., & Salerno, E. *Pharmacology in Nursing*. 17th ed. St. Louis: Mosby, 1989.

McKusick, V. A. *Mendelian Inheritance in Man*. 10th ed. Baltimore: Johns Hopkins University Press, 1992.

____. *Mendelian Inheritance in Man: A Catalog of Human Genes & Genetic Disorders*. 11th ed. Vols. 1, 2. Baltimore: Johns Hopkins University Press, 1994.

March of Dimes Birth Defects Foundation. *Genetic Series: Down Syndrome*. Pub. #09-174-00, Oct. 1985. White Plains, NY.

____. *Genetic Series: Marfan Syndrome*. Pub. #09-319-00, Nov. 1987.

____. *Genetic Series: PKU*. Pub. #09-274-00, Oct. 1986.

____. *Genetic Series: Rh Disease*. Pub. #09-179-00, Oct. 1976.

____. *Genetic Series: Spina Bifida*. Pub. #09-264-00, Nov. 1987.

____. *Genetic Series: Tay-Sachs*. Pub. #09-100-00, Oct. 1986.

____. *Genetic Series: Thalassemia*. Pub. #09-041-00, March 1986.

____. *Genetic Testing & Gene Therapy: What They Mean to You & Your Family*. Pub. #09-576-00.

Martin, L. L., & Reeder, S. J. *Essentials of Maternity Nursing: Family Centered Care*. Philadelphia: Lippincott, 1991.

Miller, C. H., & Lubs, M. L. *The Inheritance of Hemophilia*. 2d ed. National Hemophilia Foundation. New York: American Legion Child Welfare Foundation, 1986.

Miller-Keane, C. *Encyclopedia & Dictionary of Medicine & Allied Health*. Philadelphia: W. B. Saunders, 1992.

Milunsky, A. "Heredity & Your Family's Health." *Genetic Counseling* 3d ed. Maryland: Johns Hopkins University Press, 1992.

Muscular Dystrophy Asso.: Fact Sheet. Pub. #P-102. Tucson: Muscular Dystrophy Asso., 1992.

____. *Facts About Myasthenia Gravis*. Pub. #P-189-5/91-75M, 1991.

Nair, P. "Early identification of HIV infection in children." *Pediatric AIDS & HIV Infection*. (1992).

National Center for Learning Disabilities. *What's In a Name?* New York: n.d.

National Center for Nutrition & Dietetics. *Nutrition Fact Sheet: Food Allergies*. Chicago: 1992.

____. *Nutrition Fact Sheet: Triglycerides*. 1992.

National Down Syndrome Congress. *Facts about Down Syndrome*. Feb. 1988. Park Ridge, IL.

National Foundation for Jewish Genetic Diseases, Inc. *Jewish Genetic Diseases: Facts for Patients & Families*. New York: 1991.

National Institute of Diabetes & Digestive & Kidney Diseases. *Diverticulosis & Diverticulitis*. NIH Pub. #90-1163, Oct. 1989. Chicago: National Center for Nutrition & Dietetics.

National Neurofibromatosis Foundation. *Neurofibromatosis: Information for Patients & Families*. 7th ed. New York: 1990.

National Organization for Albinism & Hypopigmentation. *Ocular Albinism*. N.p., 1988.

____. Special conference edition, *NOAH News* Vol. 9 #2. Philadelphia: 1992.

____. *What Is Albinism?* 1988.

National Retinitis Pigmentosa Foundation, d/b/a RP Foundation Fighting Blindness. *Information About RP & Allied Retinal Degenerative Diseases*. Baltimore: 1991.

____. *Fighting Blindness News*. (Spring 1992).

____. *Fighting Blindness News*. (Summer 1992).

Office of Technology Assessment. *Cystic Fibrosis & DNA Tests: Implication of Carrier Screening*. 1991.

Olds, S. B., London, M. L., & Ladewig, P. A. *Maternal Newborn Nursing: A Family Centered Approach*. 3d ed. Redwood City, CA: Addison-Wesley, 1988.

Ort, S. *Tourette Syndrome & the School Nurse*. New Haven: Yale University School of Medicine, 1991.

Ostrer, H., et al. "Insurance & genetic testing: Where are we now?" *American J. of Human Genetics* Vol. 52. (1993).

O'Toole, M., et al. *Miller-Keane Encyclopedia & Dictionary of Medicine, Nursing, & Allied Health*. 5th ed. Philadelphia: W. B. Saunders, 1992.

Parkinson's Disease Foundation. *Parkinson's Disease: Progress, Promise & Hope*. New York: 1992.

Peterman, T. A., Wasserheit, J. N., & Cates, W. *Prevention of the Sexual Transmission of HIV*. Atlanta: Centers for Disease Control, 1992.

Pillitteri, A. *Maternal & Child Health Nursing: Care of the Childbearing & Childrearing Family*. Philadelphia: Lippincott, 1992.

Powers, J. "Distilling the flood of water worries." *Building Ideas* (Fall 1993) pp. 54-57.

Pyeritz, R. E., & Conant, J. *The Marfan Syndrome*. 3d ed. Port Washington, NY: National Marfan Foundation, 1989.

Rawlins, R., Williams, S., & Beck, C. *Mental Health—Psychiatric Nursing: A Holistic Life-Cycle Approach*. St. Louis: Mosby-Year Book, 1993.

Reeder, S. J., Martin, L. L., & Koniak, D. *Maternity Nursing: Family, Newborn, & Women's Health Care*. 17th ed. Philadelphia: Lippincott, 1992.

"Report of the task force on genetic information & insurance: NIH/DOE working group on ethical, legal, & social implications of human genome research." *Genetic Information & Health Insurance* (May 1993).

Resta, R. G. "The crane's foot: The rise of the pedigree in human genetics." *J. of Genetic Counseling* 2(4):235-60 (1993).

Rinzler, C. A. *Are You at Risk?* New York: Oxford, 1992.

Rubin, K. W. "Water: The forgotten nutrient." *Food Service Director*. (Jan. 1991) Chicago: National Center for Nutrition & Dietetics.

Scriver, C. R., Beaudet, A. L., Sly, W. S., & Valle, D. *Metabolic Basis of Inherited Disease*. 6th ed. New York: McGraw-Hill, 1989.

Shepard, T. H. *Catalog of Teratogenic Agents*. 6th ed. Baltimore: Johns Hopkins Univ. Press, 1989.

Seventh Special Report to the U.S. Congress on Alcohol & Health: Fetal Alcohol Syndrome & Other Effects of Alcohol on Pregnancy Outcome. RP0756. Rockville, MD: Dept. of Health & Human Services, n.d.

Shives, L. *Basic Concepts of Psychiatric-Mental Health Nursing*. St. Louis: Lippincott, 1990.

SIDS Alliance. *Facts About SIDS*. 3d ed. Columbia, MD: 1989.

____. *Sudden Infant Death Syndrome: A Family Tragedy*. Glenview, IL: 1990.

____. *The Sudden Infant Death Syndrome Alliance Greater Illinois Chapter Newsletter* Vol. 7 #4 (Spring 1992) Glenview, IL.

Smeltzer, S. C., & Bare, B. G. *Brunner & Suddarth's Textbook of Medical-Surgical Nursing*. 7th ed. Philadelphia: Lippincott, 1992.

Strong, Deckelbaum, et al. *Integrated Cardiovascular Health Promotion in Childhood*. 1992. American Heart Asso. Pub. #71-0014 SA.

Sullivan, E., Bissel, L., & Williams, E. *Chemical Dependency in Nursing*. Redwood City, CA: Addison-Wesley, n.d.

Surgeon General's Report. *Cancers Associated with Smoking* (1982).

TAP Pharmaceuticals. *Advanced Prostate Cancer: Treatment & Choices*. Pub. #97-9665. North Chicago: 1989.

Tapley, Morris, Rowland, et al. *The Columbia University of Physicians & Surgeons Complete Home Medical Guide*. Yonkers, NY: Consumers Union, 1989.

Taylor, C., Lillis, C., & Lemone, P. *Fundamentals of Nursing*. Philadelphia: Lippincott, 1989.

Tourette Syndrome Asso.. *Facts You Should Know About the Genetics of Tourette Syndrome*. Bayside, NY: n.d.

____. *Questions & Answers on Tourette Syndrome*. (1989) Pub. #150M89/B2.

____. *Second International Scientific Symposium on Tourette Syndrome*. (Oct. 1991) Bayside, NY.

Townsend, M. *Psychiatric Mental Health Nursing*. Philadelphia: F. A. Davis, 1993.

Treadway, D. *Before It's Too Late: Working with Substance Abuse in the Family*. Cleveland: W. W. Norton, 1989.

Tribole, E. *Eat Right America: Your Guide to Achieving a Lowfat Lifestyle*. N.p.: American Dietetic Asso., 1992.

Troyer, G. T., & Salman, S. L. *Handbook of Healthcare Risk Management*. Chicago: Aspen Press, 1986.

Twin Cities District Dietetic Asso.. *Manual of Pediatric Nutrition*. St. Paul, MN: 1990.

U.S. Dept. of Agriculture & U.S. Dept. of Health & Human Services. *Nutrition & Your Health: Dietary Guidelines for Americans*. Pub. #US GPO: 1990-273-930). Chicago: The American Dietetic Asso., 1990.

U.S. Dept. of Health & Human Services. *Adult Kidney Cancer & Wilms' Tumor.* NIH Pub. #90-2342 (Nov. 1989). Bethesda: National Cancer Institute.

____. *Advances in Alcohol Treatment Research.* Pub. #13-PH297 (July 1991).

____. *Bone Marrow Transplantation.* NIH Pub. #92-1178 (April 1991).

____. *Cancer of the Bladder.* NIH Pub. #90-722 (April 1990).

____. *Cancer of the Colon & Rectum.* NIH Pub. #92-95 (Oct. 1991).

____. *Cancer of the Lung.* NIH Pub. #93-526 (Feb. 1993).

____. *Cancer of the Pancreas.* NIH Pub. #92-2941 (Aug. 1992).

____. *Cancer of the Uterus: Endometrial Cancer.* NIH Pub. #91-171 (Jan. 1991).

____. *Cancer Rates & Risks* (3d ed.) NIH Pub. #85-691 (April 1985).

____. *Diet, Nutrition & Cancer Prevention: The Good News.* NIH Pub. #87-2878 (Sept. 1987).

____. "Epidemiology" (Ch. 2), "Genetics & Environment" (Ch. 3), & "Adverse Social Consequences" (Ch. 7). *Seventh Special Report to the U.S. Congress on Alcohol & Health.* (Jan. 1990) Rockville, MD.

____. *Fact Sheet: What Is SIDS?* (Aug. 1989) McLean, VA: National SIDS Clearinghouse.

____. *Health Care Financing Administration.* 42 CFR, Ch. IV., Sec. 482.24.

____. *The Immune System: How It Works.* NIH Pub. #92-3229 (June 1992) Bethesda: National Institute of Allergy & Infectious Diseases & the National Cancer Institute.

____. *Oral Cancers.* NIH Pub. #92-2876 (Dec. 1991).

____. *Sexually Transmitted Diseases: Treatment Guideline.* (Sept. 1989) U.S. GPO: 1990-732-160.

____. *Skin Cancers: Basal Cell & Squamous Cell Carcinomas, Research Report.* NIH Pub. #91-2977 (Sept. 1990).

____. *Smart Advice for Women 40 & Over: Have a Mammogram.* NIH Pub. #90-1581 (Jan. 1990) Bethesda: National Cancer Institute.

____. *Testicular Cancer.* NIH Pub. #90-654 (March 1990).

____. *Understanding the Immune System.* NIH Pub. #92-529 (Oct. 1991) Bethesda: National Institute of Allergy & Infectious Diseases & the National Cancer Institute.

____. *U.S. Dept. of Agriculture: Dietary Guidelines for Americans* 2d ed. (1985).

____. *What You Need to Know About Breast Cancer.* NIH Pub. #93-1556 (March 1993) Bethesda: National Cancer Institute.

____. *What You Need to Know About Cancer of the Colon & Rectum.* NIH Pub. #88-1552 (Dec. 1987) Bethesda: National Cancer Institute.

____. *What You Need to Know About Cancer of the Pancreas.* NIH Pub. #88-1552 (March 1990).

____. *What You Need to Know About Non-Hodgkin's Lymphoma.* NIH Pub. #89-1567 (Nov. 1988) Bethesda: National Cancer Institute.

Varcarolis, E. *Foundations of Psychiatric Mental Health Nursing.* Philadelphia: W. B. Saunders, 1990.

Weaver, D. D. *Catalog of Prenatally Diagnosed Conditions.* Baltimore: Johns Hopkins University Press, 1989.

Wertzm, D. C., & Fletcher, J. C. "Disclosing genetic information: Who should know?" *Technology Review* (July 1989).

Whitley, D. E. *STDs: Sexually Transmitted Diseases.* 3d ed. Arlington, TX: Fairview Publications, 1991.

Williams, C. "Marfan Syndrome: The Silent Killer." *USA Today.* (Nov. [n.d.] 1989).

Williams, D. B., & Windebank, A. "Subject review: Motor neuron disease (amyotrophic lateral sclerosis)." *Mayo Clinical Procedures* 66:54-82 (1991).

Wilson, H., & Kneisl, C. *Psychiatric Nursing.* Redwood City, CA.: Addison-Wesley, 1992.

Winkelstein, M. L. *Primary Immune Deficiency Diseases: A Guide for Nurses.* Baltimore: University of Maryland School of Nursing, 1992.

Winter, R., & Baraitser, M. *London Dysmorphology Database.* Oxford University Press, 1992.

Wong, D. L. *Whaley & Wong's Essentials of Pediatric Nursing.* 4th ed. St. Louis: Mosby-Year Book, 1993.

PART 2 — ADDITIONAL READING ABOUT CONFIDENTIALITY OF GENETIC INFORMATION

Alper, J., & Natowicz, M. "Genetic discrimination & the public entities & public accommodations titles of the Americans with Disabilities Act." *American J. of Human Genetics* 53:26-32 (1993).

____. "Genetic testing & insurance." *British Medical Journal* Vol. 307 (Dec. 1993).

American Asso. for the Advancement of Science, Committee on Scientific Freedom & Responsibility. *The Genome, Ethics & the Law: Issues in Genetic Testing: AAAS-ABA National Conference of Lawyers & Scientists, AAAS Committee on Scientific Freedom & Responsibility.* American Bar Asso. Conference (1992).

American Council of Life Insurance. *Genetic Test Information & Insurance: Confidentiality Concerns & Recommendations.* N.p., n.d.

American Council of Life Insurance Subcommittee on Privacy Legislation & the Task Force on Genetic Testing. Report. Washington, DC: American Council of Life Insurance, 1991.

Billings, P., et al. "Discrimination as a consequence of genetic testing." *American J. of Human Genetics* 50:476-82 (1992).

Billings, P., & Hubbard, R. "Fragile X testing: Who benefits? School-sponsored genetic screening program raises specter of discrimination." *geneWATCH* Vol. 9 #3-4 (Jan. 1994).

Casey, C. T. "Fragile X syndrome: Improving understanding & diagnosis." *J. American Medical Asso.* Vol. 271 (Feb. 1994).

Chapman, M. "Predictive testing for adult-onset genetic disease: Ethical & legal implications of the use of linkage analysis for Huntington disease." *American J. of Human Genetics* 47: 1-4 (1990).

Duster, T. *Back Door to Eugenics.* New York: Routledge, Chapman & Hall, 1990.

Genetic Discrimination: Position Paper. Cambridge, MA: Council for Responsible Genetics, n.d.

Genetic Tests & Health Insurance: Results of a Survey: Background Paper. (1992) Office of Technology Assessment, Congressional Board of the 102d Congress.

Holtzman, N. *Proceed with Caution: Predicting Genetic Risks in Recombinant DNA Era.* Baltimore: Johns Hopkins University Press, 1989.

Holtzman, N., & Rothstein, M. "Eugenics & genetic discrimination." *American J. of Human Genetics* 50:457-9 (1992).

Kapp, M. B. "Don't ask, don't tell? Ethical & legal implications of advances in genetic testing technology." *Legal Medicine.* (1994).

Kevles, D., & Hood, L., eds. *The Code of Codes: Scientific & Social Issues in the Human Genome Project.* Cambridge, MA: Harvard University Press, 1992.

Light, D. "The practice & ethics of risk-rated health insurance." *J. American Medical Asso.* Vol. 267 #18: 2503-508 (May 1992).

McEwen, J. R., & Reily, P. R. "State legislative efforts to regulate use & potential misuse of genetic information." *American J. of Human Genetics* Vol. 51 #3 (Sept. 1992).

Natowicz, H., Alper, J[ane], & Alper, J[oseph]. "Genetic discrimination & the law." *American J. of Human Genetics* 50:465-75 (1992).

Nelkin, D., & Tancredi, L. *Dangerous Diagnostics: The Social Power of Biological Information.* N.p.: Basic Books, 1989.

Ostrer, H., et al. "Insurance & genetic testing: Where are we now?" *American J. of Human Genetics* Vol. 52 (1993).

Weiss, R. "Predisposition & prejudice." *Science News* Vol. 135 (Jan. 1989).

Wertz, D. C., & Fletcher, J. C. "Disclosing genetic information: Who should know?" *Technology Review* (July 1989).

Wilkie, T. *Perilous Knowledge: The Human Genome Project & Its Implications.* Berkeley: University of California, 1993.

GLOSSARY OF MEDICAL TERMS

Abortion The interruption of pregnancy through expulsion of the fetus before it can survive outside the uterus (generally before the twentieth week of pregnancy). Abortion may be either induced (also called therapeutic) or spontaneous.

Abscess A localized build-up of pus due to the breakdown of tissue by bacteria.

Acidosis A disrupted acid/alkaline balance due to a depletion of the body's alkali supplies or a production of acid. The condition is linked with several disorders, such as diabetes.

Acne The inflammation of the sebaceous (oil) glands due to a build-up of sebum, a fatty substance discharged through the pores to lubricate the skin. The condition is associated with the hormonal changes of adolescence, but may occur at any age.

Addiction Physical and emotional dependence on a drug due to the body's adaptation to its presence.

Addison anemia See Pernicious anemia.

Addison disease A disorder caused by insufficient secretion of aldosterone and cortisol from the adrenal glands, resulting in a variety of serious symptoms.

Adhesion The abnormal union of body surfaces caused by fibrous scars formed when tissues heal.

Adolescence The stage of development between puberty and full maturity.

Adrenal glands Endocrine glands that are situated just above the kidneys and which secrete important hormones. Among the hormones secreted are epinephrine (adrenaline), which affects heart rate and blood circulation and is instrumental in the body's response to physical stress, and cortisone, a natural anti-inflammatory. See also Epinephrine, Cortisone.

Adrenaline See Epinephrine.

Adrenocorticotrophic hormone (ACTH) A hormone produced by the pituitary gland in order to induce the secretion of corticoids from the adrenal glands.

Afterbirth The collection of special tissues which are associated with fetal development and which are expelled after the delivery of the baby. See also Placenta.

Agalactia The inability to produce milk after childbirth.

AIDS (Acquired Immune Deficiency Syndrome) An incurable disease that attacks and weakens the body's immune system, leaving the patient open to opportunistic infections and disorders that normally would be warded off.

Albumin A protein found in animals, plants, and egg whites; the presence of albumin in the urine could indicate kidney disease.

Alcoholism Dependence on or addiction to alcohol. A poisoning of the body with alcohol. Physical damage can occur in the liver, heart, and kidneys as a result of alcohol poisoning. It can also lead to decreased resistance to infections.

Alkali Opposite of acid and acid neutralizer. Bicarbonate is the body's chief alkali.

Allergen Any agent that produces an allergic reaction. Common allergens include animal fur, pollen, dust, and certain foods. See also Allergy.

Allergy A hypersensitive or exaggerated reaction to exposure to certain substances (see also Allergen) or conditions such as sun rays. Manifestations of allergies include rashes, cold-like symptoms, headaches, gastrointestinal symptoms, and asthma.

Alveoli The microscopic air sacs in the lungs through which oxygen and carbon dioxide are exchanged.

Amenorrhea The failure to menstruate. Amenorrhea is a symptom of many diseases and conditions.

Amino acid The nitrogen-containing components of protein used by the body to build muscle and other tissue. Some essential amino acids must be supplied by eating high-protein foods while others are synthesized in the body.

Amnesia Memory loss.

Amniocentesis The extraction and examination of a small amount of the amniotic fluid in order to determine genetic and other disorders in the fetus. See also Amniotic fluid.

Amnion The bag of waters in which the fetus and the amniotic fluid are contained during pregnancy.

Amniotic fluid The fluid surrounding the fetus.

Amphetamine A drug that stimulates the central nervous system.

Analgesic Any substance that gives temporary relief from pain.

Androgens Hormones, such as testosterone and androsterone, which are produced in the testes and are responsible for male characteristics. They are also produced normally in small amounts in females.

Androsterone One of the male sex hormones.

Anemia A deficiency in the hemoglobin, the number of red blood cells, or in the amount of blood. Anemia is usually a symptom of an underlying disorder.

Anesthesia Loss of sensation or feeling. General anesthesia involves the whole body whereas local anesthesia involves only a particular area.

Anesthesiology The branch of medicine dealing with anesthesia and the application of anesthetic agents in surgery and pain relief.

Aneurysm A sac filled with blood which forms as a result of an abnormal widening of a vein or artery.

Angina Intense pain that produces a feeling of suffocation. The term is commonly used to refer to chest pains (angina pectoris) that are usually a result of an interruption of the oxygen supply to the heart muscle.

Angiography Examination of the interior blood vessels by injecting radiopaque substances so that any disorder or abnormality shows up on x-ray film. The record of pictures is called an angiogram.

Anoxia Oxygen deficiency.

Antacid An acid-neutralizing substance.

Antibiotic An antibacterial substance derived from bacteria, molds, and other substances. Penicillin is a common antibiotic.

Antibody The components of the immune system which eliminate or counteract foreign substances (antigens) in the body.

Anticoagulant An agent that retards the blood clotting process.

Antidote An agent that counteracts the effects of a poison.

Antigen A substance, usually a protein found in germs or foreign tissue, which stimulates the production of antibodies.

Antihistamine A drug that blocks histamine action. Since histamines are often produced in large amounts in response to allergens, they cause many of the symptoms associated with allergies; antihistamines are often used to relieve allergic reactions, such as hay fever or hives. Antihistamines also may be prescribed to counter nausea.

Antihypertensive Any drug that lowers blood pressure.

Antiseptic Any substance that prevents or slows the proliferation of germs or bacteria.

Antitoxin An antibody produced by or introduced into the body to counteract a poison.

Anus Opening at end of the rectum (last segment of the large intestine) through which fecal waste passes.

Anvil One of the tiny bones in the middle ear (also called the incus).

Anxiety Feelings of apprehension and undue uneasiness. Appropriate anxiety may occur in the face of identifiable danger. In contrast, clinical anxiety is the feeling of apprehension or fear even in the face of no identifiable hazards.

Aorta The body's largest artery, it carries blood from the left ventricle of the heart and distributes it to all parts of the body.

Aphasia Loss of the ability to speak or to understand speech due to brain damage. The organs of speech may be unimpaired.

Apnea The absence of breathing.

Appendicitis An inflammation of the appendix which results in severe pain on the lower right side, fever, and nausea or vomiting. Appendicitis calls for immediate medical attention, usually requiring removal of the appendix.

Aqueous humor The fluid in the anterior part of the eyeball.

Areola A round pigmented area around a raised center, such as the nipple of a breast.

Arrhythmia Any deviation from the regular heartbeat rhythm.

Arteriole A tiny artery that joins another artery to the capillaries.

Arteriosclerosis Also called hardening of the arteries, this condition involves a thickening of the walls of the arteries resulting in a loss of elasticity. See also Atherosclerosis.

Artery A blood vessel that transports oxygenated blood away from the heart to the rest of the body.

Arthritis Inflammation of a joint.

Ascorbic acid Vitamin C.

Asphyxia Suffocation due to lack of oxygen or overabundance of carbon dioxide.

Aspiration The removal of fluids from the lungs or other body cavities. A suction or siphoning implement is used.

Aspirin Acetylsalicylic acid. A drug used to relieve

Source: *The Columbia University College of Physicians and Surgeons Complete Home Medical Guide* (1989). With permission.

pain and lower fever. It is also an anti-inflammatory drug and anticoagulant.

Asthma A disorder of the respiratory system due to bronchial spasm that results in breathing difficulties.

Astigmatism A defect in one of the eye's surfaces that leads to an inability to focus the eye correctly.

Atherosclerosis A form of arteriosclerosis in which, in addition to the thickening and reduced elasticity of the arteries, a fatty substance (plaque) forms on the inner walls of the arteries and obstructs the flow of blood.

Athlete's foot See Tinea pedia.

Atrophy Wasting; degeneration of a body part through lack of activity or nourishment.

Auscultation A method of examining the body by listening, usually using a stethoscope.

Autoimmune disease Any disease in which the body manufactures antibodies against itself. The body regards its own tissue as a foreign substance and acts accordingly to eliminate it.

Bacilli Rod-shaped bacteria.

Bacteria One-celled microscopic organisms. Some cause disease, some are harmless, some are beneficial.

Bag of waters See Amnion.

Barbiturate A drug that produces a sedation, hypnosis, anesthesia, or sleep.

Barium tests Diagnostic tests using barium, a metallic element which does not permit x-rays to pass through and therefore makes internal organs visible on X-ray films. Common barium tests are the barium swallow (upper GI series) and the barium enema (lower GI series).

B cell A specialized type of white cell (lymphocyte) that works as part of the immune system by providing antibodies that attack foreign agents, such as bacteria or viruses.

Bedsore Decubitus ulcer, an ulcer-like sore on the skin as a result of the pressure of the bed against the body.

Bell's palsy A paralysis of the face muscles due to the inflammation of the facial nerve.

Benign Harmless or innocent. Term is used to describe a nonmalignant tumor which will not spread or grow back after removal.

Bile The bitter alkaline fluid secreted by the liver to aid in digestion. Bile is greenish yellow until it is stored in the gall bladder where it becomes concentrated and darker in color.

Biofeedback A behavior modification therapy by which a patient is taught to control involuntary body functions such as blood pressure.

Biopsy The examination of a small sample of tissue, taken from a patient's body, usually used to determine if a growth is cancerous.

Birth control See Contraception.

Birthmark A colored patch or skin blemish which is present at birth.

Blackhead An open comedo, in which a follicle is clogged by fatty substances secreted by the sebaceous glands. Its black coloration is caused by exposure to air, not dirt as is commonly assumed.

Bladder A sac containing fluid or gas.

Bladder infection See Cystitis.

Blastomycosis A fungal disease usually affecting the lungs but sometimes the whole system.

Blind spot The spot where the optic nerve and the retina connect. It is not light sensitive.

Blister An accumulation of fluid causing a raised sac under the surface of the skin.

Blood The body fluid circulated by the heart through a network of arteries, veins, and capillaries to provide oxygen and nutrients to all body cells and to remove carbon dioxide and wastes from them.

Blood clotting The process of blood coagulation in which blood platelets and proteins join together to close up a break in the circulatory system.

Blood corpuscle Either a red blood cell (erythrocyte) or a white blood cell (leukocyte).

Blood count The amount of red and white blood cells in the blood.

Blood plasma The part of the blood composed mostly of water (over 9%). The other constituents include electrolytes, nutrients, wastes, clotting agents, antibodies, and hormones.

Blood pressure The force exerted by the blood against the arterial walls. A sphygmomanometer measures both the systolic pressure (when the heart is at maximum contraction) and diastolic pressure (when the heart is relaxed between beats).

Blood serum The liquid that separates from the blood when it clots. It is the plasma without the clotting agents and is yellowish in color.

Blood sugar The glucose that is circulated in the blood. It is the end product of carbohydrate metabolism (although protein and some fat also may be converted to glucose) and is the body's major fuel.

Blood transfusion The intravenous replacement or replenishment of a patient's blood with healthy, compatible blood from an outside source.

Blood type Grouping of hereditary factors in the blood. The four major groupings are A, B, O, and AB. It is essential to determine if the donor's and recipient's blood types are compatible before a transfusion is administered.

Blood vessel A vein or artery.

Boil A round, painful, pus-filled bacterial infection of a hair follicle, usually caused by staphylococci (also called furuncle).

Bone The hard tissue of the skeleton.

Bone graft Transplantation of bone from one person to another or from one part of the body to another.

Boric acid A mild antiseptic powder which is poisonous if swallowed. It was once considered a useful household first-aid item, but it is no longer recommended because of its limited effectiveness and potential toxicity.

Botulism A dangerous form of food poisoning caused by the toxin produced by botulinus bacteria. The toxin attacks the nervous system causing headache, weakness, constipation, and paralysis. The causative bacterium grows in anaerobic (without oxygen) conditions and therefore is found in improperly canned or improperly refrigerated fresh foods.

Bowel Intestine, gut.

Brain The central organ of the nervous system consisting of the cerebrum, cerebellum, pons varolii, midbrain, and medulla.

Breast The mammary (milk-producing) gland and the fat and connective tissue around it.

Breech delivery (or presentation) Delivery of a baby with either the feet or buttocks, instead of the head, emerging first.

Bright's disease A term formerly used to describe nephrosis, a disease affecting the kidney's filtering units (nephrons).

Bromides A group of drugs once used as anticonvulsants because of their sedative effects on

the central nervous system. They have been replaced by newer, more effective drugs that do not have as high a risk of adverse reaction.

Bronchi The two tubes branching off at the lower part of the trachea (singular: bronchus).

Bronchiole Subdivision of a bronchus which leads to the alveoli in the lungs.

Bronchitis Inflammation of the bronchi.

Bronchopneumonia Bacterial infection that results in the inflammation of the bronchioles.

Bruise Damage to the subcutaneous blood vessels resulting in the escape of blood into other tissues. Characteristic features are pain, swelling, and discoloration of the skin. A bruise in which the outer layer of skin is not broken is called a contusion. An abrasion or laceration is a bruise in which the skin is broken.

Bulimia Excessive appetite. Also refers to the binge-purge syndrome in which deliberate overeating is compensated for through self-induced vomiting, laxative use, excessive exercise, or starvation.

Bunion A deformity of the big toe resulting from an inflammation of the joint that connects the toe to the foot.

Bursa A fibrous, fluid-filled sac in the joints which aids movement by decreasing friction.

Bursitis A painful condition involving inflammation of the bursa, a fluid-filled sac in a joint.

Caffeine A substance that stimulates the central nervous system. It is present in coffee, tea, chocolate, and certain soft drinks.

Calamine lotion A compound containing zinc oxide used to treat skin rashes, irritations, and other skin disorders.

Calcium An essential mineral. Calcium is the main material in teeth and bones and is vital to proper function of the heart, other muscles, and other body tissues.

Calculus Abnormal stone formation in certain parts of the body such as the gall bladder or kidneys. Calculi are composed of minerals, cholesterol, bile pigments, or other substances, depending upon their location (plural: calculi).

Callus (1) An area where the skin has become thick in order to protect itself against repeated friction. (2) The partly calcified tissue that forms around a broken bone in the healing process.

Calorie Measure of energy (heat) used in physics and in nutrition.

Cancer A general term referring to the abnormal reproduction of cells in the body. The term covers many malignant tumors affecting many parts of the body.

Candidiasis A yeast infection caused by the candida fungus. Also called moniliasis or thrush.

Canker sore An ulcer-like sore on the mucous membrane of the mouth or lips.

Capillary A minute thin-walled blood vessel, in a network which facilitates the exchange of substances between surrounding tissues and the blood.

Carbohydrates Organic compounds of carbon, hydrogen, and oxygen. They include starches, cellulose, and sugars and are divided into three groups: monosaccharides (simple sugars), disaccharides (containing two different sugars), and polysaccharides (complex sugars).

Carcinogen Any agent that is capable of causing cancer.

Carcinoma The type of cancer which originates in the epithelial cells located in glands, skin, and mucous membranes.

Cardiac Pertaining to the heart.

Cardiograph A device for tracing the movements of the heart. The record produced is called a cardiogram or electrocardiogram.

Cardiopulmonary Pertaining to the heart and lungs.

Cardiovascular Pertaining to the heart and blood vessels.

Carditis Inflammation of the heart.

Caries Tooth or bone decay.

Cartilage The white, elastic tissue located in joints, the nose, and the outer ear.

Cast Fibrous material that has collected in body cavities and hardens to the shape of them.

Castor oil An oil derived from a poisonous bean plant and which acts as a purgative or cathartic.

Castration The removal of ovaries or testes.

Cataract An opacity or clouding of the eye lens, which can eventually lead to loss of vision as progressively less light is filtered through the lens to the retina.

Cathartic Any substance that stimulates rapid intestinal activity resulting in bowel evacuation (also called purgative).

Catheterization Any procedure in which a small flexible tube is inserted into the body for the purpose of withdrawing or introducing substances.

Caustic Having the ability to destroy or corrode organic tissue.

Cauterization The application of caustic chemicals or electrically heated devices for the purpose of eliminating infected, unwanted, or dead tissue.

Cavities (1) Dental caries. (2) Hollow spaces.

Cell A minute mass of protoplasm containing a nucleus; the structural unit of body tissue.

Cellulose A polysaccharide carbohydrate (starch) found in plant cells. It is indigestible by humans but aids in the overall digestive process by providing roughage.

Cerebellum The movement-coordinating part of the brain.

Cerebral cortex The convoluted outer surface of the brain.

Cerebrum The largest part of the brain, containing two hemispheres and the cerebral cortex. The cerebrum controls thinking, feeling, and voluntary activities.

Cervix The neck or narrow part of the uterus.

Cesarean section Delivery of a baby through the abdominal wall by means of a surgical procedure.

Chancre The highly infectious ulcerated sore that is the first sign of syphilis.

Chemotherapy The use of chemicals to treat disease with minimal damage to the patient. Its use in the treatment of cancer is widespread and has increased life expectancy of patients.

Chilblains Painful and itchy swelling of the skin due to exposure to the cold.

Cholera An epidemic disease characterized by diarrhea, vomiting, thirst, and cramps. It is spread through polluted water.

Cholesterol A crystalline fat-like substance found in the brain, nerves, liver, blood, and bile. It is synthesized in the liver and is essential in the production of sex hormones, nerve function, and a number of other vital processes. Excessive consumption of dietary cholesterol (found only in animal products, such as fat, red meat, whole milk, and egg yolks) is thought to contribute to heart disease.

Chorea A disease of the nervous system manifested by spasmodic movements of the body.

Chromosome Any one of the rod-shaped bodies in the nucleus of a cell which carry hereditary factors.

Cirrhosis Chronic inflammation and hardening of an organ, usually the liver, but occasionally the heart or kidneys.

Cleft palate Congenital defect of the mouth in which the palate bones fail to fuse and result in a groove in the roof of the mouth. Cleft lip is often associated with cleft palate.

Climacteric Menopause.

Clitoris A small organ situated at the front of the vulva that is a source of female orgasm. It contains erectile tissue.

Colic Spasmodic pain in the abdomen.

Colitis Inflammation of the colon (large intestine), characterized by bowel spasms, diarrhea, and constipation. Ulcerative colitis is a more serious form of the disease, and is characterized by open sores in the lining of the colon and the passage of diarrhea streaked with blood and mucus.

Colon Large intestine extending from the small intestine to the rectum. Undigested food that is not absorbed by the body passes from the small intestine into the colon; water is extracted from the waste, which is eventually eliminated from the body in the form of a bowel movement.

Colostomy Surgical procedure to create an artificial anus in the abdominal wall.

Colostrum The pale yellow first milk secreted by women in the late stages of pregnancy and just after delivery.

Colposcope A magnifying device used to examine the cervix and vagina.

Coma State of unconsciousness from which one cannot be awakened.

Comedo See Blackhead.

Communicable disease Transmissable to other persons. Contagious.

Conception Impregnation of ovum by a sperm.

Concussion Injury resulting from a severe blow or shock to the head.

Congenital Existing at birth or before.

Congestive heart failure A condition in which weakened heart muscles are unable to pump strongly enough to maintain normal blood circulation. As a result, blood backs up in the lungs and veins leading to the heart. Often accompanied by accumulation of fluid in various parts of the body.

Conjunctiva The transparent membrane lining the front of the eyeball and eyelid.

Conjunctivitis Inflammation of the conjunctiva.

Constipation A condition of infrequent and difficult bowel movements.

Contraception Prevention of conception. Birth control.

Contraceptive An agent used in preventing conception.

Contusion A bruise; bleeding under the skin.

Convulsions Involuntary spasms due to abnormal cerebral stimulation.

Cornea Transparent membrane that protects the outer surface of the eye.

Corn A patch of thickened skin (callus) usually occurring around the toes and caused by friction or pressure.

Coronary Related to the coronary arteries, the blood vessels that supply the heart muscle with blood.

Coronary artery disease Progressive narrowing of the coronary arteries, usually due to a build-up of fatty plaques (atheromas) along the vessel walls. The most common cause of angina pectoris and heart attacks. See also Heart attack.

Coronary thrombosis The blockage of a coronary artery with a clot (thrombus), a common cause of heart attacks.

Corpuscle A small mass of protoplasm. Red corpuscles are called erythrocytes and white corpuscles are called leukocytes.

Cortisol A principal hormone produced by the adrenal gland.

Cortisone Hormone preparation closely related to cortisol which acts as an anti-inflammatory agent and is used in treating various diseases. Corticosteroid.

Coryza Acute upper respiratory infection lasting only a short while. Head cold.

Cowpox A viral disease of cattle used to vaccinate against smallpox in humans. Since the worldwide elimination of smallpox, vaccination against this disease is no longer necessary.

Cranium The section of the skull that encases the brain.

Curettage A scraping out of tissue from an organ (particularly the uterus) for diagnostic purposes with a fork-like instrument called a curette.

Cuspid Canine tooth; having only one point.

Cuticle The epidermis (outer layer of skin); dead skin, especially that which surrounds fingernails and toenails.

Cyanosis A condition in which tissue takes on a bluish tinge due to lack of oxygen.

Cyst An abnormal cavity or sac enclosing a fluid, gas, or semisolid substance.

Cystic fibrosis A hereditary respiratory disease occurring in early childhood. It is characterized by the build-up of mucus in the lungs and other abnormalities affecting the exocrine system (glands that secrete directly into their target organs, such as the sweat glands).

Cystitis A bladder infection that is more common in women, but which also occurs in men.

Cystoscopy A diagnostic procedure involving examination of the bladder with a cystoscope inserted through the urethra.

Cytology The study of the origins, structures, and functions of cells.

Dandruff A common condition in which white scales and flakes of dead skin appear on the scalp.

Debility Lessened ability; weakness.

Decubitus ulcer Bedsore.

Defibrillation Cessation of fibrillation (tremor or twitching of cardiac muscle) and resumption of normal heart rate through electric shock (defibrillator) or drugs.

Deficiency disease Disorder resulting from a nutritionally deprived diet or inability of the body to absorb needed nutrients.

Degenerative disease A group of diseases characterized by deterioration of body part(s) and resulting in progressive disability.

Dehydration Inadequate amount of fluids in the body caused by the removal or abnormal loss of fluids from the body, or from the failure to ingest sufficient fluids.

Delirium Mental disorder characterized by delusions or hallucinations. May be caused by disease, high fever, or drug use.

Delirium tremens Delirium suffered by chronic alcoholics as a result of withdrawal. Characterized by vivid hallucinations, uncontrollable trembling of hands, confusion, and nausea.

Delusion A false belief that persists even in the presence of contrary evidence.

Dementia Deterioration of mental faculties due to irreversible organic causes.

Dementia praecox Schizophrenia.

Dendrite One of the thread-like branches of the nerve cell that transmit impulses to the cell body.

Dentin The calcified tissue that encloses the tooth's pulp cavity.

Deoxyribonucleic acid (DNA) The fundamental component of all living matter, which controls and transmits the hereditary genetic code.

Depilatory Hair-removing agent.

Depressant An agent that produces a calming, sedative effect, slowing down body functions.

Depression An organic disease characterized by profound feelings of sadness, despair, and worthlessness unexplained by life's events. Depression is often recurring and interrupted by feelings of extreme euphoria, a condition referred to as bipolar depression or manic-depressive state.

Derma or **dermis** The skin.

Dermatitis Inflammation of the skin.

Desensitization (Immunotherapy) Neutralization of allergies by periodic exposure to progressively larger doses of the allergen.

Dextrose A form of glucose, a simple sugar.

Diabetes mellitus A chronic condition characterized by an overabundance of blood sugar due to insufficient insulin production in the pancreas or inability of the body to utilize insulin.

Dialysis A technique for separation of waste products or toxins from the bloodstream. Used in cases of kidney failure and overdose.

Diaphragm (1) The large muscle between the chest and the abdomen. (2) A dome-shaped rubber cap inserted vaginally to cover the cervix in order to prevent conception.

Diastole The interval between contractions of the heart (heartbeat) in which the heart relaxes. The diastolic reading obtained in blood pressure measurement is the lower number.

Diethylstilbestrol (DES) Synthetic estrogen hormone once used to prevent miscarriage. Its use is believed to have resulted in a higher incidence of vaginal and reproductive abnormalities, including difficulty in achieving or maintaining a pregnancy, among daughters born to women who took it. Sons may also suffer reproductive abnormalities. DES is also used to prevent conception if given promptly after unprotected intercourse (the so-called morning-after pill). Since it causes severe nausea and vomiting and other adverse effects, its use is limited primarily to rape victims.

Digestion The process by which food is transformed into absorbable nutrients.

Digit Finger or toe.

Dilation Enlargement or expansion of an organ or passageway (e.g., blood vessel, uterine cervix, or the pupil of the eye). May be artificially induced for therapeutic or diagnostic purposes.

Diplopia Double vision.

Disk (vertebral) The cartilage cushions between the vertebrae.

Dislocation The displacement of a bone from its normal position in a joint.

Diuretic Any substance that increases the flow of urine and excretion of body fluid.

Diverticulitis Inflammation of diverticula.

Diverticulosis A disorder in which diverticula, pouch-like sacs protruding from the wall of an organ, develop. Most commonly seen in the intestinal tract.

Dominant A term used in genetics to describe the stronger of two hereditary traits.

Dorsal Pertaining to the back.

Down syndrome A congenital condition that may include mental retardation and physical malformations caused by abnormal chromosomal distribution. Also called Trisomy 21. Formerly called mongolism.

Dropsy See Edema.

Duodenum The portion of the small intestine closest to the stomach.

Dura mater The outermost layer of fibrous membrane covering the brain and spinal cord. One of three types of meninges.

Dysentery Infectious inflammation of the bowel characterized by diarrhea, with passage of blood and mucus and severe abdominal cramps.

Dyslexia Learning disability characterized by impaired reading ability and tendency to reverse characters.

Dysmenorrhea Painful menstruation or cramps.

Dyspareunia Painful sexual intercourse.

Dyspepsia Indigestion.

Dysphagia Difficulty in swallowing.

Dyspnea Difficulty in breathing.

Dystrophy Wasting (decrease in size or mass) of body tissues, usually due to defective metabolism or nutrition.

Dysuria Painful urination.

Echography The use of ultrasound waves in detecting and diagnosing abnormalities. The result is called an echogram.

Eclampsia A sudden convulsive attack caused by toxemia during pregnancy.

Ectopic pregnancy Pregnancy in which the fertilized egg begins to develop outside the uterus, usually in a fallopian tube.

Eczema Skin rash characterized by itching and scaling.

Edema Swelling of body tissue caused by a build-up of fluid.

Effusion An accumulation of fluid between body tissues or in body cavities.

Ejaculation Emission of semen from the penis during the male orgasm.

Electrocardiography A diagnostic procedure in which metal plates (electrodes) are placed on body surfaces for the purpose of detecting and tracing electrical impulses from the heart. The resulting graph is called an electrocardiogram (EKG or ECG).

Electroencephalography A diagnostic procedure in which electrical impulses from the brain are traced and recorded through metal plates (electrodes) attached to the head. The resulting graph is called an electroencephalogram (EEG).

Electrolysis Decomposition or destruction by means of electricity.

Electroshock therapy (EST) The use of a controlled amount of electric current in treatment of severe depression. The electric shock is administered through electrodes placed on the head. It is not used as often today as in the past, but in selected patients it is still considered the most effective and fastest treatment for certain forms of depression.

Elephantiasis Enlargement and swelling of body parts as a symptom of a tropical disease caused by a parasitic worm in the lymphatic system.

Embolism Obstruction of a blood vessel by a solid body, called an embolus. Common emboli include blood clots, fat globules, or air bubbles.

Embryo The term used to refer to the fetus in the first 8 weeks after conception.

Emetic Agent that induces vomiting.

Emission Discharge of fluid.

Emphysema A respiratory disease characterized by progressive loss of elasticity of lung tissue, making it difficult to exhale stale air fully. Most commonly caused by smoking.

Empyema Accumulation of pus in a body cavity, usually the lungs.

Encephalitis Inflammation of the brain due to virus infection, lead poisoning, or other causes.

Endocrine system The physiological network of ductless glands which secrete hormones into the bloodstream to control the digestive and reproductive systems, growth, metabolism, and other processes.

Endometriosis A gynecological disease in which tissue normally found in the uterus grows in other areas.

Endometrium The lining of the uterus in which the fertilized ovum is implanted but which is shed during menstruation if conception has not taken place.

Endoscopy Diagnostic procedure using an illuminating optical instrument to examine a body cavity or internal organ.

Enema Fluid injected through the rectum to the lower bowel. Used to induce bowel movement or diagnose bowel disorders (barium enema).

Enteritis Inflammation of the intestine.

Enuresis Inability to control urination while sleeping. Bed-wetting.

Enzyme A substance, usually protein, which causes a chemical reaction. A catalyst.

Ephedrine Chemical used to dilate breathing passages and shrink mucous membranes. It also increases blood pressure and heart rate and therefore should be administered to heart patients only with discretion.

Epidermis Outermost layer of skin.

Epiglottis The flap of cartilage which covers the larynx in the act of swallowing and aids in directing food to the esophagus.

Epilepsy A disease of the nervous system characterized by convulsive seizures as a result of an imbalance in the electrical activity of the brain.

Epinephrine (also called adrenaline) The hormone produced by the medulla (inner core) of the adrenal glands. It is secreted in stressful situations in order to increase the body's capacity to respond or to speed up bodily processes.

Episiotomy An incision made in the final stages of childbirth from the vagina downward toward the anus.

Erection The stiffening or swelling of the penis or other erectile tissue as it becomes filled with blood.

Erysipelas A severe infectious skin disease caused by a streptococcal organism and characterized by swelling and redness.

Erythema Reddening of the skin from dilation of capillaries under the skin.

Erythroblastosis fetalis The anemic condition in infants due to Rh incompatibility between mother and child. The condition is seen in Rh positive babies born to Rh negative women. The mother builds antibodies against the baby's blood, destroying the red blood cells. It is seen only rarely in first babies because the mother usually is not exposed to the baby's blood until delivery. The condition can now be prevented by giving the mother a shot of Rh immune globulin shortly after the birth of an Rh incompatible baby. Some doctors also administer the shot to an Rh negative woman during the last trimester of pregnancy if there is a chance that the baby may be Rh positive; e.g., if the father has Rh positive blood.

Erythrocyte Red blood corpuscle.

Esophagus Tube that transports food from the mouth to the stomach.

Estrogen A primarily female sex hormone produced by the ovaries, adrenal glands, and placenta. In women it controls development of secondary sex characteristics, menstruation, and pregnancy. A small amount of estrogen is produced in the testes of men, and also in fat tissue.

Eustachian tube The tube that connects the middle ear to the pharynx.

Exophthalmos Protruding eyeballs, sometimes due to diseases of the thyroid gland.

Expectorant A drug that promotes the coughing of sputum.

Faint Brief loss of consciousness due to insufficient blood in the brain.

Fallopian tubes The two tubes extending one from each side of the uterus through which an egg must pass after release from the ovary. Also called oviducts.

Farsightedness Also called hyperopia. A disorder of the eyes which causes difficulty in focusing on close objects.

Fascia Thin connective tissues that join the skin to underlying tissues.

Fat An essential nutrient of animal or plant origin. May be saturated or unsaturated.

Fauces The opening from the throat to the pharynx.

Feces The waste matter discharged from the bowels.

Femur Thigh bone.

Fertility The ability to conceive.

Fertilization Impregnation of ovum by sperm cell.

Fetus The stage in human development after the eighth week of pregnancy.

Fever Abnormally high body temperature. Generally above 98.6°F or 37°C.

Fiber (1) Body tissue composed mainly of fibrils, tiny thread-like structures. (2) The plant cell components that are indigestible by humans. Dietary fiber. Roughage.

Fibrillation Uncoordinated tremors or twitching of cardiac muscle resulting in an irregular pulse.

Fibrin Protein formed in blood during clotting process.

Fibroid A benign tumor of fibromuscular tissue, usually occurring in the uterus.

Fibula The long, thin bone found in the lower leg.

Fission Splitting.

Fistula An abnormal connection between two body cavities.

Flat foot A congenital or acquired deformity in which there is only a slight, or no, arch between the toes and the heel of the foot.

Flatulence An overabundance of gas in the stomach or intestines.

Fluorine A chemical that in small amounts prevents tooth decay.

Fluoroscope A special X-ray that projects images on a screen. Used to observe the organs or bones while in motion.

Folic acid A B-complex vitamin, used to promote blood regeneration in cases of folate deficiency. Occurs naturally in liver, kidney, green vegetables, and yeast.

Follicle A small sac or tubular gland.

Fontanel A membranous spot on a baby's head where skull bones have not yet come together.

Foramen An opening. Usually used in reference to the opening in a bone through which blood vessels or nerves pass.

Forceps Surgical instrument used to grasp or compress tissues.

Fracture A crack or break in a bone.

Frontal Pertaining to the front of a structure.

Frostbite Freezing of the skin as a result of exposure to extreme cold. Affected area may become red and inflamed.

Fulminating Developing quickly with great severity.

Fungicide Any substance that eliminates fungi.

Fungus A low form of vegetable life including some which can cause disease. Fungal infections.

Furuncle (boil) A round, painful, pus-filled bacterial infection of a hair follicle.

Gall bladder A membranous sac that is situated below the liver and condenses and stores the bile drained from the liver.

Gallstones Stone-like masses that form in the gall bladder. May be composed of calcium, bile pigment, and/or cholesterol.

Gammaglobulin The type of blood protein that contains antibodies to fight infection. Gamma-globulin can be separated from other constituents in blood and used to prevent or treat infections.

Ganglion (1) A mass of nerve tissue, a nerve center. (2) A cystic tumor in a tendon sheath.

Gangrene Death of body tissue usually due to loss of blood supply. Affected area becomes shrunken and black.

Gastrectomy Surgical removal of a part or all of the stomach.

Gastric Pertaining to the stomach.

Gastric juice Acidic secretion of the stomach containing enzymes and hydrochloric acid to aid in digestion.

Gastric ulcer A peptic ulcer that forms in the stomach.

Gastritis Inflammation of the stomach.

Gastroenteritis Inflammation of the mucous membranes of the stomach and intestines.

Gastroenterology Study of the stomach and intestines and the diseases affecting them.

Gastrostomy Surgically formed fistula between the stomach and abdominal wall.

Gene A part of the chromosome that determines hereditary characteristics.

Genetics The study of heredity.

Genitals/genitalia Reproductive organs.

Geriatrics The branch of medical science devoted to diseases of the aged.

Germ Microorganism usually associated with causing disease.

Germicide Germ-killing agent.

Gerontology The study of aging and the diseases associated with it.

Gestation Pregnancy.

Gingivitis Inflammation of the gums.

Gland Any organ that produces and secretes a chemical substance used by another part of the body. Ductless, or endocrine, glands secrete into the bloodstream. Exocrine glands transport the secretion directly to a particular location.

Glandular fever Infectious mononucleosis.

Glans penis The head of the penis.

Glaucoma A disease of the eye in which increased pressure within the eye damages the retina and optic nerve. Leads to impaired sight and sometimes blindness.

Globulin The portion of blood protein in which antibodies are formed.

Globus hystericus The feeling of a lump in the throat due to hysteria, anxiety, or depression. Sometimes accompanied by difficulty in swallowing.

Glomerulus (glomeruli) A small tuft of blood capillaries in the kidney, responsible for filtering out waste products.

Glucose (dextrose or blood sugar) The most common monosaccharide (simple sugar) and the main source of energy for humans. It is stored as glycogen in the liver and can be quickly converted back into glucose.

Glucose tolerance test Test to determine body's response to a glucose challenge. Used to detect hypoglycemia or diabetes.

Glycogen Animal starch. The form in which glucose is stored in the liver. Glycogen is easily converted into glucose for body use as energy.

Glycosuria Sugar in the urine.

Goiter Enlargement of the thyroid gland which causes swelling on the front of the neck.

Gonad Primary sex gland. Ovary in the female; testis in the male.

Gonococci Kidney-shaped gonorrhea-causing bacteria.

Gonorrhea A common venereal disease caused by the gonococcus bacterium and characterized by inflammation of the urethra, difficulty in urination (in males), and inflammation of the cervix (in females).

Gout A metabolic disorder in which an overabundance of uric acid causes urate crystals to form in the joints and sometimes elsewhere.

Graafian follicles Tiny vesicles in the ovaries which contain ova before release (ovulation).

Graft Transplantation of tissue or skin from one part of the body to another.

Gram-negative or **gram-positive** Method of classifying bacteria according to how they are affected when stained with alcohol.

Grand mal A severe epileptic attack in which convulsions are accompanied by loss of consciousness.

Granulation The new skin tissue containing capillaries, blood vessels, and reparative cells that forms in a wound's healing process.

Granulocytes White blood cells (leukocytes) containing granules. They are manufactured in the bone marrow to digest and destroy bacteria.

Granuloma A tumor or growth containing granulation tissue.

Granuloma inguinale A contagious venereal disease characterized by ulcers on the genitals.

Gravel Fine, sand-like particles composed of the same substance as kidney stones but usually passed in the urine without notice.

Graves disease One form of hyperthyroidism or an overactive thyroid gland, usually accompanied by abnormalities of the eyes and skin.

Gravid Pregnant.

Greenstick fracture Incomplete fracture due to the pliability of the bone. Usually occurs in children whose bones are still growing.

Grippe Influenza.

Gristle See Cartilage.

Groin The lower abdominal area where the trunk and thigh join. Also called the inguinal area.

Gumma A fibrous tumor filled with a rubber-like substance which occurs in the brain, liver, or heart in the late stages of syphilis.

Gynecology The branch of medical science that deals with the normal functioning and diseases of women's reproductive organs.

Gynecomastia Abnormal enlargement of the male mammary glands (breasts).

Halitosis Technical term for bad breath.

Hallucination A false perception believed to be real but actually having no basis in fact.

Hallucinogen Agent capable of producing hallucinations. Psychedelic drug.

Hallus valgus See Bunion.

Hallux The big toe.

Hammertoe A permanent hyperextension of the toe which cannot be flattened.

Hamstring Group of tendons at the back of the knee.

Hangnail A piece of skin partly detached from the side of a nail which becomes irritated and inflamed.

Hansen's disease Leprosy.

Harelip Congenital defect of the lip due to a failure of bones to unite, causing a split from the margin of the lip to the nostril. Cleft lip.

Hay fever An allergic reaction to pollen in which mucous membranes of the eyes, nose, and throat become inflamed.

Hearing aid Device used to amplify sounds for those with hearing difficulties.

Heart The muscular organ that pumps blood through the body. It is situated between the lungs and behind the sternum (breastbone).

Heart attack Myocardial infarction. Damage to part of the heart muscle caused by interruption of the blood circulation in the coronary arteries.

Heart block A condition of varying degree in which an abnormality in the tissues connecting the auricles (atria) and ventricles interferes with the normal transmission of electrical impulses. It may lead to disturbances in the heart's rhythm or pumping action.

Heartburn Burning sensations in the upper abdomen or behind the sternum. Usually caused by the regurgitation of gastric juices into the esophagus.

Heart failure See Congestive heart failure.

Heart-lung machine An apparatus that takes over for the heart during open heart surgery. The blood bypasses the heart, is oxygenated in the machine, and is pumped back into the body.

Heart murmur Any of various sounds heard in addition to the regular heartbeat. Often associated with a diseased heart valve, but may also have a benign or harmless cause.

Heat exhaustion Collapse, with or without loss of consciousness, due to extreme heat conditions and loss of salt through sweating. In attempts to cool the body surface, blood accumulates close to the skin, thus depriving the vital organs of full blood supply.

Heat stroke An emergency condition in which the sweating mechanism of the body fails, resulting in an extremely high body temperature.

Hemangioma A malformation of blood vessels which appears as a red, often elevated mark on the skin. It may be present at birth and may require treatment if it fails to disappear on its own.

Hematemesis Vomiting of blood.

Hematology The scientific study of blood.

Hematoma A blood-filled swelling resulting from blood vessels injured or ruptured by a blow.

Hematuria The presence of blood in the urine.

Hemiplegia Paralysis affecting one side of the body.

Hemochromatosis (bronzed diabetes) Abnormal accumulation of iron deposits in the body as a result of a metabolic disturbance. Symptoms include a bronzing of the skin, diabetes, and cirrhosis of the liver.

Hemodialysis Removal of waste materials from the blood. The artificial kidney was designed to perform this function.

Hemoglobin The red pigmented protein in red blood cells that contains iron. Hemoglobin is responsible for transporting oxygen to body tissue and removing carbon dioxide from body tissue.

Hemolysis Breaking down of red blood cells.

Hemophilia An inherited blood disorder in which the blood is unable to clot, causing severe bleeding from even minor wounds. The disease affects only males but is passed on by female carriers.

Hemoptysis Spitting up blood.

Hemorrhage Abnormal bleeding due to rupture of a blood vessel.

Hemorrhoids (piles) Varicose veins in and around the rectal opening. Hemorrhoid symptoms include pain, bleeding, and itching.

Hemostat An instrument that prevents bleeding by clamping a blood vessel.

Heparin Anticoagulant substance that is found in the liver and other tissues. It is sometimes administered to prevent blood clots. It also may be used to treat a threatened stroke, thrombophlebitis, and various clotting diseases.

Hepatitis Inflammation of the liver, usually due to a viral infection but can be the result of alcoholism and other conditions. Hepatitis B is transmitted through blood contact (e.g., contaminated hypodermic needles or transfused blood from a hepatitis B carrier). Hepatitis A is transmitted through fecal contact, usually contaminated food. A third type, non-A, non-B, is not as well understood as the other two.

Hepatoma Tumor of the liver.

Heredity The transmission of traits from parents to offspring. Genetic information is carried by the chromosomes.

Hermaphrodite An individual possessing both the male and female sex organs.

Hernia The abnormal protrusion of part or all of an organ through surrounding tissues.

Heroin An addictive narcotic derived from opium.

Herpes simplex Recurring infection caused by herpes virus. Type I involves blister-like sores usually around the mouth, referred to as cold sores or fever blisters. Type 2 usually affects the mucous membranes of the genitalia and can be spread by sexual contact. In unusual circumstances, either type can cause damage to other parts of the body, such as the eyes or brain. Also, the distinction between Type I and Type 2 herpes is not as clear as once thought; either virus can cause genital or oral sores.

Herpes zoster (shingles) A painful viral infection resulting in inflammation and blisters following the path of a nerve. It is caused by the same virus that causes chickenpox, which remains in the body in a latent form and may erupt many years later in an attack of shingles.

Heterosexuality Sexual orientation to persons of the opposite sex.

Hiatus hernia A disorder in which a portion of the stomach protrudes through the esophageal opening of the diaphragm. May cause symptoms of indigestion, heartburn, or regurgitation of food.

Hiccups (hiccoughs) An involuntary spasm of the diaphragm followed by the sudden closing of the glottis which coincides with the intake of a breath.

High blood pressure See Hypertension.

Histamine A chemical found in body tissue and released to stimulate production of gastric juices for digestion. In an allergic reaction, excessive amounts of histamine are produced and cause surrounding tissue to become inflamed. Antihistamines are thus prescribed for relief from allergic attacks.

Hives (urticaria) Itchy red and white swellings that appear on the skin, usually in an allergic reaction.

Hodgkin disease A serious disorder of the lymphatic system in which the lymph nodes enlarge. Type of cancer.

Homograft Tissue or organ transplantation from one individual to another of the same species.

Homosexuality Sexual orientation to persons of one's own sex.

Hormone Secretion from an endocrine gland transported by the bloodstream to various organs in order to regulate vital functions and processes.

Hyaline A glass-like substance that occurs in cartilage or the eyeball.

Hyaline membrane disease (respiratory distress syndrome) A condition affecting newborn premature infants in which the air sacs in the lungs are immature and clogged with hyaline, a crystalline material that makes effective breathing difficult or impossible.

Hydrocele An abnormal accumulation of fluid, usually in the sac of the membrane that covers the testicle.

Hydrocephalus (water on the brain) Abnormal increase in cerebral fluid resulting in enlarged head.

Hydrochloric acid An acid, composed of hydrogen and chlorine, secreted by the stomach in the process of digestion.

Hydrolysis Division into simple substance(s) by the addition of water.

Hydrophobia See Rabies.

Hydrotherapy Treatment of disease or injury by use of baths or wet compresses.

Hymen The membrane partially covering the entrance to the vagina.

Hyperchlorhydria Excessive hydrochloric acid in the gastric juice.

Hypercholesterolemia Excessive amounts of cholesterol in the blood, due to a metabolic disorder in which the body manufactures too much cholesterol or cannot process it correctly.

Hyperemesis Excessive vomiting.

Hyperemesis gravidarum Excessive vomiting during pregnancy, commonly referred to as morning sickness.

Hyperglycemia Excessive amounts of sugar in the blood. One of the indications of diabetes.

Hyperhidrosis Excessive sweating.

Hyperinsulinism A condition in which excessive amounts of insulin cause abnormally low blood sugar. Similar to insulin shock.

Hyperkinesis Hyperactivity. Excessive movement or activity.

Hyperopia Farsightedness.

Hyperplasia Overgrowth of an organ caused by an increase in the number of normal cells.

Hypertension High blood pressure. A condition in which the arterioles constrict and cause the heart to pump harder in order to distribute the blood to the body, thus elevating blood pressure.

Hyperthyroidism Overactivity of the thyroid gland. Symptoms include weight loss, restlessness, and sometimes goiters.

Hypertrophy Increased size of a body tissue or organ usually in response to increased activity.

Hypnosis A trance-like state in which a person's consciousness is altered to make him or her susceptible to suggestion.

Hypnotic A drug that induces sleep.

Hypochondria Excessive anxiety about and preoccupation with illness and supposed ill health.

Hypoglycemia Low blood sugar. Hypoglycemic shock due to insulin overdose is another term for insulin shock.

Hypophysis The pituitary gland.

Hypospadias A congenital malformation of the urethra.

Hypotension Low blood pressure.

Hypothalamus The part of the brain just above the pituitary gland. It has a part in controlling basic functions such as appetite, procreation, sleep, and body temperature and may be affected by the emotions.

Hypothyroidism Abnormal inactivity or decrease in activity of the thyroid.

Hysterectomy Surgical removal of the uterus.

Hysteria A neurosis, usually due to mental conflict and repression, in which there is uncontrollable excitability or anxiety.

Iatrogenic disease Any disorder or disease caused as an unintentional side effect of a physician's prescribed treatment.

Ichthyosis A congenital disorder in which the skin is dry and scaly.

Icterus Jaundice.

Idiopathic Peculiar to an individual or originating from unknown causes.

Ileitis Inflammation of the ileum (lower portion of the small intestine). Crohn disease.

Ileum The lower portion of the small intestine.

Ilium Broad upper part of the hip bone.

Immobilization Making a bone or joint immovable in order to aid in correct healing.

Immunity State of resistance to a disease. Active immunity is acquired by vaccination against it or by previous infection. Passive immunity is acquired from antibodies either from the mother through the placenta during gestation or from injection of serum from an animal that has active immunities.

Immunization The procedure by which specific antibodies are induced in the body tissue.

Impacted Wedged in tightly and abnormally immovable.

Imperforate Without normal opening.

Impetigo Highly contagious inflammatory pustular skin disease caused by staphylococci or streptococci.

Impotence Inability of the male to achieve penile erection and engage in sexual intercourse.

Incisors The 8 sharp cutting teeth, 4 in each jaw.

Incontinence Inability to control release of urine or feces.

Incubation period The interval of time between contact with disease organisms and first appearance of the symptoms.

Incubator A temperature- and atmosphere-controlled container in which premature or delicate babies can be cared for. Also a container in which bacteria or other organisms are grown for cultures.

Incus The small bone of the middle ear which conducts sounds to the inner ear.

Indigestion An abnormality in the digestive process. Dyspepsia.

Induration Hardening of tissue.

Infarct An area of dead tissue as a result of a total blockage of the blood supply.

Infertility Inability to reproduce.

Inflammation The reaction of tissue to injury, infection, or irritation. Affected area may become painful, swollen, red, and hot.

Influenza (flu) A contagious viral infection that occurs in epidemics.

Inguinal Pertaining to the groin.

Inoculation The intentional introduction of a disease agent to the body to cause a mild form of the disease and thereby induce immunity to it.

Inoperable Not treatable by surgery.

Insemination Introduction of semen into the vagina either through sexual intercourse or artificially.

Insomnia Inability to sleep. Can be chronic or occasional.

Insulin The hormone produced and secreted by the beta cells of the pancreas gland. Insulin is needed for proper metabolism, particularly of carbohydrates, and the uptake of sugar (glucose) by certain body tissues.

Insulin shock Loss of consciousness caused by an overdose of insulin.

Integument The skin.

Intention tremor Involuntary trembling triggered or intensified when movement is attempted.

Interferon A complex natural protein that causes cells to become resistant to infection.

Intertrigo (chafing) Superficial inflammation of opposing skin surfaces that rub together.

Intestines The section of the digestive tract extending from the stomach to the anus.

Intima Innermost lining of an artery.

Intracutaneous test Introduction of allergens into the skin in order to test sensitivity to particular substances.

Intrauterine contraceptive device (IUD) Device made of stainless steel, silkworm gut, or plastic which is inserted by a physician into the uterus to prevent pregnancy.

Intravenous Into or within a vein.

Intravenous feeding Nourishment through a glucose solution and other nutrients injected directly into a vein.

Involution of uterus Shrinking of the uterus to normal size after childbirth.

Iris The round, colored portion of the eye that surrounds the pupil.

Iritis Inflammation of the iris.

Iron The essential mineral micronutrient of hemoglobin.

Iron lung A respirator. A machine that artificially expands and contracts to facilitate breathing for patients with paralyzed respiratory muscles.

Irreducible Incapable of being replaced to normal position. Applied to fractured bones or to hernia.

Ischemia Localized blood deficiency, usually as a result of a circulatory problem. For example, cardiac ischemia results when a coronary artery is so occluded that it cannot deliver sufficient blood to the heart muscle.

Islets of Langerhans The groups of cells (alpha and beta) in the pancreas that secrete endocrine hormones; the alpha cells produce glucagon, and the beta cells produce insulin.

Isotope A chemical element similar to another chemical element in structure and properties but differing in radioactivity or atomic weight.

Jaundice Yellow discoloration of the skin and eyes caused by excessive amounts of bile pigments in the bloodstream.

Jejunum Part of the small intestine situated between the duodenum and the ileum.

Jigger Sand flea that burrows into skin to lay eggs, causing itching and inflammation (also called chigger).

Jock itch See Tinea cruris.

Joint The point where two or more bones connect.

Jugular veins The two veins on the sides of the neck that carry blood from the head to the heart.

Kala-azar A chronic infection transmitted by sand flies that occurs mainly in the tropics and Asia. Symptoms include anemia, fever, and emaciation.

Keloid An overgrowth of scar tissue after injury or surgery.

Keratin Substance that is the chief constituent of the horny tissues, such as the outer layer of skin, nails, and hair.

Keratitis Inflammation of the cornea.

Ketogenic diet A diet that results in the excessive burning of fat, which can lead to ketosis.

Ketosis The buildup of ketone bodies, highly acidic substances, in the body. Often associated with diabetes, the condition can lead to a fatal coma.

Kidneys The two bean-shaped glands that regulate the salt, volume, and composition of body fluids by filtering the blood and eliminating wastes through production and secretion of urine.

Kinesthesia Perception of movement, position, and weight. Muscle sense.

Klinefelter syndrome Chromosomal abnormality in which an individual has two X and one Y sex chromosomes. As a result, the individual appears to be male but has oversized breasts, underdeveloped testes, and is sterile.

Kneecap Patella.

Knee jerk Reflex reaction in which the foot kicks forward in response to a tap on the ligament below the kneecap.

Kwashiorkor A disease caused by protein deficiency due to malnutrition. It occurs most often in underdeveloped countries where children do not receive enough protein (through milk or meat) in their diets. Symptoms include growth retardation, apathy, anemia, and abnormal distension of the abdomen.

Kyphosis A rounding of the shoulders or hunchback caused by poor posture or disease, such as osteoporosis.

Labia Lip-like organs. Labia majora: two folds of skin and fatty tissue that encircle the vulva. Labia minora: the smaller folds inside the labia majora that protect the clitoris.

Labor (parturition) The rhythmic muscle contraction of the uterus in the process of childbirth.

Laceration A wound caused by the tearing of tissue.

Lacrimal ducts (lacrimal or tear glands) Glands at the upper edge of the eyes which secrete tears.

Lactation Production and secretion of milk by the breasts.

Lactic acid Acid produced by the fermentation of lactose; a waste product from the muscles.

Lactose A sugar contained in milk.

Lactovegetarian Vegetarian who eats dairy products.

Lancet Small double-edged knife used in surgery.

Lanolin Fat derived from wool and used as an ointment or lotion base.

Laryngitis Inflammation of the larynx characterized by hoarseness or complete loss of voice.

Larynx Voicebox. A cartilaginous structure containing the apparata of voice production: the vocal cords and the muscles and ligaments which move the cords.

Laser Light Amplification by Stimulated Emission of Radiation.

Laser beam A beam of intense controlled light which can sever, eliminate, or fuse body tissue.

Laxative Any agent that encourages bowel activity by loosening the contents.

Lead poisoning Intoxication from ingestion of lead.

Lecithin A waxy, fatty compound found in cell protoplasm.

Lens The transparent tissue of the eye which focuses rays of light in order to form an image on the retina.

Leprosy An infectious skin disease caused by bacteria and affecting the nerves and skin with ulcers.

Leptospirosis (infectious jaundice) An infectious disease spread to humans by urine of infected animals. Symptoms include jaundice.

Lesion Any breakdown of tissue, i.e., wound, sore, abscess, or tumor.

Leukemia A group of diseases of the blood-forming organs in which a proliferation of bone marrow and lymphoid tissue produces an over-abundance of white blood cells (leukocytes) and disrupts normal production of red blood cells. A form of cancer.

Leukocytes White blood cells instrumental in fighting infection.

Leukocytosis Abnormal increase in the number of white blood cells in the body, often due to the physiological response to infection.

Leukopenia Abnormal deficiency of white blood cells.

Leukorrhea Vaginal discharge of mucus. When discharge is heavy, it may be a sign of infection or disease.

Libido Term used by Freud for the desire for sensual satisfaction. Commonly used to mean sexual desire.

Ligament The tough, fibrous band of tissue that connects bones.

Ligature A thread of silk or catgut on wire used to tie off blood vessels to prevent bleeding during surgery.

Lipid Fat or fat-like substance such as cholesterol or triglycerides.

Lipoma A benign tumor composed of fat cells.

Lithiasis Formation of gallstones or kidney stones (calculi).

Litholapaxy Method of crushing a stone and removing its fragments from the urinary bladder through a catheter.

Lithotomy Removal of stone by cutting into the bladder.

Lithuresis Elimination of gravel in the urine.

Liver The largest internal organ of the body. Among its many functions are secreting bile and digestive enzymes, storing glycogen, neutralizing poisons, synthesizing proteins and several blood components, and storing certain vitamins and minerals.

Lobotomy Surgical disconnection of nerve fibers between the frontal lobe and the rest of the brain. Once commonly used to calm uncontrollable mental patients.

Lochia Vaginal discharge of blood, mucus, and tissue after childbirth.

Lockjaw See Tetanus.

Lordosis Swayback. Condition in which the inward curve of the lumbar spine is exaggerated.

Low blood sugar Hypoglycemia.

Lues Syphilis.

Lumbago Lower back pain.

Lumbar Lower back between the pelvis and the ribs.

Lungs Two organs of sponge-like tissue which surround the bronchial tree to form the lower respiratory system. Vital to oxygenation of blood and expulsion of gaseous waste from the body.

Lupus erythematosus An inflammatory auto-immune disease. Systemic lupus erythematosus involves deterioration of the body's connective tissues.

Lymph Transparent yellowish fluid containing lymphocytes and found in lymphatic vessels. Lymphatic fluid.

Lymph nodes Oval-shaped organs throughout the body that manufacture lymphocytes and filter germs and foreign bodies from the lymph.

Lymphocytes A disease-fighting type of leukocyte manufactured in the lymph nodes and distributed in the lymphatic fluid and blood.

Lymphogranuloma venereum A sexually transmitted viral disease that causes sores around genitals and swollen lymph nodes in the male groin.

Lymphosarcoma Malignant tumor of lymphatic tissue.

Maceration The softening of tissue in contact with fluid.

Macula Spot of discolored skin.

Macula lutea The small, yellow round spot on the retina. Center of color perception and clearest vision.

Madura foot Mycetoma; fungus infection of the foot characterized by swelling and development of cyst-like nodules. Occurs mostly in India and the tropics.

Malabsorption Defective absorption of nutrients in the small intestine. Malabsorption syndrome is characterized by steatorrhea (loose fatty stool) or diarrhea, weight loss, weakness, and anemia.

May be caused by lesions on the intestine, metabolic deficiencies, or surgery.

Malacia Softening of a part.

Malaise A general feeling of illness and discomfort. Tiredness, irritability, and listlessness.

Malaria A tropical parasitic disease spread by mosquitoes. Symptoms include chills, fever, and sweating.

Mal de mer Seasickness.

Malignant Harmful, life-threatening. Used mostly in reference to a cancerous tumor.

Malingering Deliberate feigning of illness.

Malleus The largest of the three bones in the inner ear.

Malnutrition Insufficient nourishment due to poor diet or defect in body's assimilation.

Malocclusion Failure of the upper teeth to mesh properly with lower teeth.

Malpresentation Any abnormal position of the fetus in the birth canal.

Mammary gland Milk-secreting gland of the breast.

Mammography Diagnostic x-ray examination of the breasts.

Mandible Lower jawbone.

Mania Mood of undue elation and excitability often accompanied by hallucinations and increased activity.

Manic-depressive psychosis Mental illness characterized by alternating periods of depression and mania.

Manubrium The handle-shaped upper part of the breastbone.

Marijuana The hemp, or cannabis, plant. A hallucinogenic drug.

Marrow The soft substance present in bone cavities. Red marrow is responsible for red blood cell production. Yellow marrow is marrow which is no longer involved in making blood cells.

Massage Rubbing, kneading, and pressing the parts of the body for therapeutic purposes. Massage can stimulate circulation, reduce tension, relax muscles, and reduce pain.

Mastectomy Surgical removal of breast tissue.

Mastication Chewing.

Mastitis Inflammation of the breast.

Mastoid cells Hollow areas (air cells) located in the middle ear.

Mastoiditis Inflammation of the mastoid cells usually as a consequence of an untreated ear infection.

Masturbation Manipulation of the genitals for the purpose of deriving sexual pleasure.

Materia medica The study of the origin, preparation, and use of medicinal substances.

Maxilla Upper jaw.

Measles An acute infectious disease characterized by fever, rash, and inflammation of mucous membranes. It is caused by a virus.

Meatus A passage or opening.

Meconium The greenish pasty discharge from the bowels of a newborn baby.

Mediastinum The space that separates the two lungs and contains the heart, thymus, esophagus, and trachea.

Medicine (1) Science of healing. (2) A therapeutic substance.

Medulla The center of an organ, gland, or bone.

Medulla oblongata The brain part connected to the spine.

Megalomania Delusions of grandeur. Symptom of insanity characterized by an exaggerated self-image.

Melanin Dark pigment found in hair, skin, and choroid of the eye.

Melanoma Tumor composed of cells containing melanin. Mostly benign, but malignant melanoma is a rare and serious form of skin cancer.

Membrane A thin layer of lining of tissue.

Menarche Commencement of first menstrual period.

Meninges Membrane covering the brain and spinal cord.

Meningitis Inflammation of the meninges.

Menopause The end of the female reproductive cycle. Commonly referred to as the change of life.

Menorrhagia Unusually heavy menstrual bleeding.

Menstruation The discharge of blood and tissue from the uterus every 28 days and lasting 4 or 5 days.

Mescaline A hallucinogen.

Mesencephalon The midbrain. The region between the cerebrum and the cerebellum.

Mesentery The folds in the abdominal lining between the intestine and the abdominal wall. They support the abdominal organs and supply them with blood and nerves.

Metabolism The combination of chemical and physical changes in the body essential for maintaining life processes. Basal metabolism is the minimum amount of energy required to sustain life while resting.

Metastasis The spread of disease from one body part to another, usually by transfer of cells or germs through the blood or lymph.

Methadone An addictive synthetic narcotic used instead of morphine and administered in drug treatment centers to heroin addicts. Also may be used as a painkiller under some circumstances.

Metritis Inflammation of the uterus.

Metrorrhagia Bleeding from the uterus between menstrual periods.

Microtome A surgical instrument for cutting thin slices of body tissue for study.

Micturition Urination.

Migraine headache Periodic severe headaches usually affecting only one side of the head and often accompanied by nausea or vomiting, inability to look at light, and fluid retention. Also referred to as vascular headaches.

Miliaria Prickly heat, heat rash. Sweat trapped under skin because of gland obstruction. Produces itching, prickling pimples on the skin.

Miosis Contraction of the pupil of the eye.

Miscarriage See Abortion.

Mitosis Cell division.

Mitral valve The valve that allows oxygenated blood into the left ventricle from the left atrium.

Molars Grinding teeth at the back of both jaws.

Mongolism See Down syndrome.

Moniliasis Yeast infection usually caused by candida albicans and affecting the mucous membranes such as the lining of the vagina, mouth, and gastrointestinal tract, and the skin and nails.

Monocyte The largest type of white blood cell.

Mononucleosis, infectious A communicable disease in which the number of monocytes in the bloodstream increases. Symptoms include fever, swollen lymph nodes, and general malaise.

Mons veneris (or mons pubis) The pad of fatty tissue that covers the pubic bone of the female.

Morning sickness Nausea during the early stages of pregnancy.

Morphine A pain-relieving narcotic derived from the opium plant.

Motor Pertaining to movement, action.

Mountain sickness A temporary onset of symptoms of difficult breathing, headache, thirst, and nausea brought on by decreased oxygen in air at high altitudes.

Mucous Pertaining to mucus.

Mucous colitis Usually a functional disorder of the bowel characterized by mucus in the stool.

Mucous membrane Thin layers of tissue containing mucus-secreting glands.

Mucus The viscid secretion of mucous glands which moistens body linings.

Multiple sclerosis A degenerative disease affecting the central nervous system and brain, characterized by increasing disability.

Mumps A contagious disease affecting mostly children. Symptoms include painful swollen glands.

Muscle Body tissue that has the ability to contract.

Muscular dystrophy A disease appearing in childhood characterized by a wasting of muscles.

Myalgia Pain in the muscles.

Myasthenia Muscle fatigue or weakness. Myasthenia gravis is a chronic, progressive disease characterized by weakness of the voluntary muscles, especially those of the eyelids.

Mycetoma See Madura foot.

Mydriasis Abnormal dilation of the pupil.

Myelin The white fatty substance that covers most nerves like a sheath.

Myelitis Inflammation of the spinal cord or bone marrow.

Myeloma Malignant tumor of the cells derived from the bone marrow.

Myocardial infarction See Heart attack.

Myoma A tumor of muscle tissue.

Myopathy Any disease of the muscle.

Myopia Nearsightedness.

Myringitis Inflammation of the eardrum.

Myxedema Thyroid deficiency characterized by a slowdown in metabolism and body function. See Hypothyroidism.

Myxoma A tumor of the connective tissue containing mucoid cells.

Narcolepsy Neurological disorder characterized by an irresistible tendency to sleep.

Narcosis Unconsciousness and insensibility to pain brought on by a drug (narcotic).

Narcosynthesis A method for treating psychoneurosis in which a hypnotic drug is injected into the patient for the purpose of reviving suppressed memories.

Nares Nostrils.

Nasopharynx The part of the pharynx situated over the roof of the mouth.

Nausea A feeling of sickness in the stomach. Sometimes followed by vomiting.

Navel Umbilicus.

Nearsightedness (myopia) A defect of the eye in which the eyeball is too convex. This causes light rays to focus in front of the retina resulting in an inability to see objects clearly at a distance.

Necropsy Autopsy. Examination after death.

Necrosis Death and deterioration of tissue surrounded by living healthy tissue.

Neonatal Pertaining to the newborn (up to 1 month old).

Neoplasm A new and abnormal growth.

Nephrectomy Surgical removal of a kidney.

Nephritis Inflammation of a kidney.

Nephrolith Kidney stone.

Nephron The unit of the kidney in which waste is removed from the blood and urine is formed.

Nephrosis Kidney degeneration without inflammation.

Nerve A bundle of fibers which carries impulses between the nerve center (the brain and spinal cord) and the other parts of the body. There are five kinds of nerves: cranial, mixed, motor, sensory, and spinal.

Neuralgia Sharp, stabbing pain in a nerve or along its course. The pain is short-lived but recurring.

Neurasthenia A nervous condition in which one suffers from fatigue and loss of initiative. Usually accompanied by oversensitivity, restlessness, and uncalled-for irritability.

Neuritis Inflammation of a nerve.

Neurofibroma Tumor of nervous and connective tissues.

Neurofibromatosis A condition in which multiple tumors (neurofibroma) form under the skin or along the course of a nerve.

Neurology The branch of medicine dealing with the nerves and the central nervous system.

Neuron A nerve cell.

Neurosis A nervous disorder, usually related to anxiety, in which there is no functional degeneration of tissue.

Nevus A congenital pigment or elevated portion of skin. Birthmark.

Nictation (or nictitation) Wink. Rapid blinking of eyelid.

Nightblindness (nyctalopia) Reduced ability to see at night.

Nitrous oxide Laughing gas; an inhalant that induces euphoria and dulls the sensation of pain. Often used in dentistry.

Nocturia Urination at night.

Node A small protuberance or swelling. A knoblike structure. Nodule.

Nucleus The center part of any cell that is essential for cell growth, nourishment, and reproduction. Except for red blood cells, all human body cells have nuclei.

Nutrient A substance that provides materials the body needs; provides nourishment.

Nutrition The combination of processes by which the body or organism receives and uses materials essential for growth and maintenance.

Nystagmus Involuntary and repetitive oscillation of the eyeballs.

Obesity Excessive weight; body weight more than 20% above the average for one's age, height, and bone structure.

Obstetrics The branch of medical science dealing with pregnancy, childbirth, and neonatal care.

Occipital Pertaining to the back of the head.

Occlusion Used in reference to a closure of ducts and blood vessels. In dentistry, it refers to the fitting together of the upper and lower teeth.

Occult Undetectable by the naked eye.

Ocular Pertaining to the eye.

Olfactory Pertaining to the sense of smell.

Oligomenorrhea Infrequent or scanty menstrual flow.

Oligospermia Abnormally deficient spermatazoa in the semen.

Oliguria Deficient urine production.

Omentum A fold of the peritoneum (membrane lining of the abdomen) that covers and connects the abdominal organs.

Omphalitis Inflammation of the navel.

Oncology The scientific study of tumors.

Onychia Inflammation of the nail matrix, the tissue from which the nail grows.

Onychopagy Nail biting.

Ophthalmitis Inflammation of the eye.

Ophthalmology The branch of medical science dealing with the eyes and their care.

Ophthalmoplegia Paralysis of eye muscles.

Ophthalmoscope An instrument for examining the interior of the eye.

Opiate Narcotic containing opium. Opiate drugs are used as painkillers, sedatives, or to slow gastric motility.

Optic nerve The fiber that transmits optic impulses from the retina to the brain.

Orbit Eye socket.

Orchiectomy (or orchectomy) Surgical removal of the testicles.

Orchitis Inflammation of the testicles.

Orgasm Climax of sexual intercourse.

Orthodontics The branch of dental science dealing with prevention and correction of teeth irregularities and malocclusions.

Orthopedics The branch of surgery dealing with diseases, disorders, and injuries to the locomotor system.

Orthopnea Condition in which breathing can only be facilitated when sitting or standing up.

Orthostatic Exacerbated by standing erect.

Osmosis The transfer of a substance from one solution to another through a porous membrane that separates them.

Osseous Composed of or resembling bone tissue.

Ossicle A tiny bone. The three bones in the inner ear are ossicles.

Ossification The process of becoming bone or the change of cartilage to bone.

Osteitis Inflammation of bone.

Osteochondritis Inflammation of bone and cartilage.

Osteoma Tumor of bone tissue.

Osteomalacia A condition in which bones become soft, brittle, flexible, and painful due to a lack of calcium and vitamin D. Similar to childhood rickets.

Osteomyelitis Inflammation of the bone and marrow resulting from infection.

Osteopathy A system of treating disease that emphasizes massage and bone manipulation.

Osteoporosis A condition in which bones become porous resulting in increased fragility. Associated with the aging process.

Otitis Inflammation of the ear.

Otorhinolaryngology Branch of medical science that deals with the ear, nose, and throat.

Ovariectomy Surgical removal of an ovary.

Ovary The female reproductive glands whose function is to produce the eggs (ova) and the sex hormones estrogen and progesterone.

Oviduct See Fallopian tubes.

Ovum The egg cell. The female sex cell which, when fertilized by the male sperm, grows into a fetus. The egg contains 23 chromosomes that pair off with 23 chromosomes in the sperm to make a complete set needed to start a new life.

Oxygen The colorless, odorless gas essential for life. Oxygen makes up about 21% of the air.

Oxygenation The saturation of a substance with oxygen.

Oxyhemoglobin Oxygen-carrying hemoglobin.

Oxytocin A pituitary hormone that is secreted during childbirth for the stimulation of uterine contractions and milk secretion. A synthetic form of oxytocin is administered sometimes to induce or hasten labor.

Ozone A form of oxygen used as a disinfectant.

Pacemaker (sino-atrial node) A small knot of tissue (node) in the right atrium of the heart from which the contraction of the heart originates. Artificial or electronic pacemakers are small, battery-operated devices that can substitute for damaged pacemaker tissue.

Pachydermia Abnormal thickening of the skin.

Paget disease (1) A type of breast cancer in which the nipple becomes sore and ulcerated. (2) Osteitis deformans. A chronic bone disease in which rates of bone production and bone loss are increased, leading to thickened, softened bones.

Palate The roof of the mouth.

Palliative Any agent that relieves pain and symptoms of disease without actually curing it.

Palpate Examine by feeling with the hand.

Palpitation Rapid, throbbing heartbeat.

Palsy Paralysis.

Pancarditis Inflammation of all the structures of the heart.

Pancreas The gland situated behind the stomach. It secretes pancreatic juice containing enzymes to aid in food digestion, and also contains groups of specialized cells (islets of Langerhans) that secrete insulin and glucagon to regulate blood sugar levels.

Pancreatitis Inflammation of the pancreas.

Pantothenic acid One constituent of the vitamin B complex.

Papanicolaou smear (Pap test) The microscopic examination of cells shed from body surfaces; used routinely to screen for cancer of the cervix or uterus.

Papilla Small conical or nipple-shaped elevation.

Papilloma A tumor, usually benign, of the skin or mucous membrane.

Papule Small abnormal solid elevation on the skin.

Paralysis Loss of nervous function or muscle power due to injury or disease of the nervous system.

Paranoia A mental illness characterized by delusions of being persecuted or conspired against.

Paraplegia Paralysis affecting both legs, usually due to disease of the spinal cord or injury.

Parasite An organism that lives in or on another organism (host).

Parathyroid glands Four small glands embedded in the thyroid gland. The hormones secreted by the parathyroids control the body's calcium and phosphorus levels.

Paratyphoid fever An infectious disease whose symptoms resemble those of typhoid fever but are less severe.

Paregoric An opium compound that slows gastric action, thereby relieving cramps or diarrhea.

Parenchyma The parts of an organ that are directly related to the function of the organ (as opposed to supporting or connective tissues).

Parenteral A substance administered by injection or directly in the bloodstream rather than orally.

Paresis Slight paralysis.

Parkinson disease (Parkinsonism) A disorder in which the person suffers from tremors, stiffness, and slowness of movement.

Paronychia Infection of the tissues surrounding a nail.

Parotid gland One of the salivary glands located near the ear.

Parotitis Mumps. A viral disease characterized by the swelling of the parotid glands.

Paroxysm A sudden but temporary attack of disease or symptoms.

Parrot fever See Psittacosis.

Parturition Childbirth.

Pasteurization A process in which disease-causing bacteria in milk or other liquids are destroyed by heat.

Patch test A diagnostic procedure in which a suspected allergen is injected (in a diluted form) into the skin.

Patella Kneecap.

Pathogen Any disease-causing agent.

Pathology The science dealing with disease, its nature, and causes.

Pectoral Pertaining to the chest.

Pediatrics The branch of medical science dealing with children and the diseases affecting them.

Pedicle Stem of a tumor.

Pediculosis Lice infestation.

Pellagra A disease due to a lack of vitamin B_2 (nicotinic acid). Symptoms include skin rashes, weakness, and mental confusion.

Pelvis (1) A basin-shaped cavity, such as that of the kidney. (2) The bony basin-shaped cavity formed by the hip bone and the lower bones of the back.

Pemphigus A serious skin disease in which groups of large blisters on the skin rupture.

Penis The external male sex organ through which urine is passed and semen is ejaculated.

Pepsin A protein-digesting enzyme secreted by the stomach in gastric juices.

Peptic Pertaining to pepsin.

Peptic ulcer Ulcer in the stomach, duodenum, or esophagus.

Percussion A method of physical diagnosis by tapping or thumping a body part to produce sounds that indicate the size, density, and position of organs.

Perforation A hole or puncture. Usually made by injury or infection (as of the eardrum) or by an ulcer.

Pericarditis Inflammation of the pericardium.

Pericardium The two-layer membranous tissue covering the heart. The layer closest to the heart is the visceral layer; the other is the parietal layer.

Perineum The area between the anus and the genitals.

Periodontal membrane Tissue around the teeth covering the roots and connecting to the jaw.

Periodontitis Inflammation of the periodontal membrane.

Periosteum The tough, fibrous membrane covering nearly all bone surfaces.

Peristalsis A wave of muscular contractions which push materials along the digestive tract.

Peritoneum The serous membrane that lines the abdominal organs.

Peritonitis Inflammation of the peritoneum.

Perlèche A condition in which the corners of the mouth become cracked, raw, and thickened due to vitamin deficiency, bacterial infection, or other causes.

Pernicious Deadly, life-threatening.

Pernicious anemia Anemia caused by a deficiency of vitamin B12 or an inability of the body to absorb vitamin B12.

Perspiration Sweat; the secretion of the sweat gland through the pores of the skin.

Pertussis Whooping cough.

Pessary (1) A device placed in the vagina to support the uterus or correct uterine displacements. (2) A vaginal suppository.

Petechiae Small hemorrhages under the skin.

Petit mal A form of epilepsy or seizure in which the person does not lose consciousness.

Phagocyte A cell that is capable of engulfing bacteria and debris.

Phalanx One of the bones in the finger or toe.

Phallus Penis.

Pharyngitis Sore throat. Inflammation of the pharynx.

Pharynx Mucous membrane-lined cavity at the back of the mouth. It extends to the esophagus.

Phimosis A condition in which the foreskin tightens so it prevents retraction over the head of the penis.

Phlebectomy Surgical removal of a vein.

Phlebitis Inflammation of a vein.

Phlegm Mucus, sputum.

Phobia An abnormally excessive and irrational fear. Some common phobias are acrophobia, fear of high places; agoraphobia, fear of open places; algophobia, fear of pain; claustrophobia, fear of closed places; ocholophobia, fear of crowds; triskaidekaphobia, fear of the number 13; and xenophobia, fear of strangers.

Physiology The study of cells, tissues, and organs and their functions and activities.

Pia or pia mater The innermost layer of the meninges which covers the brain and spinal cord.

Pica The craving or consumption of unusual substances that ordinarily are not food, such as dirt, chalk, or paint chips.

Pigment Any coloring matter.

Piles See Hemorrhoids.

Pimple Common term for a pustule or papule.

Pineal body A small gland, conical in structure, located on the back of the midbrain. Its function is not fully understood but it may be concerned with regulation of growth or of the sex glands.

Pinkeye Contagious conjunctivitis.

Pituitary gland The pea-sized gland located at the base of the brain. It is controlled by the hypothalamus and it, in turn, controls the hormone production in many other endocrine glands.

Pityriasis A skin disease in which patches of skin become red and scaly.

Placebo A substance without medicinal properties which is administered for psychological benefit or as part of a clinical research study.

Placenta The structure developed on the uterine wall about the third month of pregnancy. Through the placenta, the fetus receives nourishment and oxygen and eliminates waste products. It is expelled from the mother after childbirth. The afterbirth.

Plague Any deadly contagious epidemic disease.

Plantar Pertaining to the sole of the foot.

Plaque patch Film of organic substance on tissues, such as teeth or in arteries.

Plasma The fluid part of blood. See Blood plasma.

Platelet (thrombocyte) The colorless bodies in the blood instrumental in blood clotting.

Pleura The membrane lining the chest cavity and covering the lungs.

Pleurisy Inflammation of the pleura.

Plumbism Lead poisoning.

Pneumococcus The oval-shaped bacterium responsible for diseases such as pneumonia, meningitis, and otitis media.

Pneumonia Infection of the lungs.

Pneumonitis Inflammation of lung tissue.

Pneumothorax Lung collapse due to air or gas in the chest cavity.

Pollinosis An allergic reaction to plant pollens inhaled with the air.

Polyarteritis Inflammation of a number of arteries.

Polycythemia An overabundance of red blood cells in the blood.

Polydipsia Excessive thirst, such as that which occurs in untreated diabetes.

Polyopia Seeing multiple images of a single object.

Polyp A nodular tumor, usually benign, that grows on a mucous membrane.

Polyphagia Excessive eating.

Postpartum After childbirth.

Pre-eclampsia A toxic condition of pregnancy characterized by high blood pressure, edema, and kidney malfunction.

Premenstrual syndrome (PMS) A variety of symptoms, both physical and emotional, associated with the menstrual cycle.

Prepuce The foreskin of the penis.

Presbycusis The normal decrease in hearing ability as one gets older.

Presbyopia Increasing inability to see objects close up. Normal condition of midlife and getting older.

Prickly heat (miliaria) Skin irritation or rash caused by perspiration.

Proctitis Inflammation of the membranes of the rectum.

Proctoscope A tubular instrument for examination of the interior of the rectum.

Progesterone The female sex hormone that causes the thickening of the uterine lining and the other body changes that occur in preparation for conception.

Prognosis Prediction or forecast of the probable course and/or results of a disease.

Prolactin Hormone secreted by the pituitary that stimulates the breasts to produce milk.

Prolapse Downward displacement of an organ from its usual position.

Prophylaxis Prevention of disease or its spread.

Prostaglandins Hormone-like substances, secreted by a wide range of body tissues, that perform varying functions in the body. They are instrumental in stimulating uterine contractions during labor and birth and are also important in muscle function.

Prostatectomy Surgical removal of all or part of the prostate gland.

Prostate gland The male sex gland located at the base of the bladder.

Prosthesis An artificial replacement for a missing body part.

Proteins Complex nitrogen compounds made up of amino acids. Most of the tissues of body, especially the muscles, are composed primarily of protein.

Prothrombin A substance in the blood which forms thrombin, an enzyme essential to blood coagulation.

Protoplasm The stuff of life in cells. The essential jelly-like substance in all living cells.

Protozoa One-celled organisms, the smallest type of animal life. Amoeba and paramecia are protozoa. Some protozoa can cause disease.

Prurigo A chronic skin disease characterized by small papules and intense itching.

Pruritis Itching.

Psittacosis (parrot fever) A disease similar to pneumonia and transmitted to humans by birds, such as pigeons.

Psoriasis A chronic skin disease characterized by an overgrowth of the epidermis in which scaly lesions appear on various parts of the body.

Psychiatry The branch of medical study dealing with mental health.

Psychoanalysis A method developed by Sigmund Freud for the diagnosis and treatment of mental illness. The patient recalls past, perhaps forgotten, events to gain insight into the unconscious mind.

Psychogenic Originating from the mind.

Psychology The study of the mind and behavior.

Psychomotor Voluntary movement.

Psychoneurosis A mild emotional or mental disturbance, usually a defensive overreaction to unresolved conflicts.

Psychopathy Any disease of the mind.

Psychosis A mental illness originating in the mind itself rather than from environmental factors.

Psychosomatic Any condition either caused or exacerbated by emotional factors.

Psychotherapy Treatment of mental disorders based on verbal communication with the patient.

Ptomaine A poisonous substance produced by the decay of protein.

Ptosis A drooping, especially of the eyelid.

Ptyalin An enzyme contained in the saliva which initiates the breakdown of starch.

Puberty The age at which secondary sex characteristics develop and reproductive organs become functionally active. In girls, puberty is marked by the onset of menstruation; in boys, by the discharge of semen and the change of voice.

Puerperium The period of time directly after childbirth until the time the uterus returns to its usual state.

Pulmonary Pertaining to the lungs.

Pulse The expansion and contraction of an artery as a response to the expansion and contraction of the heart.

Pupil The opening in the middle of the iris of the eye which allows the passage of light to the retina.

Purgative A drug inducing evacuation of the bowels. A cathartic or strong laxative.

Purpura A disorder in which hemorrhages of tiny blood vessels cause purple patches to appear on the skin and mucous membranes.

Purulent Containing pus.

Pus A thick, yellowish fluid containing bacteria and white blood cells. Formed in some types of infection.

Pyelitis Inflammation of the kidney pelvis.

Pyorrhea The discharge of pus, usually from the teeth sockets.

Pyrexia Fever.

Pyrosis Heartburn.

Pyuria Pus in the urine.

Q fever A mild infectious disease caused by a rickettsia germ. It is usually transmitted from cows and sheep to humans by contaminated milk, tick bites, or contaminated food products.

Quadriplegia Paralysis of the arms and legs.

Quarantine Isolation of persons who might be sick from or have come in contact with a communicable disease.

Quickening The stage of pregnancy in which the first fetal movements are felt by the mother, usually around the eighteenth week of pregnancy.

Quinsy Acute inflammation of the tonsils accompanied by abscess.

Rabbit fever See Tularemia.

Rabies Hydrophobia. A deadly disease of the central nervous system caused by the rabies virus and spread by the bite of an infected (rabid) dog or other animal.

Radiation sickness Nausea and diarrhea caused by exposure to moderate radiation. Exposure to massive doses is extremely serious and perhaps fatal.

Radioactive Giving off penetrating energy waves to produce electrical or chemical effects.

Radioisotope An element whose atomic number is the same as another but whose atomic weight differs. Radioisotopes can be injected into the body and traced with monitors for diagnostic purposes.

Radium A highly radioactive metal used to treat cancer.

Rales Abnormal sounds from lungs or bronchi.

Rash Eruption on the skin.

Rat-bite fever An infectious disease caused by bacteria spread to humans by rat bites.

Raynaud disease A disease in which blood vessels of the fingers and toes constrict on exposure to cold, causing numbness and pallor. Blood vessels then expand causing the area to tingle and become red or purple as the blood returns.

Recessive A term used in genetics to describe the weaker of two hereditary traits.

Rectum The portion of the large intestine closest to the anal opening. It consists of the rectal and anal canals.

Reflex An unconscious, automatic response to a stimulus.

Refractory Not reacting to treatment.

Regeneration Repair or renewal of tissue.

Regurgitation Backflow.

Relapsing fever Recurrent fever as a symptom of infection caused by bacteria carried by lice and ticks.

Remission An easing of the symptoms of disease.

Renal Pertaining to the kidneys.

Renin An enzyme found in the kidney and capable of raising blood pressure.

Rennin The enzyme contained in the gastric juice that digests milk.

Repression Refusal of the conscious mind to acknowledge unacceptable or conflicting thoughts, feelings, or ideas.

Resection Removal of a part of an organ or tissue by means of surgery.

Respiration Breathing.

Respiratory distress syndrome See Hyaline membrane disease.

Resuscitation Restoration of breathing or heartbeat to one who is apparently dead or threatened with death.

Reticuloendothelial system A network of tissues containing cells (phagocytes) capable of taking up bacteria and foreign bodies in the bloodstream.

Retina The layered lining of the eye which contains light-sensitive receptors (the rods and cones) and conveys images to the brain.

Retinoblastoma A malignant tumor of the retina occurring in infants and children only.

Retinopathy An injury or disease of the retina, particularly common in insulin-dependent diabetes.

Retractors Devices used to pull back the edges of a wound.

Rh factor A group of antigens in the blood. Some people lack the Rh factor and are therefore designated as Rh negative. Complications can occur if an Rh negative mother conceives and has an Rh positive baby. See Erythroblastosis fetalis.

Rheumatoid factor Abnormal protein in the blood of most people afflicted with rheumatoid arthritis or other autoimmune diseases.

Rhinitis Inflammation of the mucous membrane of the nose; usually as a symptom of the common cold or allergies.

Rhinoplasty Plastic surgery of the nose.

Rhinovirus Any of the more than 100 viruses which cause the common cold.

Rhodopsin The visual purple in the rods of the retina. It becomes bleached when exposed to light and requires vitamin A for regeneration.

Riboflavin Vitamin B2.

Rickets A childhood disease caused by a deficiency of vitamin D. Symptoms include improper development of bones and teeth because of a calcium/phosphorus imbalance.

Rickettsia Disease-causing microorganisms, smaller than bacteria but larger than viruses. Usually transmitted to humans by the bites of fleas, lice, and ticks.

Rickettsial pox A rickettsial disease spread by the bites of mites. Symptoms include a pox-like rash, headache, and fever.

Ringworm A fungal infection affecting the tissues of the skin, hair, nails, and scalp. Dermatophytosis is the general medical name; examples of ringworm infections are tinea pedis (athlete's foot) and tinea capitis of the scalp.

Rocky Mountain spotted fever A rickettsial disease spread by ticks. Symptoms include fever, headache, muscle pain, and rash.

Rods Cylindrical nerve structures in the retina. They contain rhodopsin; together with the cones, they perceive the images of light, dark, and color which are transmitted to the brain.

Roentgen rays X-rays.

Root canal The nerve-containing passageway through the root of the tooth.

Rose fever An allergic reaction to roses; term often used to describe pollen and/or mold allergies that occur during the spring as opposed to hay fever, which is in the fall.

Roseola Any pink eruption on the skin.

Roughage Indigestible matter (such as fiber).

Roundworms Parasites found in contaminated feces. In humans, roundworms cause ascariasis, a condition whose symptoms include disruption of the digestive system and abdominal pain.

Rubella German measles.

Rubeola Measles.

Rupture A tearing or bursting of a part. Also, a hernia.

Saccharin Sugar substitute derived from coal tar.

Sacroiliac The joint connecting the base of the spine to the upper part of the hip bone.

Sacrum The triangular bone just above the coccyx, near the lower end of the spine. It is composed of five vertebrae that have fused together. Together with the bones of the pelvis it forms the sacroiliac joint.

St. Anthony's fire See Erysipelas.

St. Vitus' dance See Chorea.

Saline Salty.

Saliva The secretion of the salivary glands. Lubricates the mouth and throat and initiates the digestion of food with enzymes.

Salivary glands The three glands on each side of the face. The sublingual gland and submaxillary gland secrete saliva onto the floor of the mouth. The parotids are situated near the ears and secrete saliva through passageways in the back of the mouth.

Salmonella A group of bacteria primarily responsible for the gastrointestinal disturbances of food poisoning.

Salpingectomy Surgical removal of the fallopian tubes. Tubal ligation. A method of sterilization.

Salpingitis Inflammation of the fallopian tubes.

Sarcoma A malignant tumor from connective tissue.

Scabies Infestation of the skin by parasites (scabies mites) that burrow under the skin surface to lay their eggs. The itch.

Scapula The shoulder blade.

Schick test A skin test for immunity to diphtheria.

Schizophrenia Dementia praecox. A group of mental illnesses classified as psychotic (rather than neurotic). Patient's thought patterns become disturbed and disorganized; hallucinations or delusions are common symptoms.

Sciatica Pain extending along the path of the sciatic nerve. Can be caused by a slipped disk or by a muscle spasm.

Sciatic nerve The largest nerve in the body. It branches out from the base of the spinal cord (where it is attached) to form the motor and sensory nerves of the legs and feet.

Sclera The fibrous outer coat of the eye.

Sclerosis Abnormal hardening or thickening of a tissue.

Scoliosis Curvature of the spine.

Scorbutus Scurvy.

Scotoma Any (normal or abnormal) blind spot in the field of vision.

Scrofula Tuberculosis of the lymph nodes in the neck.

Scrotum The pouch that holds the testicles in the male.

Scurvy A disease caused by a deficiency of vitamin C. Symptoms include anemia, weakness, and bleeding gums.

Sebaceous glands The oil glands that secrete sebum, a fatty substance to lubricate the skin.

Seborrhea Overactivity of the sebaceous glands resulting in a greasiness of the skin.

Sebum The fatty substance secreted by the sebaceous glands.

Secretion Any substance formed or emitted by glands or tissue. Various secretions perform various functions for the body.

Sedative A calming agent that reduces excitability.

Semen The thick, whitish secretion produced by the male testes and sex glands and containing the male reproductive cells, the spermatozoa.

Semicircular canals The three membranous canals of the inner ear that control the sense of balance.

Seminal vesicles The two glands that store the spermatozoa.

Senescence The process of aging, growing old.

Senility Abnormal deterioration of mental function associated with increasing age. Many physical diseases, such as arteriosclerosis, may be associated with senility.

Sepsis The state of being infected by germs in the blood or tissues.

Septicemia Blood poisoning. The presence of living bacteria in the bloodstream.

Septum A dividing wall between two compartments or cavities.

Serum The fluid formed in the clotting of blood. Contains antibodies and is injected in vaccines to build up immunities to specific diseases.

Serum sickness An allergic reaction (usually hives and fever) to the injection or administration of serum.

Shingles (Herpes zoster) A virus infection of nerve endings characterized by pain and blisters along the course of the nerve. Caused by a latent form of the same virus that causes chickenpox, usually years after that disease.

Shock A condition in which the body processes slow down in response to injury or extreme emotion. Symptoms include rapid pulse, low blood pressure, paleness, and cold, clammy skin.

Sickle cell anemia A hereditary type of anemia caused by malformed (crescent-shaped) red blood cells.

Siderosis Chronic inflammation of the lungs caused by inhaling iron particles. An excess of iron in the circulating blood.

Silicosis Inflammation and damage of the lung caused by silicon dioxide. It is an occupational disease associated with sand blasting and stone cutting.

Sinus A cavity or hollow space, especially of the nasal passages.

Sinusitis Inflammation of a sinus.

Smegma Thick sebaceous secretion that accumulates beneath the prepuce and clitoris.

Solar plexus A network of nerves in the abdomen.

Somnambulism Sleepwalking.

Somniloquy Talking in sleep.

Spasm Sudden and severe involuntary contraction of a muscle.

Speculum An instrument used to dilate a body passage in order to examine the interior, such as the examination of the vagina and cervix during pelvic examination.

Spermatocele Enlargement of the scrotum due to the development of a fluid-filled sac (cystic dilation) of the tubules.

Spermatozoa Male reproductive cell. See Ovum.

Spermicide An agent that kills spermatozoa.

Sphincter A ring of muscle which encircles and controls the opening of an orifice.

Sphygmomanometer An instrument used to measure blood pressure.

Spina bifida A congenital defect in which some of the vertebrae fail to close, thereby exposing the contents of the spinal canal.

Spinal canal The central hollow formed by the arches of the vertebrae which contains the spinal cord.

Spinal column The structure formed from the 33 vertebrae (spinal bones). The backbone.

Spinal cord The cord or column of nerve tissue extending from the brain, enclosed in the spinal canal.

Spinal nerves 31 pairs of nerves that pass out of the spinal cord and carry impulses to and from all parts of the body.

Spinal tap The withdrawal of cerebrospinal fluid for the purpose of diagnosis or relief of pressure on the brain. Lumbar puncture.

Spirochete Spiral-shaped bacterium. Syphilis is caused by a spirochete.

Spleen A large lymphoid organ behind the stomach on the lower left side of the rib cage. Its function includes cleansing the blood of parasites and manufacturing lymphocytes. It is, however, not an essential organ to life since these functions can be performed elsewhere in the body.

Spondylitis Inflammation of the spine.

Spore A life stage in the cycle of certain microorganisms in which it becomes inactive and highly resistant to destruction. A spore can become active again.

Sprain Injury to the soft tissue around a joint.

Sprue A chronic malabsorption disorder in which the body cannot absorb fats. Symptoms include diarrhea, indigestion, weight loss, and soreness in the mouth.

Sputum Discharge from the lungs and throat composed of mucus and saliva.

Stapes A tiny stirrup-shaped bone in the inner ear.

Staphylococci Spherical bacteria occurring in clusters. Responsible for food poisoning and skin infections, staph infections.

Steapsin Fat-digesting enzyme produced in the pancreas.

Steatorrhea Pale, bulky stools containing undigested fats.

Stenosis A narrowing of a body passage, tube or opening.

Sterile (1) Germ-free. (2) Unable to reproduce.

Sternum The breastbone. The bone in the middle of the chest.

Steroids (corticosteroids, cortisone) Natural hormones or synthetic drugs that have many different effects. Some steroids are anti-inflammatory and are used to treat arthritis, asthma, and a number of other disorders.

Stethoscope An instrument that amplifies bodily sounds.

Stillborn Term used to describe a baby born dead after the twentieth week of pregnancy.

Stomach The pouch-like organ into which food flows from the esophagus, where digestion takes place by means of enzymes, hydrochloric acid, and the churning action of the stomach muscles.

Stomatitis Inflammation of the soft tissues of the mouth.

Stool Feces. Evacuation of the bowels.

Strabismus An eye disorder in which both eyes are unable to focus simultaneously. Cross-eyedness.

Strain Injury caused by misuse or overuse of a muscle.

Strawberry tongue A bright red tongue with enlarged papillae. Associated with scarlet fever.

Streptococci Spherical bacteria that grow in chains. They are responsible for infections like scarlet fever and strep throat.

Striae Stripes, narrow bands. Stretch marks are a common example.

Stroke An interruption of the blood flow to the brain causing damage to the brain. Depending on the severity and location of the stroke, it may result in partial or complete paralysis or loss of some bodily function, or death.

Stroma The supporting tissue of an organ as opposed to the functioning part. See Parenchyma.

Stupor A state of impaired but not complete loss of consciousness and responsiveness.

Sty Infection of one of the sebaceous glands of the eye.

Subconscious The mind's contents not in the range of consciousness.

Subcutaneous Under the skin.

Sulfonamides Sulfa drugs. A group of medicines that were the first antibiotics.

Sunstroke Failure of the body's temperature control system as a result of overexposure to high heat and humidity. Body temperature rises to a very high degree, leading to coma and death. See also Heat stroke.

Suppository Medicated substance in solid form for insertion into a body opening, usually the vagina or rectum. It melts inside the body to release the medicine.

Suppuration Pus formation.

Suprarenal glands See Adrenal glands.

Surgery The branch of medical science that deals with disease, deformity, or injury by means of operation or manipulation.

Suture (1) To join two surfaces by stitching. (2) The thread-like substance used to join two surfaces.

Sympathectomy Surgical removal of part of the sympathetic nervous system.

Sympathetic nervous system Part of the autonomic nervous system. A chain of spinal nerves whose functions include contraction of blood vessels, increase of heart rate, and regulation of glandular secretions.

Synapse The point of communication between nerve endings.

Syncope Fainting.

Syndrome A group of symptoms occurring together, presumably from the same cause.

Synovia The viscid fluid that lubricates joints.

Systole The contraction of the heart muscle. Systolic pressure is the greater of the two blood pressure readings (the other is diastolic).

Systolic murmur An abnormal sound heard during contraction of the heart.

Tachycardia Excessively rapid heartbeat.

Talipes (clubfoot) Congenital deformity in which the foot is twisted out of the normal position.

Tampon A plug of cotton or other absorbent material that is inserted into a body cavity in order to soak up discharge, such as vaginal tampons to absorb menstrual flow.

Tartar Calcified deposits on the teeth from a buildup of plaque.

Tay-Sachs disease A congenital disease affecting the fat metabolism in the brain and characterized by progressive weakness, disability, and blindness, leading to death. Also known as Amaurotic familial idiocy.

T cell A specialized type of white blood cell (lymphocyte) that works as part of the immune system by attaching itself directly to an invading organism, such as a parasite or fungus, and destroying it. See also B cell.

Temple Area of the head between the eye and ear.

Tendonitis Inflammation of a tendon.

Tendon A white fibrous band that connects muscle to bone.

Tenesmus Urgent desire to evacuate the bowel or bladder with painful and ineffectual straining to urinate or to move the bowels.

Tensor A muscle that stretches or tenses.

Testicles, testes The pair of primary male sex glands enclosed in the scrotum. They produce spermatozoa and the male sex hormone testosterone.

Testosterone The male sex hormone which induces secondary sex characteristics.

Tetanus (lockjaw) A serious and acute infection caused by the invasion of toxic microorganisms into an open wound.

Tetany Muscular spasms and cramps due to muscular hypersensitivity. Causes include gastrointestinal disorders or calcium deficiency.

Thalamus An egg-shaped mass of gray matter at the base of the cerebrum.

Thermometer Instrument used to measure temperature.

Thiamine (vitamin B₁) One of the B-complex vitamins.

Thoracic Pertaining to the chest.

Thorax The chest.

Thrombin An enzyme that converts fibrinogen into fibrin, which is necessary for blood to clot.

Thrombocyte Blood platelet, necessary for the process of blood clotting.

Thrombosis The formation of a blood clot that partially or completely blocks the blood vessel.

Thrombus A blood clot formed in a blood vessel.

Thrush A fungal infection (candidiasis) of the mouth, often occurring in infancy, but also in immunocompromised people whose resistance to disease is low.

Thymus A gland active in childhood and located behind the breastbone. It plays a part in defending the body against infection.

Thyroidectomy Surgical removal of the thyroid.

Thyroid gland The ductless gland located in the neck. The secretions of the thyroid gland control the rate of metabolism, among other functions.

Thyroxin The primary hormone secretion of the thyroid gland.

Tibia The shin bone. The larger (inner) of the two bones of the lower leg.

Tic Involuntary spasmodic movement or twitching.

Tick A blood-sucking parasite that is associated with the spread of disease.

Tincture A medicinal mixture of alcohol and a drug.

Tinea (ringworm) Fungus infection of the skin, and depending upon the location, the cause of barber's itch, jock itch, scalp ringworm, or ringworm of the foot.

Tinea curis Fungal infection of the groin area. Commonly called jock itch.

Tinea pedia (athlete's foot) A fungal infection of the foot characterized by itching, small sores, and cracks on the skin.

Tinnitus Ringing, buzzing, or other perceived noises that originate inside the head rather than from outside stimuli.

Tissue A group of cells or fibers which perform similar functions and together form a body structure.

Tonsillectomy Surgical removal of the tonsils.

Tonsillitis Inflammation of the tonsils.

Tonsils (Palatine) The two masses of lymphoid tissue covered by mucous membrane that are located one on each side of the back of the throat.

Topical Local; pertaining to a surface area of the body.

Torticollis (wryneck) A condition in which the sternocleidomastoid muscle on one side of the neck contracts and pulls the head into an abnormal position.

Toxemia (blood poisoning) A condition in which poisonous compounds (toxins) are present in the bloodstream. Toxemia of pregnancy is another term for eclampsia.

Toxic Poisonous.

Toxic shock syndrome (TSS) An acute form of blood poisoning caused by the Staphylococcus aureus bacteria. Associated with the use of super-absorbent tampons during menstruation, it has been identified in children and men as well.

Toxin Poisonous substance produced by bacteria that may have serious effects in humans. Examples include toxic shock syndrome or botulism.

Toxoid A toxin that has been altered so that it is no longer poisonous but still stimulates antibody production. Used in vaccinations.

Toxoplasmosis A disease transmitted from animals (especially cats) to humans who come in contact with parasite-infected feces or who eat undercooked meat containing the parasite. Infection during pregnancy can cause birth defects or fetal death.

Trachea Windpipe. The tube extending from the larynx to the bronchi.

Tracheitis Inflammation of the trachea.

Tracheobronchitis Inflammation of the trachea and the bronchi.

Tracheotomy A surgical operation in which a new slit is made in the trachea in order to bypass an obstruction and allow air into the lungs.

Trachoma Contagious virus disease of the eye in which the conjunctiva and other mucous membranes become infected. May lead to blindness.

Traction Continuous pulling of a body part using weights and pulleys. Used in treatment of dislocations, deformity, and severe muscle spasm.

Tranquilizers A category of drugs used to relieve anxiety or calm disturbed behavior. Minor tranquilizers (such as Valium) are used to alleviate anxiety in stressful situations. Major tranquilizers (such as Thorazine) are used to reduce symptoms of mental illness (abnormal thought patterns, hallucinations) and make the patient more receptive to psychiatric treatment.

Transfusion The injection of fluids (usually blood or its components) into the circulatory system.

Transplantation The transference of an organ or tissue from one part of the body to another or from one individual to another.

Trauma Injury to the body or emotional shock.

Tremor Involuntary quivering or trembling. May have nervous, congenital, or organic origin or may result from certain drugs.

Triceps Muscle that extends forearm.

Trichinosis A disease caused by ingestion of parasites often found in raw or insufficiently cooked pork.

Trichomoniasis Inflammation, usually of the vagina but also may affect the urethra in males. Caused by a protozoan (single-celled) parasite, *Trichomonas vaginalis*.

Tricuspid valve The heart valve through which blood passes from the right atrium to the right ventricle.

Trigeminal nerve The fifth cranial nerve. Its three branches serve the face, the tongue, and the teeth.

Triglycerides The most common lipid found in fatty tissue. A high level of triglycerides may increase the risk of blood vessel or heart disease.

Truss A device used to hold a hernia or organ in place.

Trypsin An enzyme produced in the pancreas to digest proteins.

Tsutsugamushi disease A rickettsial disease found in Asia. Scrub typhus.

Tubal ligation (salpingectomy) Method of sterilization that ties or cuts a woman's fallopian tubes so that sperm is unable to reach an ovum.

Tubal pregnancy The most common form of ectopic pregnancy in which a fertilized egg starts to develop in the fallopian tubes instead of the uterus.

Tubercle (1) A nodule on a bone. (2) Lesion characteristic of tuberculosis.

Tuberculin test A skin test to detect tuberculosis or tuberculosis sensitivity. An extract of tubercle bacilli is injected into the skin; a positive reaction indicates possible tuberculosis or previous exposure to it.

Tuberculosis An infectious disease affecting the lungs most often but also other parts of the body. It is caused by the tubercle bacillus. Symptoms include cough, chest pains, fatigue, sweating, and weight loss. Commonly referred to as TB.

Tubule A small tube.

Tularemia Rabbit fever. A disease of small animals that spreads to humans by direct contact (e.g., handling the meat of an infected animal) or by the bite of a vector such as a tick or flea. Symptoms include chills, fever, and swollen lymph nodes.

Tumefaction Swelling.

Tumor An abnormal growth of tissue similar to normal tissue but without function. May be benign (harmless) or malignant (cancerous).

Tympanic membrane The eardrum.

Tympanum The middle ear.

Typhoid fever Bacterial infection spread through contaminated water, milk, or food, especially shellfish. Symptoms include fever and diarrhea; the disease may cause fatal dehydration.

Typhus A rickettsial disease transmitted by lice to humans. Symptoms include headache, chills, pain, and fever.

Ulcer An open sore on the skin or in a body cavity. Term commonly refers to intestinal or peptic ulcers, which form in the digestive tract.

Ulcerative colitis An inflammation of the colon and rectum in which ulcers in the digestive tract cause bloody stool.

Ulna The larger bone of the forearm.

Ultrasound Sound waves of very high frequency used for diagnostic purposes. The echoes of the ultrasound are registered with devices that construct pictures showing internal organs.

Umbilical cord The tube that connects the fetus to the placenta and through which the fetus is nourished and wastes are disposed of.

Umbilicus The navel. The round scar in the middle of the abdomen marking the entry site of the umbilical cord.

Undulant fever (brucellosis, or Malta fever) A disease transmitted from animals to humans through contaminated, unpasteurized milk products. Symptoms include fatigue, chills, joint pains, and a fever that alternates between near normal and extremely high (104°F).

Urea The nitrogen-containing waste product of protein breakdown that is excreted as the main component of urine.

Uremia A condition in which toxic substances remain in the blood due to the failure of the kidneys to filter out and excrete them.

Ureter One of the two tubes connecting the kidneys to the bladder and through which urine passes (by means of muscle contractions) into the bladder.

Urethra The tube through which the urine passes from the bladder to the outside.

Urethritis Inflammation of the urethra.

Uric acid An acid that is the waste product of metabolism. It is usually excreted in the urine, and a buildup of it is characteristic of gout.

Urinalysis Examination and analysis of the urine for diagnostic purposes.

Urination (micturition) The discharge of liquid waste through the urethra.

Urine The amber-colored liquid produced in the kidneys from waste products filtered out of the blood. It is released through the ureters to the bladder where it is stored temporarily before excretion. The urine is discharged from the bladder through the urethra during urination.

Urogenital Pertaining to the urinary and genital organs.

Urology The branch of medical science that deals with disorders of the urinary tract of the female and the urogenital system of the male.

Urticaria (hives) An allergic reaction in which itchy elevations (wheals or welts) appear on the skin. May be due to a food allergy, drugs, or other substances. Antihistamines may be prescribed in serious or recurring cases, but most hives disappear in a few days with no treatment.

Uterus (womb) The hollow pear-shaped muscular organ where the fertilized ovum develops during pregnancy. It normally weighs about 2 ounces but enlarges to 30 ounces in pregnancy.

Uvea The pigmented parts of the eye.

Uvula The small tag of tissue that hangs from the center of the soft palate at the back of the throat.

Vaccination Inoculation of an antigenic substance in order to stimulate immunity to disease.

Vaccine Dead or weakened microorganisms that prevent disease by stimulating artificial immunity.

Vaccinia Cowpox.

Vagina The muscular canal lined with mucous membrane which extends from the vulva to the uterus. Sometimes referred to as the birth canal.

Vaginismus Painful contractions of the muscles of the vagina; often responsible for painful intercourse.

Vaginitis Inflammation of the vagina, accompanied by discharge and discomfort.

Vagus The tenth cranial nerve that extends from the brain to serve the stomach, intestines, esophagus, larynx, lungs, and heart.

Varicella Chickenpox.

Varicocele Varicose or swollen veins in the spermatic cord.

Varicose veins Abnormally swollen, dilated veins in which the valves are weakened and thereby allow the backflow of blood. Areas most commonly affected are the lower legs and the rectum. See also Hemorrhoids.

Variola Smallpox.

Vas deferens The duct of the testes through which the spermatozoa must pass in ejaculation.

Vascular Pertaining to, or supplied with, vessels, usually blood vessels.

Vasectomy A method of sterilization of the male. The passageway of the vas deferens is cut off so that the spermatozoa cannot enter the semen.

Vasoconstrictor Any agent that causes the blood vessels to narrow or to contract.

Vasodilator Any agent that causes the blood vessels to widen or enlarge.

Vasomotor Having the ability to contract or enlarge the blood vessels.

Vector An animal, insect, or person that carries disease.

Vein The vessels that carry deoxygenated blood from all parts of the body back to the heart.

Venereal diseases Diseases transmitted through sexual contact.

Venesection (bloodletting) Cutting a vein for the withdrawal of blood.

Venipuncture Puncturing a vein for the withdrawal of blood.

Venous Pertaining to the veins.

Ventral Pertaining to the front of the body, the abdomen.

Ventricle A small cavity, especially the two lower muscular chambers of the heart and the four cavities of the brain.

Venule A small vein that serves as a link between the arterial and venous systems.

Verruca A wart.

Vertebra One of the 33 flat, roundish bones that make up the spinal column.

Vertigo Dizziness.

Vesicle A small sac or bladder.

Viable Capable of survival.

Vibrios Hook-like bacteria.

Villus A microscopic finger-shaped projection such as those found in the mucous lining of the stomach walls.

Viral Pertaining to a virus.

Virulent Poisonous, disease-producing.

Virus A submicroscopic organism that causes disease and is capable of reproduction only within the living cells of another organism (such as a plant, animal, or human). Viruses cause many diseases of humans ranging from mild ailments (such as the common cold) to serious, even fatal, diseases.

Viscera The internal organs (singular: viscus).

Visual purple See Rhodopsin.

Vitreous humor The jelly-like substance found between the lens and the retina that supports the interior parts of the eye.

Vocal cords Two ligaments in the larynx, the vibrations of which produce the sounds of the human voice.

Volvulus A twist or knot in the intestine that blocks passage.

Vomit Ejection of matter from the stomach through the mouth.

Vulva The external genitalia of the female, including the clitoris and vaginal lips.

Vulvovaginitis Bacteria-caused inflammation of the vulva and the vagina.

Walleye An eye condition in which the cornea is whitish and opaque instead of clear; term also used to describe a form of divergent strabismus (crossed eyes) in which the images are slanted in different directions instead of merging into one.

Wart Small, harmless growths on the skin caused by a virus.

Wasserman test Blood test used to detect syphilis.

Wen A sebaceous cyst caused by the obstruction of an oil gland of the skin.

Wheal A temporary skin elevation, usually the result of an allergic reaction.

White blood cell See Leukocytes.

Widal test Blood test used to detect typhoid fever.

Windpipe See Trachea.

Womb See Uterus.

Xanthoma An accumulation or nodule of cholesterol that forms under the skin and appears as an elevated yellow patch.

Xeroderm Dry skin.

Xerophthalmia A dryness of the membranes of the eyelids and eye, associated with vitamin A deficiency.

Xerosis Abnormal dryness.

Xiphoid The sword-shaped piece of cartilage at the lower edge of the breastbone.

X-rays Electromagnetic radiation waves of very short length that are capable of penetrating some substances and producing shadow pictures showing structures of differing densities.

Yaws (frambesia) A tropical disease very similar to syphilis and caused by a spirochete resembling syphilis organisms.

Yellow fever An acute disease caused by a virus spread by insect bites. Usually seen in South America and Africa.

Zoonoses Any disease transmitted by an animal to humans.

Zoster See Herpes zoster; Shingles.

Zygote The fertilized egg before division.

INDEX

Definitions of technical terms are found in the Glossary of Medical Terms, which is not indexed.

coarctation of the aorta 119
cocaine 26, 37, 66
cochlea 87
codeine 66
coffee 63
colectomy 152
collagen 226, 230
colon 139, 142, 144, 148, 151, 152; *see also*
    gastrointestinal system
colonoscopy 148
color discrimination 82
colorectal cancers 144
coma 96, 99, 100, 104
comedones 235
common bile duct 140
common variable immunodeficiency
    disease 209
communicable diseases 72, 96
complement system 201, 209, 210
complexion, ruddy 133
complications of delivery 34, 37–39
compulsion 111
conception 14, 23
conductive hearing loss 87, 88
cones 82
confidentiality 3, 7–10, 248, 265
congenital
    adrenal hypoplasia 186
    heart disease 118
    hip dislocation 221
    immune deficiencies 209
    megacolon 141
    muscular dystrophy 225
    nephrosis 160
congestive heart failure 118, 120, 131
conjunctiva 83
conjunctivitis 83
consciousness, loss of 96, 98, 100
constipation 112, 142, 144, 146, 171, 204, 208
contact lenses 83, 84
contaminated water 63
contraceptives 117
contraction, heart 121
control, loss of 112
controlled substances, effects 66
conversion tables, metric 51
convulsive disorder 96
Cooley anemia 207
coordination, impaired 96, 101, 105
copper deficiency 100
cornea 82, 83, 238
coronary artery 117, 12, 121, 124
coronary atherosclerotic heart disease 121
cortex, adrenal 187
corticosteroids 150, 185
cortisol 186, 187, 188
cortisone 188
Corynebacterium diphtheriae 69
cough 71, 121, 122, 128–34, 141, 145
    barky or brassy 132, 133
counseling, preconceptional 23
cramping 144, 151, 178, 179
cranial nerves 86, 93
creosote 236
cretinism 192
cri du chat 44
crib death 76
Crohn disease 144, 151
crossed eyes 86, 235
croup 132
crying 132
cryosurgery 85, 170, 177, 236, 238
cryptorchidism 168, 170
curvature of cornea 84

curvature of spine 221, 226, 229
Cushing disease 187
Cushing syndrome 187, 188
cyanosis 41, 118, 121, 130, 131, 141
cystic fibrosis 132
cystic mastitis 178
cystine 160
cystinuria 160, 163
cystitis 160, 163
cysts 149, 158, 178, 235
cytomegalovirus 27, 48

D

D and C 35
dactylitis 207
dander, animal 74, 129
daydreams 111
deafness 87, 104, 159
death certificate 248
deceased family members 265, 267
dehydration 112, 142, 162, 186, 187, 189
delivery 42
    complications 34, 38, 39
delusions 113
dementia 95
demineralizing bones 191
dental care 73
deoxyribonucleic acid 13
depressants 65, 66
depression 102, 104, 111, 112, 113, 186,
    188, 191
dermatitis 235
dermis 234
DES, see diethylstilbestrol
detergents 235, 236
deviated eye 86
diabetes insipidus 188
diabetes mellitus 188, 189, 190, 205
    cardiovascular system 117, 118, 120
    eye disorders 82, 83, 84
    gastrointestinal system 146, 149, 150
    obesity 55
    pregnancy 24, 32, 33, 34, 38
    type I 189
    type II 189
dialysis 160
diaphragm 138, 140, 148
diaphragmatic hernia 140
diarrhea 48, 98, 143, 144, 148, 151, 162,
    186, 187, 204, 208, 210
diastolic blood pressure 123
diet
    blood system 204, 207, 208
    cardiovascular system 117, 121–23
    cravings 206
    endocrine system 187, 192
    fiber 62
    gastrointestinal system 143–45, 149–51
    general health 55, 60, 61, 62
    male system 169
    mental illness 112
    musculoskeletal system 224, 227, 229
    nervous system 94, 98, 103
    urinary system 160, 162, 164
diethylstilbestrol 36, 176,
DiGeorge anomaly 209
digestion 132, 138, 139, 145
digestive tract 138
dilation and labor 36
dilation and curettage 35
dimmed vision 83
dimpling, nipple 176
diphtheria 69
discrimination, genetic 7
distal muscular dystrophy 226

diuretics 111, 112
diverticular disease 144
diverticulitis 144
diverticulosis 144
diverticulum 144
dizziness 87, 88, 96, 123, 124, 193, 213
DNA 6, 13
DNA profiling 10
DNA testing 132
dominant gene 15
dopamine 102
double vision 101
double helix 13
Down syndrome 44, 95
drooling 133, 141
drooping eyelids 226
drug addiction 66
drug dependency, *see* chemical
    dependency
dry skin, *see* skin
Duchenne muscular dystrophy 224
duodenum 139, 140, 150
dust 129, 134
dwarfism 192
dysgraphia 75
dyslexia 75
dysplasia 176
dyspraxia 75
dysrhythmias, *see* arrhythmias
dyssemia 76
dystrophin 225

E

ears 86–89
    ache 70
    drum 86, 87, 88
    infection 135
    low-set 159
    ringing in 87, 88, 193
eating
    disorders 111–13
    habits 55
eclampsia 32, 33, 37
ectopic pregnancy 36, 180
eczema 75, 103, 235, 237
edema, *see* swelling
endometrial cancer 177
Edwards syndrome 45
eggs 13, 17, 61, 174, 185
ejaculation 170
elbows, *see* extremities
electrical conduction of the heart 116, 117
electroconvulsive therapy 113
elephant man disease 101
Emery-Dreifuss muscular dystrophy 226
emotional changes 93–95, 99, 101, 111, 112
emphysema 65, 131, 133
employee health file 7, 9, 10
encephalitis 96, 99
encephalocele 94
endocarditis 124
endocrine system 184–95
endolymphatic hydrops 87
endometriosis 177, 178
endometritis 179
endometrium 177
enteropathy, glutin-induced 143
enucleation 85
environmental factors 7, 18, 54–56, 75, 94–
    95, 101, 110, 123, 128, 131–32, 150–51,
    169, 203, 211, 222, 227, 237, 241
enzymes 98, 104, 132–33, 138–39, 150,
    235, 238
eosinophils 199, 211
epidemic hepatitis 73, 147

Marfan syndrome 123
Marie-Strümpel disease 222
marijuana 66
marrow, *see* bone marrow
masculinization 186, 187
mastectomy 176
measles 70
meatus, urethral 157, 158
mechanical breathing assistance, *see* breathing
meconium 50
meconium aspiration syndrome 49
medical information, basic 7
Medical Information Bureau 9
medical records 8, 9, 265
Mediterranean anemia 207
medulla oblongata 93
medullary carcinoma 193
megacolon 141
meiosis 14
melanin 56, 102, 103, 234, 235, 236
melanocytes 56, 234, 236
melanoma, malignant 236
memory cells 201
memory loss 95, 99
menarche 174
Meniere disease 87
meninges 92, 95, 100
meningitis 69, 88, 96, 99, 100
meningocele 94, 95
meningomyelocele 95
Menkes syndrome 100
menopause 174, 175, 177, 178, 227
menstruation 13, 186
    cessation of 188
    cycle 174, 178, 179, 189
    periods, heavy 209, 214
mental illness 110–14
mental
    confusion 121
    illness 110
    impairment 95, 96, 99, 104, 105, 192
    retardation 44, 45, 46, 98, 100, 102, 105
    talent, superior 100
mescaline 66
metabolism 185, 191, 192
metastasis 85, 130, 131, 145, 148, 149, 176, 212, 213, 236
metric conversion table 51
MI, *see* myocardial infarction
MIB, *see* Medical Information Bureau
middle ear, *see* ear
migraine headache 101
military service 7, 248, 267
milk 60, 61, 63, 98, 103
milk production 175
mineralocorticoids 185, 186
miscarriage 22, 26–27, 29–30, 35, 38, 43, 94, 176, 180
mite, scabies 237
mitosis 14
molar pregnancy 36
mole 236
mongolism, *see* Down syndrome
monocytes 201, 211
monosomy X 46
mood disorders 112, 113, 188, 191
moon face 188
morphine 66
mosaic chromosome pattern 44
motor area 93
motor neuron disease 95
motor skills, delayed 224
mouth 138, 149, 236
    dry 188, 189

sores 112
tingling 192
mucocutaneous candidiasis 209
mucosa 138, 139, 143–46, 150–51
mucus
    in stool 144, 145
    respiratory system 128–32, 134–35
multifactorial disorders 7, 8, 16, 43, 94, 95, 102, 132, 140, 142, 159, 234
multiple myeloma 213
multiple sclerosis 101
mumps 70, 171
muscle 219, 224, 228
    aches 73
    atrophy 96
    control 95
    coordination 102, 104
    cramping 95
    extraocular 86
    heart 116, 125
    irritability 192
    mass, loss of 229
    movement 96, 101
    nervous system 92, 95, 97, 98, 101, 105
    paralysis 71, 98
    shortening 225
    smooth 220
    spasms 72, 104
    stiffness 72, 96
    striated 220
    weakness 71, 112, 229, 230
        facial 224, 225, 226
        arms 225, 226
        feet 224
        hands 224, 225, 226
        legs 225
        pelvis 225
        shoulder 225, 226
muscles, sphincter 157
muscular dystrophy 224
musculoskeletal system 218–231
mutant genes 7, 12, 13, 15, 104, 142
mutation 104
myasthenia gravis 101
Mycobacterium tuberculosis 135
myelin 92, 101
myclinated nerve axon 93
myelocytic leukemia 211
myelogenic leukemia 211
myelogenous leukemia 211
myeloma, multiple 210, 213
myelomeningocele 94
myocardial infarction 124
myocarditis 124
myometrium 177
myopia 84
myotonia atrophica 224
myotonic muscular dystrophy 224
myxedema 192

N

nailbeds 203, 236
narcolepsy 68
narcotics 66
nasal 128, 129
National Genealogical Society 267
natural delivery 42
nausea 69, 73, 124, 230
    ear 87, 88
    endocrine system 186, 191
    female system 178, 180
    gastrointestinal system 143–45, 147, 150–51
    nearsightedness 84, 235
    nervous system 96, 99, 100, 101

urinary system 162, 164, 171
neck 93, 96, 190, 238
necrotizing enterocolitis 50
needle aspiration 176, 178
Neisseria gonorrhoeae 31
nephritis 159
nephroblastoma 164
nephrogenic diabetes insipidus 162
nephrolithiasis 163
nephron 156, 160, 161, 162
nephrosis 160, 162
nephrotic syndrome 162
nerve
    acoustic 86
    cells 92, 93, 98, 99
    cranial nerve VIII 86
    damage 101
    deafness 159
    endings 234
    endocrine system 186, 192
    eyes 235
    messages 102
    optic 82, 83
    paralysis 163
    pathways 101, 235
    tumors 105
nervous system 92–107
neural tube defects 94
neurofibromas 102
neurofibromatosis 101
neuron 92, 93, 96, 101, 102
neurotransmitter 92
neutrophils 199, 201, 211
newborn screening 98
nicotine, *see* tobacco
night blindness 85
night sweats 212, 213, 214
night vision 82
nightmares 111
nipple 175
nitrite-processed foods 145
nodules 176, 178, 190, 235
non-A, non-B hepatitis 147
nonallergic asthma 129
nonaspirin products 104, 130
nonbreathing, *see* apnea
nonhereditary breast cancer 175
non-Hodgkin lymphoma 213
nonimmunologic asthma 129
nonketotic hyperosmolar coma 189
non-REM sleep 67
nonself 200
nonsex chromosomes 15
nontropical sprue 143
norepinephrine 186, 193
nose 128, 135
    enlarged 190
    flat 158, 159
    runny 129
nosebleeds 123, 209, 214
numbness 105, 112, 189, 192, 208, 213, 214
nutrition 18, 55
    eyes 85
    female system 177
    gastrointestinal system 138–39, 143, 151
    musculoskeletal system 226, 227, 230
    nervous system 94, 98, 100, 101, 111–12
    pregnancy 24, 32
    respiratory system 131, 132
    skin 235
nystagmus, *see* eyes

O

oats 143
obesity 55, 62, 68, 117, 143, 227

No family can afford to be without this book!
Discover Your Genetic Connections™
It just may save your life and the life of a loved one.

Genetic Connections™ is a step-by-step guide to documenting your family health history and graphing your family pedigree. Complete with illustrations, health forms, and pedigree materials, this comprehensive guide helps you understand the human body and the role genetics plays in various diseases.

Your family pedigree can reveal prevalent diseases within your family and may indicate how they have been transmitted generation to generation. Your information can help your health-care provider determine your risk of developing these same diseases so that life-saving preventive care can begin.

ORDER FORM

HOW TO ORDER:

All orders must be prepaid. Prices are subject to change without notice. Please allow four to six weeks for delivery.

(1) Fill out the order form indicating the quantity for each item.

(2) Choose your preferred method of payment and indicate on the order form.

(3) Sign your mail order, if paying by charge card. Please do not send cash.

PLEASE SEND...

Item/Version	Qty.	Unit Price	Total Price
☐ **Paperback**	_____	$34.95	_____
☐ **Hardcover**	_____	$39.95	_____
☐ **Concealed Wire-O Bound Hardcover**	_____	$44.95	_____
☐ **Completer Set***	_____	$20.00	_____

*Includes slipcase and binder, mechanical pencil, set of 4 colored pencils, photo sheets, form protectors, and acid-free health history forms. This set will hold those documents you have been gathering as you research your family health history.

	Qty.	Unit Price	Total Price
☐ **Health History Forms** Set of 10, printed on acid-free paper	_____	$6.00	_____
Tax (Missouri residents add 5.225%)			_____
Shipping & Handling Flat rate of $5.50 for each book or completer set; $7.50 for each book with completer set. Provide billing and shipping addresses			_____
Total this order			_____

METHOD OF PAYMENT:

☐ **Check**   ☐ **Money Order**   ☐ MasterCard   ☐ VISA

Card Number _____

Signature _____   Exp. Date _____

BILLING ADDRESS:

NAME _____

ADDRESS _____

CITY/STATE/ZIP _____

DAYTIME PHONE _____

EVENING PHONE _____

SHIPPING ADDRESS:

NAME _____

ADDRESS _____

CITY/STATE/ZIP _____

DAYTIME PHONE _____

EVENING PHONE _____

Telephone Orders: Call toll-free **1-800-206-5450**. Have your Visa or MasterCard ready.

Fax Orders: Credit card orders only. Fill out and fax this form to **(314) 239-9937**.

Mail Orders: Send to Sonters Publishing, PO Box 109-100, Washington, MO 63090

GUARANTEE
If not fully satisfied, you may return them at any time for any reason.
Thank You!

Form #0317-95/500